Diabetes Mellitus in Developing Countries and Underserved Communities

Sam Dagogo-Jack
Editor

Diabetes Mellitus in Developing Countries and Underserved Communities

Springer

Editor
Sam Dagogo-Jack
University of Tennessee Health
Science Center
Memphis, Tennessee
USA

ISBN 978-3-319-41557-4 ISBN 978-3-319-41559-8 (eBook)
DOI 10.1007/978-3-319-41559-8

Library of Congress Control Number: 2016959999

Printed on acid-free paper

This Springer imprint is published by Springer Nature
The registered company is Springer International Publishing AG Switzerland
The registered company address is Gewerbestrasse 11, 6330 Cham, Switzerland

This volume is dedicated to all persons who struggle with the syndrome of diabetes mellitus, the global community of clinicians who manage diabetes, and the researchers dedicated to finding better methods for the treatment, prevention, and, ultimately, cure of diabetes mellitus.

Preface

No other disorder exerts a more pervasive and catholic global burden on humanity and society than does diabetes. The current diabetes epidemic is felt on all continents, by all ethnic groups, among the rich and poor, and across gender and age groups. In the first Global Diabetes Report released in 2016, the World Health Organization noted that diabetes is "no longer a disease of predominantly rich nations" and that the "prevalence of diabetes is steadily increasing everywhere, most markedly in the world's middle-income countries." There were an estimated 108 million adults with diabetes globally in 1980. By 2014, that number had risen to 422 million adults, and the global estimate is projected to increase to 592 million adults with diabetes by 2035. Sadly, low- and middle-income countries are projected to experience the steepest increase as they transition to lower-middle and upper-middle income status. The complications of diabetes, such as blindness, kidney failure, amputations, heart disease, stroke, and mortality, are a personal tragedy as well as a threat to national and global security, through their negative effects on the vitality and economic productivity of afflicted citizens.

Low- and middle-income countries have limited resources for dealing with the costs of controlling diabetes and its complications. Even in the developed economies, the quality of diabetes control is suboptimal for approximately 50 % of the affected population. Moreover, socioeconomically vulnerable demographic subgroups have always existed in North America, Europe, Australia, and New Zealand; individuals from those groups often experience disparities in diabetes prevalence, quality of care, and outcomes. Autochthonous or aboriginal people and migrant groups predominate among the vulnerable and often underserved populations with regard to diabetes. The chronic low-grade human migration trends (usually from lower-income to upper-income regions) have escalated exponentially as a result of recent geopolitical upheavals. The flood of new immigrants to Europe and elsewhere has added to the challenges of providing optimal diabetes care in a setting of rapid cultural, linguistic, and socioeconomic metamorphosis.

Diabetes Mellitus in Developing Countries and Underserved Communities, a global textbook of diabetes, presents a detailed consideration of the epidemiology, genomic landscape, clinical presentation, complications, management, and prevention of diabetes in all regions of the world. The regions covered include sub-Saharan Africa, the Middle East and North Africa, Eastern Europe, China and the Western Pacific, India and Southeast Asia, Latin America and the Caribbean, as well as Australia, New Zealand, North

America, and Western Europe. In the latter more affluent regions, appropriate focus is placed on vulnerable indigenous and immigrant populations. Additional attention is given to a description of regional coordination of diabetes care, diabetes prevention services, preferences and imperatives regarding pharmacotherapy, and the status of diabetes research. The chapters conclude with the identification of future directions, unmet needs, unanswered questions, or even unquestioned answers, with regard to diabetes in specific regions.

The availability, in a single volume, of comprehensive information on the peculiarities of diabetes pathophysiology, genetics, and best practices in major regions of the world, crafted by leading authorities in the field, is a valuable resource for clinicians, researchers, scholars, public health leaders, students, and everyone interested in diabetes. The authors are to be commended for their hard work in creating this informed and informative treatise on global diabetes.

The conceptual insight of Kristopher Spring (editor, Clinical Medicine) and logistical support from Ms. Saanthi Shankhararaman (project coordinator), both at Springer, greatly facilitated the creation of this book. Much gratitude is owed to them for their professionalism and engagement that resulted in the successful execution of the book project.

Memphis, TN, USA Sam Dagogo-Jack

Contents

Contributors

S.R. Aravind, MBBS, DNB, FRCP, FDRC, DHA, FRSSDI Columbia Asia Hospital, Yeshwanthpur, Bangalore, India

Felix Assah, MD, PhD Faculty of Medicine and Biomedical Sciences, University of Yaoundé I, Yaoundé, Cameroon

Evan Atlantis, PhD Western Sydney University, Campbelltown, NSW, Australia

Omar Y. Bello-Chavolla Department of Endocrinology and Metabolism, Instituto Nacional de Ciencias Médicas y Nutrición Salvador Zubirán, Mexico City, Mexico

Facultad de Medicina, Universidad Nacional Autónoma de México, Mexico City, Mexico

Michael S. Boyne, MD, FRCPC Tropical Metabolism Research Unit, Tropical Medicine Research Institute, The University of the West Indies, Mona, Kingston, Jamaica

Juliana C.N. Chan, MD, FRCP The Chinese University of Hong Kong, Prince of Wales Hospital, Shatin, Hong Kong, China

Elaine Y.K. Chow, MBChB, PhD Department of Medicine and Therapeutics, Hong Kong Institute of Diabetes, Hong Kong, SAR, China

Obesity and Li Ka Shing Institute of Health Sciences, The Chinese University of Hong Kong, Prince of Wales Hospital, Hong Kong, SAR, China

Stephen Colagiuri, MD W.H.O. Collaborating Centre on Physical Activity, Nutrition and Obesity, The University of Sydney, Sydney, NSW, Australia

Sam Dagogo-Jack, MD, MBBS, MSc, FRCP, FACP, FACE Division of Endocrinology, Diabetes & Metabolism, University of Tennessee Health Science Center, Memphis, TN, USA

Vasile Fedash, MD, PhD Institute of Physiology and Sanocreatology of ASM, Chisinau, Moldova

Sherita Hill Golden, MD, MHS Department of Medicine, Johns Hopkins University School of Medicine, Baltimore, MD, USA

Vitaliy Gurianov, PhD Bogomolets National Medical University, Kyiv, Ukraine

Osama Hamdy, MD, PhD, FACE Joslin Diabetes Center, Harvard Medical School, Boston, MA, USA

Anthony J. Hanley, PhD Departments of Nutritional Sciences and Public Health Sciences, Faculty of Medicine, University of Toronto, Toronto, ON, Canada

William H. Herman, MD, MPH University of Michigan, Ann Arbor, MI, USA

Joshua J. Joseph, MD Division of Endocrinology, Diabetes and Metabolism, Johns Hopkins University School of Medicine, Baltimore, MD, USA

Shashank R. Joshi, MD, DM, FICP, FACP, FACE, FRCP Joshi Clinic, Lilavati & Bhatia Hospital, Mumbai, India

Grace Joshy, PhD Australian National University, Canberra, ACT, Australia

Mykolay Khalangot, MD, Sc D Shupyk National Academy of Postgraduate Medical Education, Kyiv, Ukraine

Yasmin Khan, MD, MPH Adult Diabetes Section, Joslin Diabetes Center, Boston, MA, USA

Victor Kravchenko, Sc D Komisarenko Institute of Endocrinology and Metabolism, National Academy of Medical Sciences, Kyiv, Ukraine

Andrea A.O. Luk, MBBS, MRCP Department of Medicine and Therapeutics, Hong Kong Institute of Diabetes, Hong Kong, SAR, China

Obesity and Li Ka Shing Institute of Health Sciences, The Chinese University of Hong Kong, Prince of Wales Hospital, Hong Kong, SAR, China

Sudaba Mansuri Department of Nutritional Sciences, Faculty of Medicine, University of Toronto, Toronto, ON, Canada

Jean Claude Mbanya, MD, PhD, FRCP Faculty of Medicine and Biomedical Sciences, University of Yaounde I, Yaounde, Cameroon

Oliver Razum Fakultät fürGesundheitswissenschaften, Universität Bielefeld, School of Public Health, Bielefeld, Germany

Carlos A. Aguilar Salinas Departamento de Endocrinologia y Metabolismo, Instituto Nacional de CienciasMédicas y Nutricion, Mexico City, Mexico

Christopher D. Saudek, MD Division of Endocrinology, Diabetes and Metabolism, Johns Hopkins University School of Medicine, Baltimore, MD, USA

David Simmons, MBBS, MA, FRACP, FRCP, MD Western Sydney University, Campbelltown, NSW, Australia

Helmut Steinberg, MD Department of Medicine, Division of Endocrinology, Diabetes and Metabolism, University of Tennessee Health Science Center, Memphis, TN, USA

Ieva Strele, MD, PhD Riga Stradins University, Riga, Latvia

Alexander Vaiserman, Sc D Chebotariov Institute of Gerontology, National Academy of Medical Sciences, Kyiv, Ukraine

Margaret Williams, PhD Auckland University of Technology, Auckland, New Zealand

About the Editor

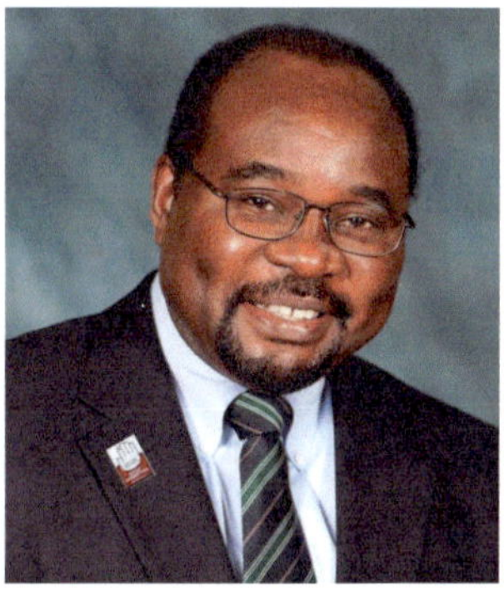

Sam Dagogo-Jack, MD, is Professor of Medicine and Chief of the Division of Endocrinology, Diabetes and Metabolism at the University of Tennessee Health Science Center, Memphis, Tennessee, where he holds the A. C. Mullins Endowed Chair in Translational Research. He is also Director of the Endocrinology Fellowship Training Program and Director of the General Clinical Research Center at UTHSC. A global citizen, Dr. Dagogo-Jack has studied, practiced, researched, and/or taught medicine and diabetology in Africa, Asia, Australia, Europe, North and South America, Caribbean countries, and the Middle East. His current research focuses on the interaction of genetic and environmental factors in the prediction and prevention of prediabetes and diabetes. Dr. Dagogo-Jack is a recipient of the *Banting Medal for Leadership* from the American Diabetes Association and the *Distinction in Endocrinology Award* from the American College of Endocrinology. He served as the 2015 President, Medicine & Science, of the American Diabetes Association.

The Global Burden of Diabetes: An Overview

1

William H. Herman

Introduction

The global burden of diabetes is enormous and growing. Between 1997 and 2010, four research groups estimated the numbers of people with diabetes globally and projected the future burden of diabetes (Fig. 1.1) [1–4]. In each instance, the previous estimate was shown to have underestimated the number of people with diabetes, and the projections painted an ever more alarming picture of the future burden of diabetes. The latest study estimated that between 2010 and 2030, the number of adults with diabetes worldwide would increase by 54 %, from 285 million to 439 million [4]. Much of the growth in the numbers of people with diabetes would occur in middle-aged working adults [4]. The number of adults with diabetes would increase by 20 % in developed countries and by 69 % in developing countries [4]. A part of the increase in the number of people with diabetes worldwide is due to increased incidence of type 2 diabetes related to urbanization, obesogenic diets, and decreased physical activity [5]. A larger part of the increase is due simply to population growth, aging of the population, and decreased mortality [5]. Whatever the causes, the estimates are conservative, and the future burden of diabetes is likely to be even greater than projected.

In 2015, the International Diabetes Federation (IDF) estimated that globally, 415 million adults 20–79 years of age or 8.8 % of the adult population have diabetes [5]. There are 321 million people of working age (20–64 years) with diabetes and 94 million people aged 65–79 with diabetes. There are slightly more men than women with diabetes (215 million men vs. 200 million women). Currently, there are more people with diabetes in urban areas (270 million) than in rural areas (145 million). Age-adjusted diabetes prevalence rates among adults 20–79 years of age vary by region and by country. In 2015, the age-adjusted diabetes prevalence was 11.5 % in North America and the Caribbean, 10.7 % in the Middle East and North Africa, 9.6 % in South and Central America, 8.8 % in the Western Pacific and Southeast Asia, 7.3 % in Europe, and 3.8 % in Africa [5]. Perhaps most alarmingly, approximately 75 % of people with diabetes live in low- and middle-income countries [5].

Diabetes prevalence rates vary greatly among indigenous communities. These communities are characterized by unique languages, knowledge systems, and beliefs [5]. Many have a special relationship with their traditional land which often has a fundamental importance for their culture [5]. In many cases, the prevalence of diabetes is greater in indigenous populations than in

W.H. Herman, MD, MPH
Departments of Internal Medicine and Epidemiology, University of Michigan,
1000 Wall Street, Room 6108/SPC 5714, Ann Arbor, MI 48105-1912, USA
e-mail: wherman@umich.edu

S. Dagogo-Jack (ed.), *Diabetes Mellitus in Developing Countries and Underserved Communities*,
DOI 10.1007/978-3-319-41559-8_1

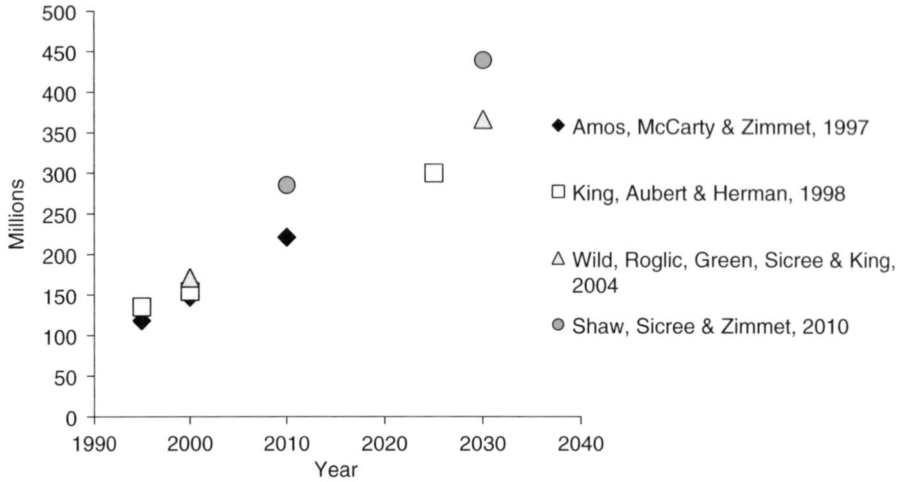

Fig. 1.1 Global estimates and projections of the number of people with diabetes

the surrounding population such as in indigenous Australian [6], New Zealand Māori [7], Greenland Inuit [8], Canadian Inuit [9], and Native American populations [10]. Some indigenous populations that still live very traditional lifestyles have a relatively low prevalence of diabetes [5].

Not every person with diabetes has been diagnosed. Globally, it is estimated that one-in-two adults with diabetes is undiagnosed [5]. In regions where healthcare resources are lacking such as in sub-Saharan Africa, the proportion of people with diabetes who are undiagnosed is as high as 67 % [5]. Even in high-income regions such as North America, slightly more than one-third of people with diabetes have not been diagnosed [5]. Globally, 81 % of people with diabetes who are undiagnosed live in low- and middle-income countries [5].

The IDF has estimated that by 2040, 642 million adults 20–79 years of age or 10.4 % of the world population will have diabetes [5]. In 2040, proportionately more people with diabetes will be 65–79 years of age. The gender difference between men and women is expected to decrease modestly by 2040, but the global difference in the number of people with diabetes in urban and rural areas is expected to widen with 478 million people with diabetes living in urban areas and 164 million living in rural areas. The largest increases in diabetes prevalence will occur in regions where economies are moving from low-income to middle-income levels. By 2040, the IDF has estimated that the age-adjusted prevalence of diabetes will be 12.0 % in North America, 9.7 % in South and Central America, 9.0 % in the Western Pacific, 9.1 % in Southeast Asia, 7.6 % in Europe, and 4.2 % in Africa [5].

The global epidemic of type 2 diabetes has major implications for healthcare expenditures. Most countries dedicate between 5 % and 20 % of their total healthcare resources to treat diabetes and its complications [5]. In 2015, the IDF estimated that total diabetes healthcare expenditures for persons 20–79 years of age were $673 billion or 12 % of total healthcare expenditures worldwide [5]. The IDF has projected that this number will increase to $802 billion by 2040 assuming constant per capita healthcare expenditures [5]. The increase in healthcare expenditures for diabetes by 2040 is projected to be proportionately less than the increase in the number of people with diabetes because countries with the largest increases in the numbers of people with diabetes are those with the lowest per capita spending for diabetes. In 2015, an average of $1,622 was spent per person with diabetes [5]. The range in expenditures for diabetes varied by almost 85-fold: from $7,859 per person per year in North America and the Caribbean, $2,610 in Europe, $1,169 in

South and Central America, $693 in the Western Pacific, $483 in the Middle East and North Africa, $243 in Africa, and $93 in Southeast Asia [5].

Not surprisingly, these dramatic differences in mean annual healthcare expenditures per person with diabetes are associated with major differences in the types of expenditures for diabetes. In developed countries where mean annual healthcare expenditures are high, a large absolute amount but a small proportion of total healthcare expenditures are for antihyperglycemic therapy [11]. The greatest proportion of healthcare expenditures for diabetes go for the treatment of complications and comorbidities. In contrast, in developing countries where mean annual healthcare expenditures are low, the greatest proportion of expenditures go for antihyperglycemic therapy [11]. Although some resources go to the treatment of acute metabolic and infectious complications, little is spent on the treatment of chronic complications and comorbidities such as renal and cardiovascular disease.

Economic development is associated with increased per capita healthcare expenditures. In a recent study, Seuring and colleagues examined the factors associated with the heterogeneity in diabetes healthcare expenditures among countries [12]. Their work demonstrated that the direct costs of diabetes are positively associated with a country's per capita gross domestic product (GDP). Healthcare expenditures increase with national economic wealth. Per capita GDP explained about one-third of the variation in diabetes healthcare expenditures among countries such that every additional dollar in per capita GDP translated into an average increase in direct diabetes expenditures of about $0.04 [12].

This phenomenon is further illustrated by a study that assessed rates of end-stage renal disease (ESRD) treatment by national wealth [13]. In low- and middle-income countries with per capita GDP less than ~$10,000, rates of ESRD treatment were very low but tended to increase with per capita GDP. In contrast, in high-income countries with per capita GDP above ~$10,000, rates of ESRD treatment were consistently higher, reflecting greater access to ESRD treatment. Economic development thus appeared to be associated with increased demand for and access to expensive but lifesaving care. As low- and middle-income countries develop economically, the demand for and per capita expenditures for the treatment of diabetes and its complications will increase substantially. The future costs of healthcare for diabetes are likely to be many times higher than projected by the IDF and, if costs remain unchecked, have the potential to bankrupt healthcare systems and indeed national economies.

What can be done? All countries, but especially low- and middle-income countries with limited resources, must carefully balance the benefits and costs of allocating scarce healthcare resources for population-level and targeted interventions for diabetes prevention, for antihyperglycemic and cardiovascular therapies to delay or prevent the development of complications among people with diabetes, and for the treatment of advanced diabetic complications. Addressing only the healthcare needs of individuals with diagnosed diabetes will leave the epidemic of type 2 diabetes and its downstream complications, comorbidities, and costs unchecked. Clearly, tailored strategies that allocate resources to prevent diabetes, to treat diabetes, and to treat its complications and comorbidities will be required.

Population-level policy interventions addressing food supply, the built environment, tax policy, and financial incentives and disincentives all offer great promise in addressing the obesogenic and diabetogenic environment at a relatively low cost. Examples abound in the area of tobacco control [14]. Unfortunately, there are many differences between smoking, diet, and physical activity and the evidence base for population-level interventions for diabetes prevention is limited.

The evidence base for targeted interventions to delay or prevent the development of type 2 diabetes is extensive, robust, and consistent. At least four trials from China [15], Finland [16], the United States [17], and India [18] have demonstrated that lifestyle interventions that achieve a 5–7 % reduction in initial body weight and increase brisk walking to approximately 150 min per week can reduce the incidence of type 2 diabetes by 29–58 % in high-risk individuals with impaired glucose tolerance. Other trials have demonstrated the efficacy of metformin [17, 18], alpha-glucosidase inhibitors [19, 20], and thiazolidinediones [21–23] for diabetes prevention. Unfortunately, such interventions required substantial resources to identify at-risk individuals, to implement interventions, and to maintain long-term adherence. In addition, the evidence that targeted interventions can be translated into long-term clinical practice in large, less highly selected populations is lacking.

The challenge is clear. As reported by the IDF, "Type 2 diabetes is a global epidemic with devastating humanitarian, social, and economic consequences" [5]. We must understand the global burden of diabetes to increase awareness, to plan for future needs, and to inform interventions. An understanding of the present and future burden of diabetes in developing countries and underserved communities is essential to this task.

References

1. Amos AF, McCarty DJ, Zimmet P. The rising global burden of diabetes and its complications: estimates and projections to the year 2010. Diabet Med. 1997;14 Suppl 5:S1–85.
2. King H, Aubert RE, Herman WH. Global burden of diabetes, 1995–2025: prevalence, numerical estimates and projections. Diabetes Care. 1998;21:1414–31.
3. Wild S, Roglic G, Green A, Sicree R, King H. Global prevalence of diabetes: estimates for the year 2000 and projections for 2030. Diabetes Care. 2004;27:1047–53.
4. Shaw JE, Sicree RA, Zimmet PZ. Global estimates of the prevalence of diabetes for 2010 and 2030. Diabetes Res Clin Pract. 2010;87:4–14.
5. International Diabetes Federation. IDF diabetes atlas. 7th ed. Brussels: International Diabetes Federation; 2015. http://www.diabetesatlas.org. Accessed 5 Jan 2015.
6. Minges KE, Zimmet P, Magliano DJ, Dunstan DW, Brown A, Shaw JE. Diabetes prevalence and determinants in Indigenous Australian populations: a systematic review. Diabetes Res Clin Pract. 2011;93:139–49.
7. Coppell KJ, Mann JI, Williams SM, Jo E, Drury PL, Miller J, et al. Prevalence of diagnosed and undiagnosed diabetes and prediabetes in New Zealand: findings from the 2008/09 Adult Nutrition Survey. N Z Med J. 2013;126:23–42.
8. Jørgensen ME, Bjerregaard P, Borch-Johnsen K, Witte D. New diagnostic criteria for diabetes: is the change from glucose to HbA1c possible in all populations? J Clin Endocrinol Metab. 2010;95:E333–6.
9. Diabetes in Canada: facts and figures from a public health perspective. Ottawa Ont: Public Health Agency of Canada; 2011.
10. Lee ET, Howard BV, Savage PJ, Cowan LD, Fabsitz RR, Oopik AJ, Yeh J, Go O, Robbins DC, Welty TK. Diabetes and impaired glucose tolerance in three American Indian populations aged 45–74 years. The Strong Heart Study. Diabetes Care. 1995;18:599–610.
11. Zhang P, Zhang X, Brown J, Vistisen D, Sicree R, Shaw J, Nichols G. Global healthcare expenditure on diabetes for 2010 and 2030. Diabetes Res Clin Pract. 2010;87:293–301.
12. Seuring T, Archangelidi O, Suhrcke M. The economic costs of type 2 diabetes: a global systematic review. Pharmacoeconomics. 2015;33:811–31.
13. Grassmann A, Gioberge S, Moeller S, Brown G. End-stage renal disease: global demographics in 2005 and observed trends. Artif Organs. 2006;30:895–7.
14. Reducing risks and preventing disease: population-wide interventions. In: World Health Organization (editor). Global status report on noncommunicable diseases 2010. Chapter 4. Geneva; 2011. http://www.who.int/nmh/publications/ncd_report2010/en/. Accessed 5 Jan 2016.
15. Pan XR, Li GW, Hu YH, et al. Effects of diet and exercise in preventing NIDDM in people with impaired glucose tolerance. The Da Qing IGT and Diabetes Study. Diabetes Care. 1997;20:537–44.
16. Tuomilehto J, Lindström J, Eriksson JG, Finnish Diabetes Prevention Study Group, et al. Prevention of type 2 diabetes mellitus by changes in lifestyle among subjects with impaired glucose tolerance. N Engl J Med. 2001;344:1343–50.
17. Knowler WC, Barrett-Connor E, Fowler SE, Diabetes Prevention Program Research Group, et al. Reduction in the incidence of type 2 diabetes with lifestyle intervention or metformin. N Engl J Med. 2002;346:393–403.
18. Ramachandran A, Snehalatha C, Mary S, Mukesh B, Bhaskar AD, Vijay V, Indian Diabetes Prevention Programme (IDPP). The Indian Diabetes Prevention Programme shows that lifestyle modification and metformin prevent type 2 diabetes in Asian Indian subjects with impaired glucose tolerance (IDPP-1). Diabetologia. 2006;49:289–97.
19. Chiasson JL, Josse RG, Gomis R, Hanefeld M, Karasik A, Laakso M, STOP-NIDDM Trail Research Group. Acarbose for prevention of type 2 diabetes mellitus: the STOP-NIDDM randomised trial. Lancet. 2002;359:2072–7.
20. Kawamori R, Tajima N, Iwamoto Y, Kashiwagi A, Shimamoto K, Kaku K, Voglibose Ph-3 Study Group. Voglibose for prevention of type 2 diabetes mellitus: a randomised, double-blind trial in Japanese individuals with impaired glucose tolerance. Lancet. 2009;373:1607–14.
21. Buchanan TA, Xiang AH, Peters RK, et al. Preservation of pancreatic beta-cell function and pre-

vention of type 2 diabetes by pharmacological treatment of insulin resistance in high-risk hispanic women. Diabetes. 2002;51:2796–803.

22. DREAM (Diabetes REduction Assessment with ramipril and rosiglitazone Medication) Trial Investigators, Gerstein HC, Yusuf S, Bosch J, et al. Effect of rosiglitazone on the frequency of diabetes in patients with impaired glucose tolerance or impaired fasting glucose: a randomised controlled trial. Lancet. 2006;368:1096–105. Erratum in: Lancet 2006; 368:1770.
23. DeFronzo RA, Tripathy D, Schwenke DC, ACT NOW Study, et al. Pioglitazone for diabetes prevention in impaired glucose tolerance. N Engl J Med. 2011;364:1104–15. Erratum in: N Engl J Med 2011;365:189. N Engl J Med 2011;365:869.

Primary Prevention of Type 2 Diabetes: An Imperative for Developing Countries

2

Sam Dagogo-Jack

Introduction

In 2015, the International Diabetes Federation (IDF) estimated that 415 million adults had diabetes worldwide (1). Type 2 diabetes mellitus (T2DM) accounts for 90–95 % of all diabetes cases. The 2015 IDF estimates for people with diabetes in regions of the world (descending order) were 153.2 million in the Western Pacific, 59.8 million in Europe, 44.3 million in North America and the Caribbean, 35.3 million in the Middle East/North Africa, and 14.2 million in sub-Saharan Africa [1]. The country-specific estimates showed that the top 10 nations with the highest numbers of people with diabetes are China (109.6 million), India (99.2 million), the United States of America (29.3 million), Brazil (14.3 million), the Russian Federation (12.1 million), Mexico (11.5 million), Indonesia (10 million), Egypt (7.8 million), Japan (7.2 million), and Bangladesh (7.1 million) [1]. Thus, countries in the developing economies contribute disproportionately to the escalating global diabetes burden (1–3). By 2040, the number of adults with diabetes is projected to increase to 642 million, again with the fastest increases occurring in developing countries. Although sub-Saharan Africa (SSA) currently has the lowest estimate for diabetes prevalence, the steepest proportionate increase in diabetes (240 %) is projected to occur in that region [1] (Fig. 2.1). In contrast, recent data indicate that the incidence of diabetes is leveling off in the United States of America, presumably as a result of increased awareness and national diabetes prevention initiatives [2]. Furthermore, major declines in the rates of diabetes complications have also occurred in the United States [3]. Unfortunately, these encouraging developments in the United States are not shared by most regions of the world, where the escalating prevalence of diabetes and ravages from the disease persist inexorably [1, 4–6].

Risk Factors for Type 2 Diabetes

Both genetic and environmental factors underlie the development of T2DM [6, 7]. To date, more than 60 gene variants associated with T2DM have been identified; however, the effect size of these individual gene variants is rather modest [8–12]. The environmental risk factors strongly associated with T2DM risk include obesity, physical inactivity, history of gestational diabetes, hypertension, and dyslipidemia, among others (Table 2.1) [6, 7, 13]. These risk factors interact with genetic predisposition (indicated by a family

S. Dagogo-Jack, MD, MBBS, MSc, FRCP, FACP, FACE
Division of Endocrinology, Diabetes & Metabolism, University of Tennessee Health Science Center, 920 Madison Avenue, Memphis, TN 38163, USA
e-mail: sdj@uthsc.edu

S. Dagogo-Jack (ed.), *Diabetes Mellitus in Developing Countries and Underserved Communities*, DOI 10.1007/978-3-319-41559-8_2

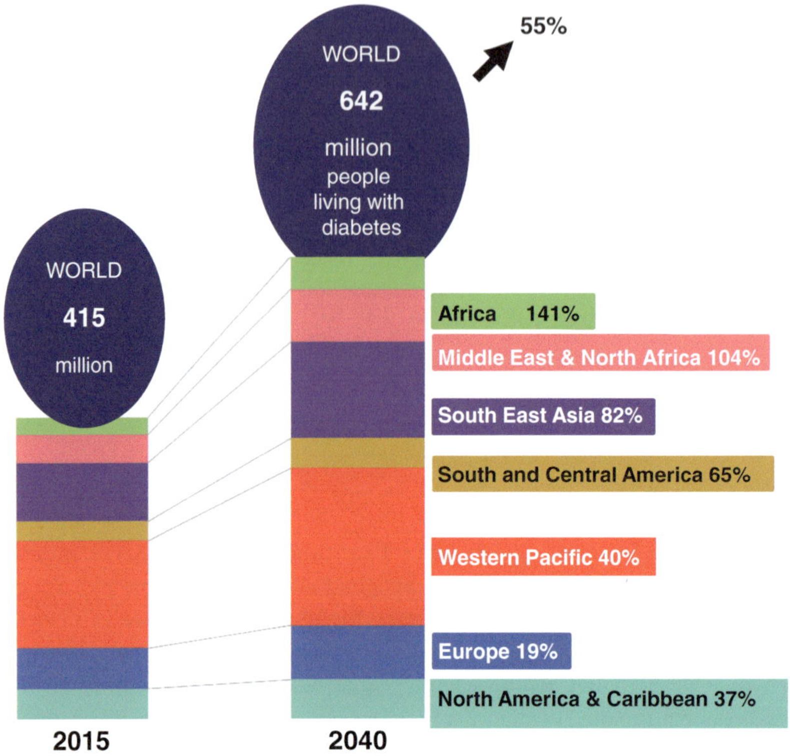

Fig. 2.1 Projected increases in diabetes prevalence in different regions of the world, 2015–2040 (Source: International Diabetes Federation [1])

history of diabetes and/or high-risk ethnic heritage) to promote the development of diabetes. Such a phenomenon was clearly demonstrated in the studies that showed a threefold increase in the rate of T2DM in recent Japanese immigrants to the United States compared with native Japanese [14]. Since a dramatic increase in disease prevalence over a relatively short time frame in humans is unlikely to be due to sudden new genetic mutations, environmental factors (notably changes in diet, physical activity, and perhaps microbial flora) probably trigger the surging diabetes rates among genetically predisposed populations. The exact mechanisms whereby these environmental triggers induce diabetes in genetically predisposed persons remain to be fully elucidated.

Table 2.1 Risk factors for type 2 diabetes

Physical inactivity
Overweight/obesity
First-degree relative with diabetes
High-risk ethnicity
Gestational diabetes or delivery of a baby weighing 9 lb or greater
HDL cholesterol <35 mg/dl ± TG >250 mg/dl
Hypertension (>140/90 mmHg or on therapy)
A1C ≥5.7, IGT, or IFG on previous testing
Conditions associated with insulin resistance: acanthosis nigricans, polycystic ovary disease, etc.
History of cardiovascular disease

Pathophysiology

Current understanding indicates that multiple pathophysiological defects underlie T2DM. Generally, at least eight unique pathophysiological defects are currently recognized in T2DM: insulin resistance, impaired insulin secretion, impaired glucagon suppression, increased lipolysis, exaggerated hepatic glucose production, incretin deficiency/resistance, maladaptive renal glucose reabsorption, and central nervous system defects (including impaired dopaminergic tone and dysregulation of satiety) [15–17] (Fig. 2.2). Insulin resistance can be inherited or acquired. Obesity, aging, physical inactivity, overeating, increased lipolysis, and accumulation of excessive amounts

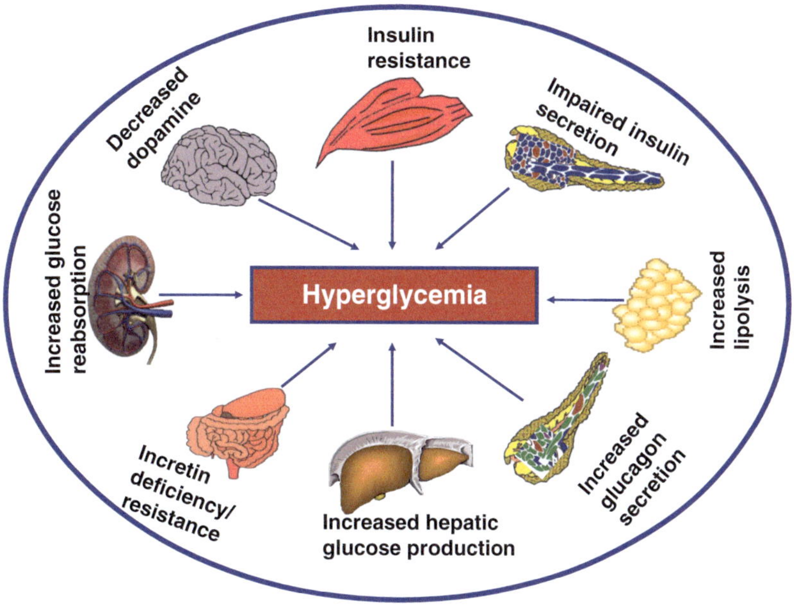

Fig. 2.2 The major pathophysiological defects that lead to the development and progression of type 2 diabetes. Many of the same defects (notably insulin resistance, impaired insulin secretion, lipolysis, and subnormal incretin response) at some degree of expression have also been described in people with prediabetes

of nonesterified (free) fatty acids are known causes of insulin resistance. Normally, cytoplasmic long-chain fatty acids are transported into mitochondria as long-chain fatty acyl coenzyme A (LCFA-CoA) for beta-oxidation, a process that is gated by carnitine palmitoyl transferase (CPT)-1 and CPT-2 (the shuttle enzymes located in the outer and inner mitochondrial membrane). This shuttle process ensures that fatty acids do not accumulate excessively in the cytoplasm. Inhibition of that process leads to intracellular accumulation of long-chain fatty acids, which can induce lipotoxicity, cellular dysfunction, and cell death [16, 17]. Further, intracellular accumulation of long-chain fatty acids along with diacylglycerol (DAG) can activate certain isoforms of protein kinase C (PKC), leading to aberrant phosphorylation of the insulin receptor and consequent insulin resistance.

Acetyl-CoA, a product of glycolysis in the Krebs cycle, can be converted to malonyl CoA by the enzyme acetyl-CoA carboxylase (ACC). Malonyl-CoA is the activated two-carbon donor required for fatty acid synthesis. Malonyl-CoA also is a potent inhibitor of CPT-1, thereby blocking the delivery and oxidation of fatty acids in the mitochondria. The result is accumulation of long-chain fatty acids in the cytosol and eventual lipotoxicity [17, 18]. Glucose abundance also increases the formation of intracellular DAG. Thus, multiple metabolic pathways link intracellular glucose abundance (usually derived from carbohydrate consumption) to impaired fat oxidation, fatty acid synthesis, accumulation of long-chain fatty acids, risk of lipotoxicity, and insulin resistance (Fig. 2.3). Among the potent interventions that have been demonstrated to ameliorate the pathological cellular and molecular processes leading to insulin resistance are caloric restriction (reduction of carbohydrate and fat intake), physical activity, and weight loss [19–27].

Prediabetes

The term "prediabetes" refers to impaired glucose tolerance (IGT) and impaired fasting glucose (IFG), two intermediate metabolic states between normal glucose tolerance and diabetes. IGT is defined by a plasma glucose level of 140 mg/dl to 199 mg/dl (7.8–11.1 mmol/l), 2 h following ingestion of a 75-g oral solution. IFG is defined by a fasting plasma glucose level of 100–125 mg/dl (5.6–6.9 mmol/l) [13] (Fig. 2.4). There is considerable overlap in the risk factors and pathophysiological defects that underlie T2DM and prediabetes. Although the exact sequence of

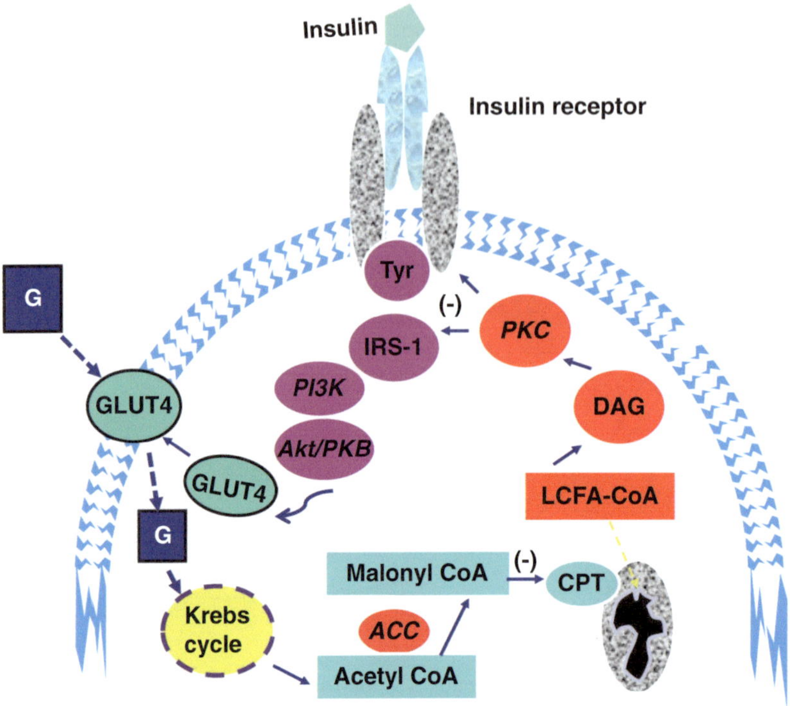

Fig. 2.3 Schematic diagram of insulin signaling pathways and interactions with glucose (*G*) and fatty acid metabolism. Increased intracellular glucose flux generates acetyl coenzyme A molecules which can be converted to malonyl coenzyme, a process catalyzed by acyl coenzyme A carboxylase (*ACC*). Malonyl coenzyme A inhibits carnitylpalmitoyltransferase (*CPT*), the mitochondrial enzyme that transports long-chain fatty acids (*LCFA*) into the inner mitochondrial space for oxidation. The resultant accumulation of LCFA in the cytosol is linked to insulin resistance via mechanisms involving protein kinase C (*PKC*) and altered phosphorylation of the insulin receptor

evolution of individual pathophysiological defects has not been determined precisely, many of the defects coevolve during the pathogenesis of T2DM and are demonstrable even at the stage of prediabetes (Fig. 2.1) [28–38]. Estimates by the Centers for Disease Control and Prevention (CDC) in the United States indicated that there were ~29 million adults with diabetes and 86 million with prediabetes in 2014 [39]. Worldwide, there are more than 400 million people with prediabetes [1]. Individuals with prediabetes progress to T2DM at an annual rate of ~10 % [31, 32].

Predictors of Progression from Prediabetes to Type 2 Diabetes

An analysis of six prospective studies [40] on progression from IGT to diabetes revealed the following features: (1) baseline fasting plasma glucose (FPG) and the 2-h OGTT glucose values are positively associated with diabetes risk; (2) the rate of progression from IGT to T2DM was exponential among subjects in the top quartile of baseline FPG but increased linearly with increasing 2-h OGTT glucose levels; (3) incident diabetes occurred at higher rates in Hispanic, Mexican-Americans, Pima, and Nauruan populations than among Caucasians; (4) the degree of obesity, as measured by the BMI, predicted T2DM risk in three studies with the lowest incidence rates of diabetes but not in the studies that recorded the highest incidence of T2DM; and (5) a family history of diabetes did not predict the risk of progression from IGT to diabetes in these studies, suggesting that genetic effects probably are fully established by the stage of IGT [40]. Thus, the magnitude of fasting and post-challenge dysglycemia (a reflection of insulin action and

Criteria for the Diagnosis of Diabetes and Prediabetes

	Normal	Prediabetes	Diabetes
Fasting Glucose	FPG < 100 mg/dl (<5.6 mmol/l)	100 – 125 mg/dl (5.6 – 6.9 mmol/l)	FPG ≥ 126 mg/dl (≥7.0 mmol/l)
OGTT	2hPG <140mg/dl (<7.8 mmol/l)	140 – 199 mg/dl (7.8 - 11.0 mmol/l)	≥200 mg/dl (11.1 mmol/l) or random BG ≥200 + typical symptoms
HbA1c	HbA1c < 5.7%	5.7 – 6.4%	HbA1c > 6.5%

Fig. 2.4 Criteria for the definition of normal glucose regulation and diagnosis of prediabetes and diabetes. *FPG* fasting plasma glucose, *2hPG* two-hour post-load plasma glucose, *OGTT* oral glucose tolerance test, using standard 75 g

insulin secretion), ethnicity, and weight gain are major predictors of progression to T2DM.

Longitudinal studies in subjects from a high-risk population (Pima Indians) [41] with baseline normal glucose tolerance (NGT) indicated that weight gain, insulin resistance, and progressive loss of insulin secretory response to glucose predicted the development of T2DM [34]. Weight gain also predicted progression from NGT to IGT (5.2 kg vs. 2.6 kg in nonprogressors) and progression from IGT to T2DM during a 6-year follow-up period [34]. The greater weight gain in the progressors was accompanied by ~ 30 % worsening of insulin resistance and >50 % decline in acute insulin secretory response to intravenous glucose [34]. Weight gain also predicted incident T2DM in African-Americans in the Atherosclerosis Risk in Communities study [42]. It follows therefore that interventions that induce weight loss (e.g., diet, exercise, medications) could prevent progression from prediabetes to T2DM. In the prospective study of Pima Indians [34], progressive impairment of first-phase insulin secretion proved to be a critical determinant of progression from NGT to IGT and from IGT to T2DM. Progression from IGT to diabetes was associated with ~75 % decline in acute insulin secretory response to intravenous glucose [34]. A high concordance rate for impaired insulin secretion has also been reported among elderly identical twins discordant for T2DM (42), which suggests a genetic basis for pancreatic beta-cell dysfunction. The role of beta-cell dysfunction in predicting progression to T2DM indicates that interventions that prevent or replenish the progressive decline in insulin secretion can be expected to prevent the development of diabetes.

Predictors of Initial Transition to Prediabetes

In contrast to the numerous studies on the transition from prediabetes to T2DM [34, 40–42], information on the incidence of prediabetes among initially normoglycemic persons is scant. In a study of 254 Pima Indians with normoglycemia, 79 subjects (31 %) progressed to prediabetes (IGT) during a mean follow-up period of 4 years [43]. Based on those results, the incidence of prediabetes among Pima Indians can be estimated at ~8 %/year [43]. Of the 468 subjects with NGT at enrollment in the Baltimore Longitudinal Study on Aging (BLSA), over half were followed for at least 10 years [44]. By 10 years, 62 % of the initially NGT participants had progressed to prediabetes, yielding an incidence rate of prediabetes 6.2 % in the BLSA cohort (96 % of whom were European-American) [44]. Dagogo-Jack et al. followed 343 healthy African-American and European-American offspring of parents with T2DM in the Pathobiology of Prediabetes in a Biracial Cohort (POP-ABC) study and observed that 100 had developed incident prediabetes (IGT and/or IFG) during a mean follow-up period of ~3 years, without evidence of ethnic disparities [45]. Thus, among black and white subjects with parental history of T2DM, the incidence of prediabetes was ~10 %/year. These data indicate that the risk of incident prediabetes among offspring of parents with T2DM in the general United States population is similar to or higher than the risk observed among Pima Indians, a group with the world's highest rate of T2DM [41]. The POP-ABC data underscore the importance of heredity, familial, and genetic T2DM. Taken together, these studies found that normoglycemic individuals develop prediabetes at an annual rate of 6–10 %, the higher rate being more likely among those with a strong family history of T2DM. Based on findings in the Pima Indian [34] and the POP-ABC [45] studies, the predictors of incident prediabetes include older age, male gender, overweight/obesity, lower insulin sensitivity, and impaired acute insulin secretory response to glucose [45]. Other predictors of incident prediabetes included food habits, physical inactivity, higher C-reactive protein, and lower adiponectin levels [45–47]. Obesity is a likely unifying factor that links the various pathophysiological mechanisms leading to dysglycemia. Comparison of several measures of adiposity indicates higher values in people who progress from normoglycemia to prediabetes compared with those who maintain normal glucose metabolism (Table 2.2).

Rationale for Primary Prevention of Type 2 Diabetes

There are compelling reasons why the primary prevention of T2DM ought to be an urgent policy priority in developing countries. Undoubtedly, the prohibitive costs of managing diabetes and its complications could easily overwhelm the budgets of many low- and middle-income countries. In many such countries, competing pressures from infectious diseases and periodic epidemics can easily relegate considerations for diabetes care to the bottom of the totem pole of noncommunicable diseases. However, the unique demographic (increased diabetes susceptibility at younger age and female preponderance) and the

Table 2.2 Selected baseline demographic and clinical characteristics of participants who developed prediabetes (progressors) compared to those who remained free of incident prediabetes during 5 years of follow-up in the POP-ABC study

Characteristic	Progressors	Nonprogressors	*P*-value
Number	111	232	–
White/black	53/58	97/135	0.3
Female/male	65/46	180/52	0.0003
Age (year)	47 ± 8.9	43.9 ± 10.7	0.0017
Age 18–40/40–65	23/88	85/147	0.0030
Weight (kg)	90 ± 20	83 ± 22	0.0036
BMI (kg/m^2)	31.4 ± 6.9	29.6 ± 7.4	0.0013
Waist (cm)	99 ± 14	92 ± 16	<0.0001
Female	98 ± 12	91 ± 16	0.0006
Male	101 ± 15	96 ± 15	0.14
Total fat mass (kg)	32.0 ± 12.6	29.9 ± 14.0	0.0025
Female	37.2 ± 12.0	32.1 ± 14.4	0.02
Male	24.2 ± 9.1	22.4 ± 9.1	0.0004
Trunk fat mass (kg)	16.6 ± 6.8	14.3 ± 7.3	<0.0001
Female	18.9 ± 6.7	15.1 ± 7.6	0.0064
Male	13.1 ± 5.4	11.5 ± 5.5	0.07

Plus–minus values are means ±SD

BMI body mass index, *POP-ABC* pathobiology of prediabetes in a biracial cohort (see [47])

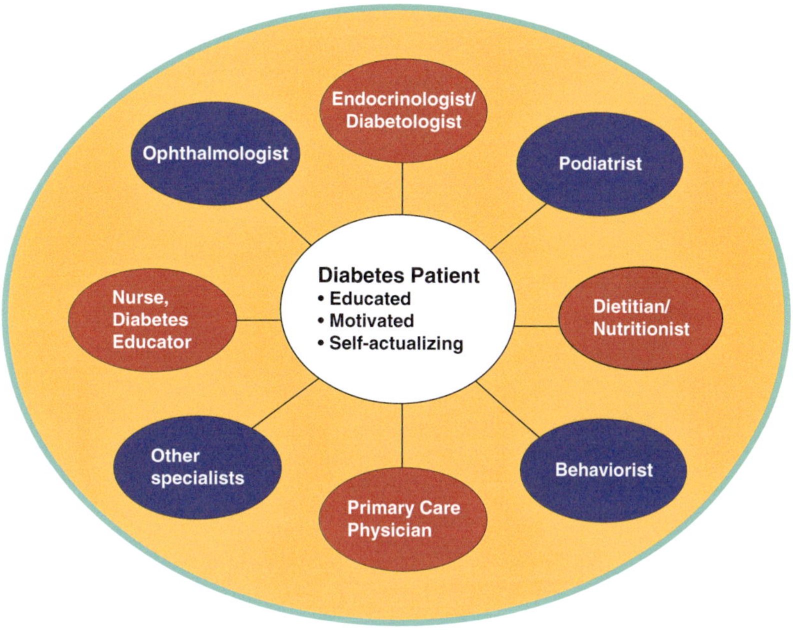

Fig. 2.5 Human capital investment in building a multidisciplinary team-based diabetes care service. A well-informed and highly motivated patient is critical to the success of diabetes care

geographical (urban vs. rural) distribution of the diabetes provide clear targets for preventive intervention. Moreover, there is interplay between diabetes and chronic infectious diseases (e.g., tuberculosis) as well as between successful control of HIV infection and iatrogenic diabetes. But, the strongest argument for prioritizing diabetes prevention is the premium availability of effective tools that have been developed in landmark studies conducted in different parts of the world that established the feasibility of preventing T2DM [48–51].

Diabetes mellitus imposes a huge drain on national health budgets. The annual diabetes-related health-care costs exceed $240 billion in the United States [52]. Although precise figures are hard to come by, on average, developing countries spent at least 5 % of their total health expenditures on diabetes in 2010 [53]. The 5 % budgetary allocation is suboptimal and could be much higher if diabetes-related medical costs were to be adjusted to account for the >50 % rate of undiagnosed diabetes in developing countries [53, 54]. Optimal control of glycemia and related comorbidities is difficult and expensive to achieve in patients with established diabetes. Availability of antidiabetes medications, diabetes testing and monitoring supplies, laboratory support, and the professional care team (comprising of physician specialists, nurses, dietitians, diabetes educators, podiatrists, and other experts) is often elusive in many countries that face challenges in health-care infrastructure (Fig. 2.5). Where some or all of these essential resources for effective diabetes control are available, their distribution often is lopsided, and most rural areas are underserved. In the absence of comprehensive national health coverage, affordability of medications and self-management supplies, even when available, cannot be guaranteed for most low-income patients. For example, in sub-Saharan Africa, insulin security and affordability have been major concerns [55, 56]. Lacking cost defrayment by government or reimbursement by third-party insurers, the limitations imposed by the significant out-of-pocket costs of diabetes care translate to chronic suboptimal care, which increases the burden of diabetes-related complications [57].

Type 2 diabetes, a global epidemic, now ranks among the leading noncommunicable public health challenges of the present era [1, 4, 5]. The public health burden imposed by diabetes is underscored by the fact that diabetes now is the leading cause of blindness, end-stage renal failure,

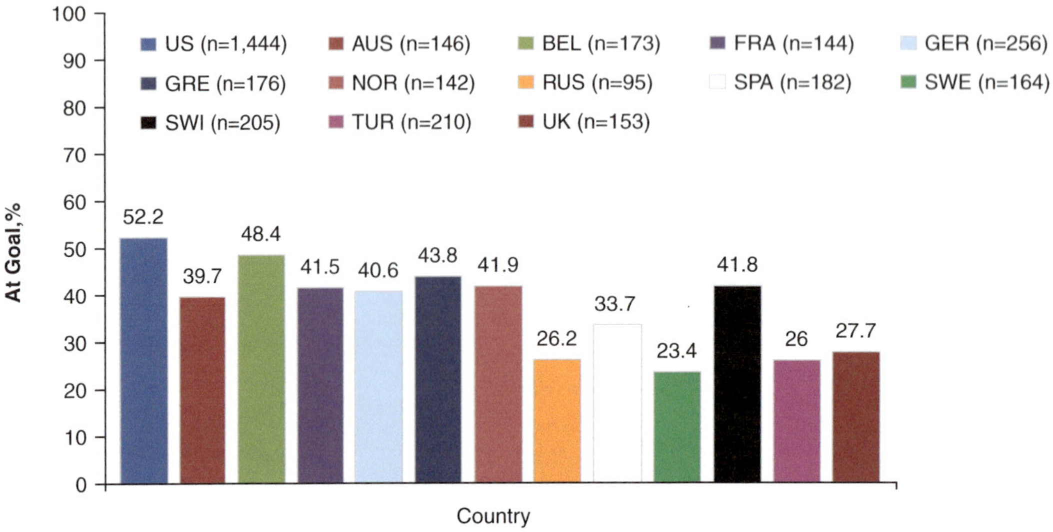

Fig. 2.6 Percentage of patients with diabetes achieving optimal control in the United States (HbA1c target <7 %) or several European countries (HbA1c target <6.5 %) (Source: see [67, 68])

and nontraumatic limb amputations and a major contributor to heart disease, stroke, and peripheral vascular disease [57–60]. These complications can be prevented or delayed by achieving and maintaining excellent control of glycemia and comorbid conditions, such as hypertension and dyslipidemia [61–64]. However, the achievement of sustained glycemic control to the level necessary for prevention of complications often proves elusive, even in countries in the developed economies [65, 66] (Fig. 2.6). Optimal glycemic control requires a highly motivated patient, working with a diabetes care team comprising physicians and several cadres of clinicians (Fig. 2.5). The care processed involves the use of multiple medications; frequent clinic visits; adherence to challenging lifestyle prescriptions; performance of demanding self-management tasks; paying for cumulative costs of home blood glucose test strips; sustained engagement by a team of physicians, nurses, dietitians, diabetes educators, ophthalmologists, podiatrists, behaviorists, and other specialized professionals; and the implementation of sundry other recommendations [13, 67] (Fig. 2.5). Lacking the requisite resources and support for excellence in diabetes care, many patients in developing countries face the specter of chronic suboptimal control of glycemia and multiple-related risk factors. Consequently, the long-term complications of diabetes flourish unchecked. Ironically, many developing countries lack the infrastructure, technology, and human resources for adequate management of diabetes complications. Services like dialysis, renal transplantation, laser surgery for retinopathy, interventional cardiology, and rehabilitation services for amputees are not routinely available. It is, thus, self-evident that primary prevention of T2DM is an imperative for developing countries [68, 69].

Unique Vulnerabilities in Developing Countries

Data from surveys in developing countries indicate that diabetes predominantly affects younger age-groups: the majority of people with diabetes fall within the age range of 40–59 years, as compared to 60 years or older in developed countries [69]. It has also been predicted that future increases in diabetes numbers would affect all age-groups in developing countries, whereas in developed countries an increase is expected predominantly among persons older than 60 years, with a slight decrease in the younger age-groups [69]. This younger age predilection means that individuals in developing countries in their prime productivity years are the ones burdened with diabetes and its complications, with dire consequences on national economies. Besides the enormous direct medical costs, the additional lost productivity from absenteeism and presenteeism inflicts compounding negative effects on current and future economic performance in the developing world. Furthermore, the preponderance of diabetes in young women of childbearing age perpetuates a vicious cycle through the effects of intrauterine fetal programming for increased susceptibility to cardiometabolic disorders in postnatal life [70, 71]. A more recent vulnerability is the unexpected association of successful antiretroviral therapy in HIV patients with treatment-emergent metabolic perturbations, including diabetes, dyslipidemia, and lipodystrophy [72, 73].

Approach to Prevention of Type 2 Diabetes

Lifestyle Modification

Three landmark studies have demonstrated the efficacy of lifestyle intervention in preventing the development of T2DM in high-risk individuals [48–51]. All studies targeted persons with prediabetes (principally IGT and high-normal fasting plasma glucose). The lifestyle counseling focused on dietary intervention and increased physical activity and a weight loss target of approximately 5 to <10 % of initial body weight. The dietary intervention was aimed at encouraging participants to adopt healthy eating patterns and to decrease caloric consumption (by ~500–700 kcal/day) through selective reduction in saturated fat calories and limitation of excessive carbohydrate intake. The physical activity component motivated high-risk individuals to accrue 150–240 min of moderate-intensity activity per week (~30–60 min daily on 5 days or more each week). The target intensity (~55 % VO_2 max) of physical activity is equivalent to walking at a brisk pace [48–51]. Compared with the control groups (who merely received passive health information), these lifestyle modifications proved remarkably efficacious in decreasing the rate of progression from prediabetes to T2DM during study periods that ranged from ~3 to 6 years [48–51].

Da Qing Study

Investigators in the Da Qing study (49) screened 110,660 men and women from 33 health-care clinics in the city of Da Qing, China, and enrolled 577 adults (mean age 45 years; mean BMI 26 kg/m^2) with IGT. The participants were randomized by clinic to a control group or to one of three active treatment groups – diet only, exercise only, or diet plus exercise – and were followed every 2 weeks during the first 3 months and quarterly thereafter for 6 years.

The primary end point, development of T2DM at 6 years, occurred in 67.7 % of subjects in the control group, 43.8 % in the diet-only group, 41.1 % in the exercise-only group, and 46.0 % in the diet-plus-exercise group. Interestingly, relative decrease in diabetes incidence in the active treatment groups was similar in lean or overweight (BMI >25 kg/m^2) subjects. After adjustments for baseline differences in BMI and fasting glucose, the diet, exercise, and diet-plus-exercise interventions produced 31 %, 46 %, and 42 % reductions in diabetes risk, compared with control [48]. However, there was apparently no additive efficacy of combined diet plus exercise versus either component of the lifestyle intervention.

Finnish Diabetes Prevention Study

In the Finnish Diabetes Prevention Study (FDPS) [49], 522 middle-aged subjects (mean age, 55 years; mean BMI 31 kg/m^2) with IGT were randomly assigned to either an intervention or control group. Each participant in the intervention group received individualized sessions with a health counselor (approximately every 2 months) and was encouraged to aim for ~5 % weight loss through reduction of total and saturated fat intake and increased intake of fiber. The lifestyle participants also were instructed to increase their physical activity by ~210 min per week. The primary end point was development of T2DM (confirmed by OGTT). The cumulative incidence of diabetes after 4 years was 11 % in the intervention group and 23 % in the control group, a significant 58 % reduction in diabetes incidence. The mean weight loss in the lifestyle group was ~3.5 kg compared with ~0.8 kg in the control group. Improvement in insulin and preservation of insulin secretion also occurred differentially in the lifestyle group compared with control [49].

Diabetes Prevention Program

The Diabetes Prevention Program (DPP) enrolled 3,234 participants with IGT and high-normal fasting glucose and assigned them randomly to intensive lifestyle intervention (ILI), metformin, or placebo treatment [50]. The enrollees included representation from all ethnic and racial groups in the US population; persons of non-European ancestry constituted 45 % of the entire cohort. The ILI targets were a minimum of 7 % weight loss/weight maintenance and a minimum of 150 min of physical activity per week. Subjects in the ILI group received a 16-lesson curriculum covering diet, exercise, and behavior modification delivered by case managers on a one-to-one basis during the first 24 weeks after enrollment. Subsequently, monthly individual sessions and group sessions with the case managers were provided, to reinforce the behavioral changes.

After an average follow-up period of 2.8 years, the participants randomized to ILI showed a 58 % reduction in the incidence of diabetes, as compared with placebo [50]. This beneficial effect of lifestyle intervention was seen in all demographic subgroups defined by age, gender, race, or ethnicity. Furthermore, reversion to normal glucose tolerance (NGT) occurred in ~40 % of subjects in the lifestyle intervention arm, as compared with ~18 % in the control arm [50]. Participants who experienced reversion to NGT (even if transiently) were 50 % less likely to develop diabetes during long-term follow-up, as compared with those who had persistent IGT status [74].

After cessation of the active phase of the studies, follow-up assessment showed continued benefit of lifestyle intervention in decreasing diabetes incidence during post-study follow-up periods spanning 10–20 years [75–77], clearly demonstrating a "legacy" effect.

Indian Diabetes Prevention Program

The Indian Diabetes Prevention Program (IDPP) randomized South Asians with IGT to four arms: control (with standard advice, $N=136$), lifestyle modification ($N=133$), low-dose metformin ($N=133$), and lifestyle modification plus low-dose metformin ($N=136$) [51]. Participants in lifestyle modification groups received counseling sessions aimed at promoting healthy eating habits (decreased intake of refined carbohydrates and fats and increased intake of dietary fiber) and boosting physical activity (at least 30 min daily). After a median follow-up of 30 months, the relative reductions in diabetes incidence were 28.5 % with lifestyle modification, 26.4 % with metformin, and 28.2 % with lifestyle modification and metformin [71]. Remarkably, these benefits of lifestyle modification occurred despite the lack of significant weight change in the two groups that focused on lifestyle change.

Translating Diabetes Prevention to Communities in Developing Countries

Collectively, the extant data show that lifestyle modification is remarkably and consistently effective in preventing the development of T2DM in high-risk populations in China, India, Europe, and the United States. To date, no large RCTs of diabetes prevention have been published from Africa, Latin America, Australia, New Zealand, the Middle East, or the Caribbean regions, although a number of pilot projects have been implemented or are ongoing. Some of these pilot projects have reported promising results among indigenous (Maori) New Zealanders [78]. There is overwhelming evidence that lifestyle modification is a more compelling approach to diabetes prevention than medications. However, the landmark lifestyle intervention programs that achieved remarkable success in preventing diabetes were designed as randomized controlled trials (RCTs) and conducted predominantly at academic medical centers. The protocols of many of the RCTs entailed frequent clinic visits, utilized specialized multidisciplinary teams (including physicians, nurses, dietitians, psychologists, exercise physiologists, and others), and consumed substantial resources and support from institutions and funding agencies. Notably, all protocol-mandated services and interventions were provided at no cost to participants in the diabetes prevention RCTs, many of whom also received incentives and stipends. Thus, the odds were stacked heavily toward success in these RCTs, and it is crucial to determine whether the sterling results obtained in the landmark RCTs could be reproduced in the community, without all of the inbuilt advantages, specialized professionals, and resources. Some community initiatives are currently underway to determine the feasibility of community programs for diabetes prevention [79, 80]. The United States Centers for Disease Control and Prevention (CDC) has been training and certifying community diabetes prevention personnel under the aegis of the National Diabetes Prevention Program [81]. Programs using trained lay persons to deliver adaptations of the DPP lifestyle intervention to groups (rather than one-on-one sessions) in the community have been shown to produce promising results [79, 80, 82].

Keys to Translation

In general, the keys to the translation of any new concept or discovery related to health consist of (1) adequate comprehension, evaluation, and acceptance of the new information within a specialized professional community; (2) processing and conversion of the new information into the professional knowledge base and dissemination to a wider circle of professionals and students; (3) diffusion of the conceptual information to the general public, through demonstrative education by convinced professionals; and (4) adoption of evidenced-based changes in practices and behaviors, triggered by the new knowledge. The preceding construct of translational cascade is somewhat akin to the sequential steps in Prochaska's transtheoretical model of behavior modification: *pre-contemplative, contemplative, preparation, action, and change* [83, 84].

Dissemination of Diabetes Prevention Knowledge

The preponderance of evidence from randomized clinical trials on the efficacy of lifestyle intervention in preventing T2DM has established the rationale for diabetes prevention as self-evident among health professionals. However, the screening for prediabetes and institution of prompt lifestyle counseling have not become routine practice, even in economically advanced countries. Bridging the hiatus between philosophical acceptance of the idea of diabetes prevention among health professionals and the adoption of pragmatic steps to detect and act upon high-risk persons requires a methodical approach.

The information and knowledge base of healthcare professional must be steered toward a more pragmatic approach to primary prevention of diabetes through a number of established approaches. First, curriculum development in primary and high schools should begin to introduce seminal data from the behavioral components of the landmark diabetes prevention studies within a wider context of instruction in wellness and health promotion. Second, students in schools of medicine, nursing, pharmacy, and allied medical fields should receive exposure to formal instruction in the design and key findings of the major diabetes prevention studies, again, within the wider context of wellness and health promotion. Third, mastery of the principles and methods of primary prevention of T2DM ought to be a priority item in the core curriculum of residency training programs for physicians. The latter can be implemented through lectures and workshops by intramural experts and invited speakers. Finally, practicing physicians in all disciplines (including internists, family physicians, endocrinologists, cardiologists, nephrologists, general and specialist surgeons), podiatrists, nurse practitioners, and other primary care providers must have their knowledge base updated to include the tenets of primary prevention of diabetes.

Operationally, the increased awareness about diabetes prevention at the primary care level should lead to increased zeal for screening and detection of individuals with prediabetes (often relatives of patients with established T2DM). Once individuals have been diagnosed with prediabetes (Fig. 2.4), appropriate referral for lifestyle counseling can follow, as recommended by the American Diabetes Association [13].

Convinced health-care workers and their families become conduits for the dissemination and diffusion of diabetes prevention ideas in targeted segments of the public (hospital communities, established patients and their relatives, schools, neighborhoods, social media and outlets, religious forums, etc.). Most human societies have encountered diabetes and are probably preconditioned for receptive attention to diabetes campaigns, having been primed by awareness of the more obvious complications, such as blindness, amputation, and end-stage kidney disease. Such a preconditioning of societal awareness of diabetes and its complications bodes well for the dissemination of ideas regarding the rationale and feasibility of diabetes prevention. Yet, the fact that T2DM can be prevented by modest caloric restriction and physical activity is yet to enter folklore. That gap in the popular consciousness (despite the raging global epidemic of diabetes) presents an enormous opportunity for leadership by health-care professionals and civic leaders. To convince and motivate large segments of society for preventive action against diabetes requires coordinated efforts at the local, regional, state, national, and international leadership levels. Creative programs anchored by ministries and departments of health, information, education, and other agencies would also be important catalysts for public education, awareness, and action. The expertise and contributions from philanthropic organizations and other nongovernmental bodies, especially local, national, and international diabetes associations, can be invaluable during the process of program building and facilitation.

Strategies for Diabetes Prevention in the Community

Five key elements can be distilled from the lifestyle intervention protocols utilized by the DPP and other major diabetes prevention trials. Most or all of these strategies can readily be adapted for widespread application in the community.

1. Selection of persons at risk
   All diabetes prevention trials targeted, screened, and enrolled a defined group of at-risk persons, using well-known risk factors for T2DM (Table 2.2). The merit of that approach is underscored by the finding that the participants randomized to placebo did in fact develop diabetes at an alarming rate (~12 % per year in DPP, ~18 % per year in IDPP) [50]. Thus, the published criteria used for selecting at-risk persons for diabetes prevention appear to be of high fidelity and can be adopted for translation of diabetes prevention in the general populace. Specifically, a positive family history of T2DM in first-degree relatives, overweight or obesity (using ethnic-specific BMI cutoffs), and a fasting plasma glucose in the range of 96–125 mg/dl predict a high yield of eligible individuals for community diabetes prevention efforts. The appropriate BMI cutoff for identifying overweight subjects appears to be >22 kg/m^2 for Asians compared with >25 kg/m^2 for most other ethnicities [85, 86]. The inclusive age range for the published diabetes prevention studies was >25 years for DPP and Da Qing studies, 40–65 years for FDPS, and 30–55 years for IDPP [48–51]. None of the published diabetes prevention studies enrolled individuals younger than age 25 years, which is a major limitation, given the increasing prevalence of T2DM in children and adolescents [87, 88]. Obesity and physical inactivity are major risk factors for T2DM in children, as in adults. Other risk factors include female gender,

ethnicity, family history of T2DM, peripubertal age, and intrauterine exposure to diabetes [89–91]. Because the long-term complications of diabetes become established over a >10-year period, the epidemic of T2DM in children and adolescents predicts dire consequences for patients at the prime of their youth [92]. Primary prevention of childhood T2DM, therefore, is of utmost public health importance. For the aforementioned reasons, it is desirable for community diabetes prevention initiatives to lower the inclusive age for screening at-risk persons well into the childhood and adolescent years. A school-based pilot study sponsored by the US National Institutes of Health showed that obesity and diabetes risk factors can be decreased by lifestyle intervention in sixth grade pupils [93].

2. Delivery of physical activity intervention
The physical activity component of lifestyle intervention in the reported diabetes prevention studies was of moderate intensity (~55 % VO2 max) and duration (~30 min daily in the DPP). Out of an abundance of caution, participants in the DPP lifestyle intervention arm underwent submaximal cardiac stress testing prior to commencement of the physical activity program [94]; however, that was not a routine requirement for physical activity in the majority of diabetes prevention trials [48, 49, 51]. It must be stressed that physical activity was well-tolerated in the DPP, and no untoward cardiovascular events or musculoskeletal injuries were reported. A routine requirement for prescreening with cardiac stress would be a serious logistical and economic hindrance to the widespread translation of diabetes prevention and may not be necessary for the majority of free-living individuals who are candidates for diabetes prevention in the community. The DPP exercise goal of 150 min per week was similar to that prescribed in the Malmo [95] and Da Qing [48] studies but lower than the 210 min per week prescribed in the Finnish study [49]. The DPP and all other landmark studies have demonstrated the efficacy, tolerability, and safety of moderate-intensity physical activity (150–210 min per week) as used for the prevention of T2DM [48–51, 95]. Walking was the preferred activity for the vast majority of participants in these studies.

Given the generally low rates of voluntary physical activity in urbanized communities [75, 76], innovative motivational strategies [96, 97] will be required to build physical activity into daily routine, especially in high-risk populations. In clinical trials, the physical activity intervention component often required exercise physiologists or other skilled staff to implement. For large-scale community translation, these specialists may not be essential, as lay persons can be trained to deliver physical activity intervention. However, the infrastructure required for effective large-scale implementation of physical activity intervention – well-lit and safe walkways, public parks, biking trail, health and fitness clubs, etc. – may not be readily available in many developing countries, especially at overcrowded urban centers. One innovative approach to the problem of space for physical activity is to establish partnerships with schools and houses of religious worship, so that their large real estate can be utilized for diabetes prevention activity after school hours and during non-worship days.

The tropical environment (especially, high temperature, humidity, and torrential rain) constitutes an additional barrier to regular outdoor exercise. Cultural barriers to exercise may also exist in some communities, where obesity may be venerated as a sign of well-being and evidence of freedom from wasting diseases (such as malnutrition, HIV/AIDS, and tuberculosis). A less obvious obstacle is a cultural mindset among blue collar workers that associates exercise with the privileged elite. These (mis)-perceptions must be confronted using education and public awareness campaigns. Such grassroots educational campaigns should emphasize the risks of obesity and the health benefits of modest increases in physical activity, thereby shifting the focus from exercise as indulgent leisure of the bourgeoisie to exercise as an engine of health promotion among the proletariat. Civic and local government leadership should collaborate to create community resources for participatory health promotion and wellness. The lowest reported dose of exercise which was effective in preventing diabetes was ~150 min/week (or ~30 min/day) [50]; however, significant metabolic benefits can be derived from shorter bouts of activity (10–15 min spread across two or three periods during the day) [98]. This specific point is worth emphasizing when counseling time-pressed subjects. Additionally, whenever appropriate, participatory physical activity and health promotion should be built into scheduled cultural festivals and other activities. The latter could include student–teacher and parent–child low- to moderate-intensity sporting events, parades, pageants, mini-carnivals, and other civic celebrations.

3. Frequent contacts
The frequency of contacts between participants in diabetes prevention programs and lifestyle interventionists was weekly, monthly, bimonthly, or quarterly, depending on the specific study protocols and phase of study. In the DPP, the greatest weight loss occurred during the initial 24 weeks of intensive individual weekly sessions with lifestyle coaches [50]. When the visit frequency was relaxed to monthly sessions, some weight regain was noted. Other studies, notably FDPS and Da Qing, used lower overall contact frequency (every 2 months to quarterly) and achieved comparable results to those achieved by the DPP [48, 49]. Clearly, regular contact at some frequency between interventionists and participants is desirable for successful diabetes prevention. Such contacts could create favorable dynamics and "bonding" between lifestyle coach and participant. Moreover, the repeated objective recording of weight, waist circumference, and other metabolic measures could have important motivational effects. However, the optimal frequency of physical contacts necessary for successful diabetes prevention in the community is unclear and could well differ by cultural and regional peculiarities. Thus, such data would need to be determined through pilot studies in different communities. Fewer face-to-face counseling sessions in group format, supplemented by virtual contacts (via SMS text messaging, e-mail, or web-based platforms) could be a less expensive approach to harnessing the power of contact in diabetes prevention efforts. Along these lines, web-based lifestyle programs have been reported to have modest but variable effects on weight loss in studies reported from Australia, the United States, Europe, and Asia [99–103]; however, extrapolation to populations with lower literacy and uncertain digital access is questionable.

4. Delivery of dietary intervention
The participants in the landmark diabetes prevention studies [48–51] were asked to reduce their daily intake of fat calories and total calories. Consumption of meals high in dietary fiber was also promoted. To help participants maintain a healthy eating pattern, additional training regarding reading and understanding food labels was provided. The nutritional counseling was delivered in person during the regular visits. As already discussed, there appeared to be a relationship between frequency of counseling visits and the magnitude of weight loss in the DPP. However, other programs that used less frequent visits achieved comparable efficacy in diabetes prevention. Thus, following initial run-in and initiation of the dietary intervention, maintenance visits at approximately 3-month intervals may be sufficient to yield desirable results in a community setting.

Pragmatically, implementing dietary intervention for diabetes prevention in local communities in sub-Saharan Africa and other developing regions would be fraught with challenges. First, of course, is the shortage of trained and culturally adapted dietitians and medical nutritionists. Second, mandatory food labeling, the result of legislation passed some decades ago in the West, is not yet a routine practice in many developing countries. In fact, nutritional information may be lacking for many staple foods. Thirdly, even where food labeling exists, low literacy rates mitigate against their comprehension. Furthermore, the popularity of informal retail markets (especially for grains, flour, corn, cereal, rice, beans, cassava powder {garri}, and other tuber-derived staples) that do not offer standardized packaging calls for creative approaches to the implementation of caloric control. Thus, effective dietary intervention strategies for diabetes prevention in developing countries must anticipate and creatively overcome or circumvent these apparent translational obstacles. In that regard, the value of local pilot and feasibility studies cannot be overemphasized. In low literacy regions, a visual (pictorial) approach to dietary modification could be an effective alternative to text-based formats. The Dietary Guidelines for Americans, issued by the United States Department of Agriculture (USDA), advocates a simple plate method: half of the plate contains fruits and vegetables; the other half is divided roughly equally into grains and protein [104]. The plate method [104, 105] is an attractive model that can be evaluated as the basis for teaching portion control and optimal dietary habits in developing countries. The visual approach uses a graphic display of a typical plate, divided into segments that contain desirable food classes in optimal proportions [105].

5. Self-monitoring
   Extensive self-monitoring of nutrient intake and minutes spent each day in physical activity (and type of activity) was an integral part of the lifestyle intervention in the DPP [50, 94]. In other studies, the frequent self-monitoring of weight and anthropometrics has been reported to be associated with long-term maintenance of weight loss [106]. The exact mechanism whereby self-monitoring of eating and exercise behavior predicts good metabolic outcome is unclear. It is plausible that such a level of involvement in one's health could have a beneficial heuristic effect by guiding food choices and lifestyle decisions. For most persons in psychic equilibrium, the potential adverse psychological impact of frequent self-monitoring of nutrient intake and physical activity is probably negligible. For these reasons, it seems prudent to incorporate some element of self-monitoring component into a community-based diabetes prevention campaign. The focus of such monitoring could be the type and amount (serving size) of food intake, daily physical activity minutes, and other lifestyle end points, as appropriate. In low literacy situations, the use of domestic surrogates (spouses, relatives, school age children, neighbors, family friends, etc.) to capture these end points could be considered. Where feasible, self-monitored data can be transmitted via SMS text to the *Community Diabetes Prevention Centers*, for tracking and real-time interventional feedback purposes.

Community Diabetes Prevention Centers

The sheer magnitude of the current and projected escalation of the diabetes epidemic in developing countries mandates the broadest possible response at the community level. One practical, efficient approach is the establishment of Community Diabetes Prevention Centers (CDPC) at several locations on the African continent, the Caribbean region, India and South Asia, the Pacific Rim, South and Central America, Australia and New Zealand, as well as in communities inhabited by high-risk populations in Europe and North America (Fig. 2.7). Such a groundswell of CDPCs can serve as essential focal points for the dissemination of diabetes prevention practices. Operationally, the CDPCs can be administered and staffed by the noncommunicable disease branch of Ministries and Departments of Health or through partnership with nongovernmental organizations. The primary purpose of CDPCs would be to test and implement culturally and regionally appropriate models for the delivery of physical activity and dietary interventions. Referral to CDPCs can be based on a risk factor approach that focuses on genetic (e.g., family history of diabetes) and other risk markers (Table 2.1). Individuals with diagnosed T2DM can be the conduits for referral of family members to CDPCs for prediabetes screening and intervention.

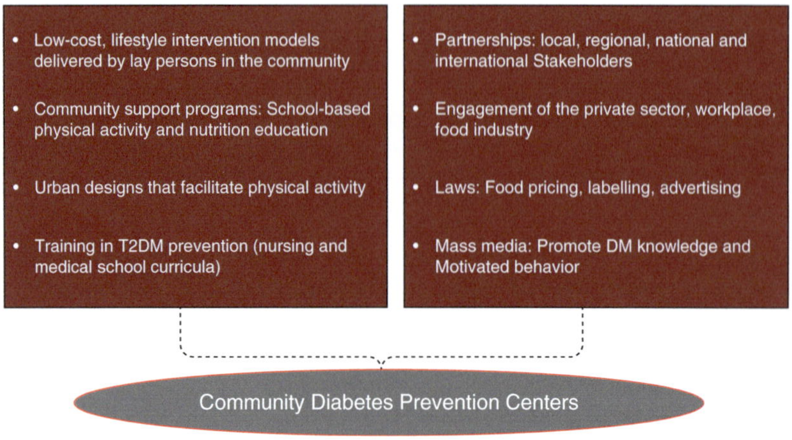

• Low-cost, lifestyle intervention models delivered by lay persons in the community
• Community support programs: School-based physical activity and nutrition education
• Urban designs that facilitate physical activity
• Training in T2DM prevention (nursing and medical school curricula)
• Partnerships: local, regional, national and international Stakeholders
• Engagement of the private sector, workplace, food industry
• Laws: Food pricing, labelling, advertising
• Mass media: Promote DM knowledge and Motivated behavior
Community Diabetes Prevention Centers

Fig. 2.7 Diabetes prevention strategies for developing countries, culminating in the creation of Community Diabetes Prevention Centers (see [68, 69])

Medications for Diabetes Prevention

Even in the most successful of the randomized controlled trials, the risk reduction for incident diabetes following lifestyle intervention was ~60 % [48–51]. That raises the argument as to whether medications could be offered to high-risk persons who are unable or unwilling to implement lifestyle changes or in whom the latter have failed to halt glycemic progression. In fact, several of the landmark diabetes prevention trials also included pharmacological arms, and additional studies have specifically tested medications for diabetes prevention. Given the linear relationship between diabetes risk reduction and the amount of weight loss (~10 % for every 1 kg weight loss) [50, 107], a medication that enhances or maintains weight loss would be a rational adjunct to lifestyle. What follows is a summary of medications that have been studied for the prevention of T2DM (Table 2.4).

The list of medications that have been tested includes sulfonylureas, metformin, acarbose, orlistat, rosiglitazone, and pioglitazone (Table 2.3). The DPP demonstrated that intervention with metformin decreased the development of diabetes in adults with impaired glucose tolerance by 31 % [50]. Curiously, the diabetes prevention efficacy of metformin was observed only in younger, obese (BMI >35 kg/m^2) individuals; among older or leaner participants, the effect of metformin in diabetes risk reduction was no better than that of placebo [50]. The STOP-NIDDM (Study to Prevent Non-Insulin-Dependent Diabetes Mellitus) employed acarbose as the intervention drug and demonstrated a 25 % decrease in the rate of progression to diabetes, compared to placebo [108]. In the XENDOS (XENical in the Prevention of Diabetes in Obese Subjects) study, the pancreatic lipase inhibitor orlistat (when prescribed in combination with lifestyle modification) resulted in a 37 % risk reduction in incident diabetes among subjects with impaired glucose tolerance, compared with lifestyle intervention alone [109].

Thiazolidinedione drugs were tested in the DREAM (Diabetes Reduction Assessment with Ramipril and Rosiglitazone Medication) [110], ACT NOW (ACTos NOW for the Prevention of Diabetes) [111], and CANOE (CAnadian Normoglycemia Outcomes Evaluation) [112] studies, which showed diabetes risk reduction rates of >50–75 %, compared with placebo. In the NAVIGATOR trial, the use of valsartan for 5 years, along with lifestyle modification, led to a relative reduction of 14 % in the incidence of diabetes among subjects with IGT, but the effect of nateglinide was not better than placebo [113]. The CANOE trial showed that low-dose combination therapy with metformin (500 mg twice daily) and rosiglitazone (2 mg daily) decreased incident type 2 diabetes by 66 % compared with placebo in IGT subjects. Of note, the low doses were well tolerated, with minimal effect on clinically relevant adverse events of the individual drugs [112].

Table 2.3 Diabetes prevention studies using lifestyle modification and medications

Year	Study acronym	Follow-up	Intervention	Outcome
1997	Da Qing	6 years	Diet + exercise	Decrease, 51 %
2001	DPS, Finland	3 years	Diet + exercise	Decrease, 58 %
2002	DPP	2.8 years	Diet+ Ex vs. Met	Decrease, 58 %
2002	STOP-NIDDM	3.3 years	Acarbose + diet	Decrease, 25 %
2004	XENdos	4 years	Orlistat + diet	Decrease, 37 %
2006	DREAM	3 years	Rosiglitazone	Decrease, 60 %
2008	ACT NOW	2–4 years	Pioglitazone	Decrease, 72 %
2006	IDPP-1	3 years	L/S ± Met	Decrease, 26–28 %
				Met not additive to L/S
2009	IDPP-2	3 years	L/S ± Pio	Pio not additive to L/S
2010	Navigator	5 years	Nateglinide	No effect
			Valsartan	Decrease, 14 %
2010	CANOE	4 years	Rosi+Met	Decrease 69 %

Ex exercise, *L/S* lifestyle, *Met* metformin, *Pio* pioglitazone, *Rosi* troglitazone

Limitations of Medications

The drugs that have been tested for diabetes prevention are associated with a range of adverse effects, the need for continuous therapy to maintain their effects, and consequent adherence barriers. In the studies that tested the effect of interruption of metformin, rosiglitazone and pioglitazone therapy for diabetes prevention, no sustained effect off medication was observed, which indicates that those medications did not fundamentally improve the underlying pathophysiology of prediabetes [114–116]. Moreover, in the Indian Diabetes Prevention Program (IDPP)-1 and IDPP-2, neither low-dose metformin nor pioglitazone, when tested in combination with lifestyle modification, achieved additive reduction of diabetes risk, compared to the effects of lifestyle modification alone [51, 117]. Clearly, the cumulative costs of long-term (probably life-long) therapy with medications (even where generic versions are available and no adverse effects occur) can be prohibitive, particularly for developing countries.

For reasons that have already been argued, the use of drugs for diabetes prevention cannot be recommended as a first-line approach in the general population. The latter conclusion is not to eschew societal expectation of safe, effective, and durable medications for diabetes prevention. Indeed, the poor human record of long-term adherence to behavioral recommendations and the known physiological adaptations that limit weight loss and trigger counter-veiling mechanisms that promote weight regain [118] create a need for such adjunctive pharmacological agents. The ideal drug for diabetes prevention (Table 2.4) should be nontoxic, well-tolerated, and at least as efficacious as lifestyle modification [28, 69].

Table 2.4 Desirable characteristics of an ideal drug for diabetes prevention

Efficacy: should equal or exceed the efficacy of lifestyle intervention
Mechanism(s): should repair the pathophysiologic defects that underlie prediabetes
Glucoregulation: should normalize glucose metabolism
Durability: effects should outlast the period of medication exposure
Adiposity: should induce weight loss or be weight-neutral
Safety: should have minimal toxicity and require no safety monitoring
Tolerability: should be well tolerated, without GI or other adverse effects
Cost: should cost less than the least expensive drug for diabetes treatment

Adapted from [28, 69]

Additionally, such a drug should repair or improve the pathophysiological defects that underlie prediabetes, so that a durable effect that outlasts the period of medication can be expected. The latter attribute would permit withdrawal of the medication after a defined period of intervention, without the risk of prediabetes relapse. Finally, the cost of such a drug must not be prohibitive, bearing in mind the large number of people with prediabetes (86 million in the United States and more than 400 million worldwide).

Current Guidelines for Use of Medication for Diabetes Prevention

The ADA consensus statement [119] recommends lifestyle modification with a weight loss goal of 5–10 % along with moderate physical activity of about 30 min daily for patients with IFG or IGT. Although no drug has been approved by the Food and Drug Administration for diabetes prevention, the ADA has suggested that treatment with metformin be considered as an adjunct to diet and exercise for the prevention of type 2 diabetes in selected high-risk persons [13, 119]. Based on the subgroup analysis of the efficacy of metformin in the DPP, metformin was most effective in preventing diabetes in high-risk, very obese (BMI >35 kg/m^2) prediabetic subjects younger than 60 years of age [50]. Additional selection criteria when considering metformin use in prediabetic subjects include a family history of diabetes in first-degree relatives, prior gestational diabetes mellitus, hypertriglyceridemia, subnormal HDL cholesterol levels, hypertension, and HbA1c 5.7–6.4 % [13, 119].

Even in persons who harbor all or most of these risk factors, active lifestyle modification is the preferred initial intervention; metformin can then be considered for individuals who fail to make significant progress. Currently, there are no clear guidelines for determining the optimal timing of metformin therapy, but failure of lifestyle intervention can be determined fairly empirically. The DPP participants assigned to lifestyle intervention lost ~7 % of their baseline body weight during the first 6 months (i.e., approximately 1 % per month). Thus, candidates for diabetes prevention who are unable to meet the lifestyle response target of losing ~1 %/month of body weight during the initial 3–6 months of behavioral intervention may be considered for adjunctive metformin therapy.

The guidelines on the management of prediabetes, issued by the Indian Health Services (IHS) and the Australian Diabetes Society/Australian Diabetes Educators Association, emphasize lifestyle intervention prior to consideration of medications. The Australian guidelines recommend trying lifestyle intervention for a minimum of 6 months before considering drugs for diabetes prevention [120]. The IHS guidelines recommend addition of either metformin or pioglitazone if initial lifestyle intervention fails to improve dysglycemia in people with prediabetes [121]. The IHS guidelines state that the decision to use medication for diabetes prevention must be made on an individual basis and with the patient's full understanding [121].

Prediabetes is diagnosed based on the presence of either IFG alone, IGT alone (determined during oral glucose tolerance test), or both IFG and IGT. Individuals who have both IFG and IGT (so-called double prediabetes) show more severe insulin resistance and impairment of beta-cell function compared to persons with a single prediabetes marker [119, 122, 123]. Nearly all persons with double prediabetes (~96 %) would qualify for metformin therapy, based on the ADA consensus criteria, whereas only ~30 % of persons with isolated IFG would be eligible for metformin treatment using the same criteria [119, 124]. This means that the use of oral glucose tolerance testing can refine and sharply tailor the selection of individuals at greatest risk (i.e., those with IFG + IGT) for metformin adjunctive treatment [119, 124]. This "maximalist" risk and "minimalist" drug intervention approach has much to commend it, as it would spare individuals and governments the huge expense of covering the costs of medications and related expenses for a much wider range of individuals from lower risk pools. Indeed, the ADA consensus statement stipulates that the presence of both IFG and IGT must be documented if metformin is to be used for diabetes prevention [119].

Costs of Preventing T2DM

Analysis of costs associated with the DPP indicates that the overall expense to society of preventing diabetes was cost-effective [125–128]. For over 3 years, the direct medical costs of the DPP interventions were US $79 per participant in the placebo group, US $2,542 in the metformin group, and US $2,780 in the lifestyle group [125, 126]. Further longer-term analysis indicated that lifestyle modification remained cost-effective, and metformin was potentially cost saving when used for preventing diabetes [128]. Cost analysis in the IDPP showed that the T2DM prevention strategies in India, especially lifestyle intervention, were cost-effective [129]. The total cost of identifying one person with IGT was US $117. The direct medical costs were US $61 per person in the control group and US $225 in the lifestyle intervention group [129]. The cost of preventing one case of T2DM through lifestyle modification in India was US $1,052 [129]. The DPP, IDPP, and other trials were by the nature of their design quite resource-intensive.

Clearly, the adaptation of diabetes prevention programs to developing countries would require extensive cost-containment and cost-shifting strategies. Reduction in contact frequency, optimization of the size of the intervention personnel, and the use of group (rather than one-on-one) counseling format should decrease costs significantly. Furthermore, the use of trained lay (nonmedical) workers to implement lifestyle modification protocols in group sessions at the Community Diabetes Prevention Centers and prorated cost sharing could be additional approaches to the implementation of affordable diabetes prevention programs in developing countries [79, 130]. Even with a markedly scaled down cost schedule, the low gross domestic product (~$500 per capita) in many developing countries suggests that these nations cannot afford to underwrite the costs of even a limited national diabetes prevention program. Given the immense future benefits to society from prevention of T2DM, novel funding sources (private, industry, international, philanthropic, and other agencies) would need to be explored and mobilized for successful implementation of diabetes prevention initiatives in most low- and middle-income countries.

Conclusion

Nearly 90 million adults in the United States and more than 400 million people around the world have prediabetes. Perhaps, one of the most significant public health advances of the present era is the demonstration that progression from prediabetes to type 2 diabetes can be interrupted by effective interventions. In addition to the compelling arguments for prioritizing diabetes prevention, there is an even more urgent need for action in low-income countries, where a narrow window of opportunity currently exists. In those countries, diabetes is currently not featured among the top ten causes of death; however, as countries emerge from poverty, the role of diabetes as a leading cause of death becomes firmly established (Fig. 2.8). This nefarious association between economic progress and death from diabetes is not inevitable; economic transition from poverty to wealth can and must be uncoupled from increased morbidity and mortality from diabetes [131]. Among the different interventions of proven efficacy in preventing diabetes, lifestyle modification is the most appealing because of its high efficacy, nontoxicity, and generalizable effects in persons from various ethnic backgrounds [48–51]. Most of the medications that have been tested for diabetes prevention fall short of the efficacy achieved by lifestyle intervention. Although the efficacy of thiazolidinedione drugs on diabetes prevention when administered to persons with prediabetes can match or somewhat exceed that of lifestyle intervention, the drug effect is not sustained and quickly dissipates following cessation of therapy [114, 115]. In contrast such a rapid "washout" effect is not seen with lifestyle intervention, where sustained benefits of diabetes prevention have been reported up to 20 years following cessation of formal intervention [75–77].

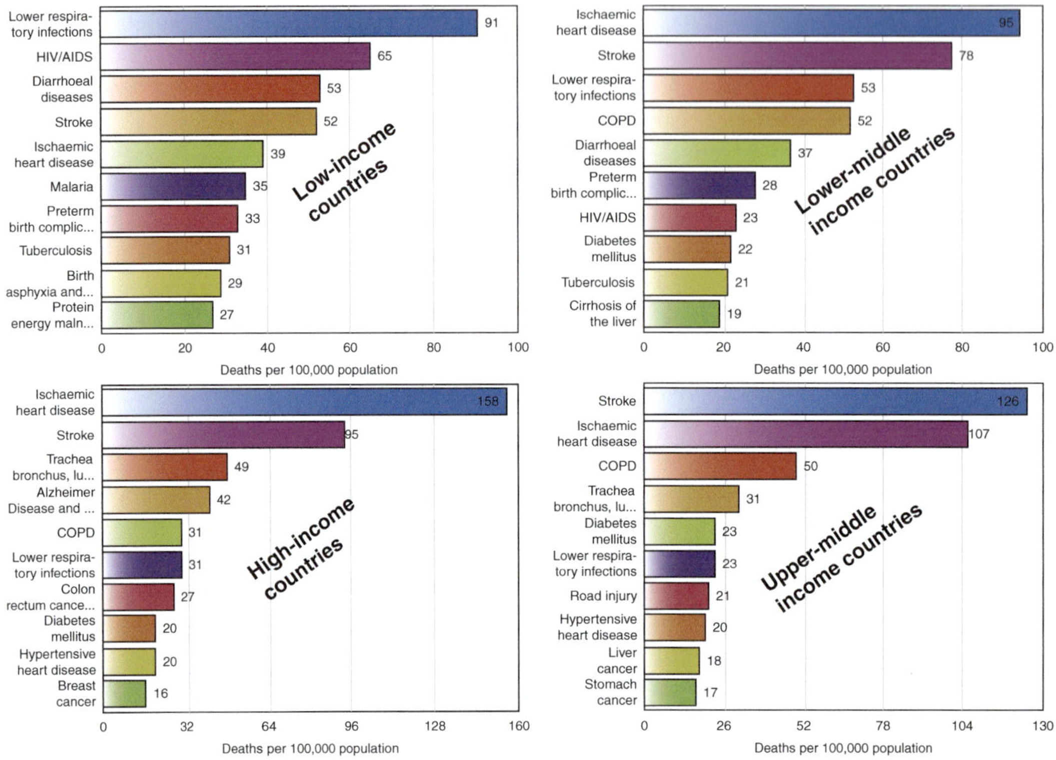

Fig. 2.8 Top ten causes of death in countries of the world grouped by income status. Diabetes does not appear among the top causes of death in low-income countries, but as countries experience upward economic transition, diabetes becomes firmly established among the top causes of death. *COPD* chronic obstructive pulmonary disease (Source: World Health Organization. Available from http://www.who.int/mediacentre/factsheets/fs310/en/index1.html. Accessed 20 May 2015)

The effective translation of diabetes prevention across global communities requires engagement and coordination at multiple levels within the health-care establishment, civic society, and government agencies. Environmental and policy changes are needed to stimulate broad societal participation in wellness and diabetes prevention activities. Pilot and feasibility projects are needed to customize generally proven methodologies to local specificities and realities in developing countries and underserved communities. Ecological improvements that result in improved access to safe walking trails, well-lit and well-kept public parks, subsidized or affordable neighborhood fitness centers, and other appurtenances for health promotion would all augur well for the practice of community diabetes prevention. The establishment of Community Diabetes Prevention Centers, to serve as a hub for harmonizing the planning, delivery, and evaluation of lifestyle intervention activities, would be an efficient approach to global diabetes prevention. Appropriate legislation that promotes food labeling, rewards healthful behavior, and redistributes revenue from "sin" tax on tobacco and alcohol to fund community diabetes prevention initiatives would be well directed. Clearly, great opportunities exist for innovative partnerships among governmental, civic, philanthropic, and other nongovernmental organizations toward a common purpose of stemming the global diabetes epidemic by focusing on primary prevention.

Acknowledgments SD-J is supported, in part, by grants (R01 DK067269, DK62203, DK48411) from the National Institutes of Health.

Disclosures The author has no conflicts of interest with regard to the content of this chapter.

References

1. International Diabetes Federation. IDF diabetes atlas 2015. 7th ed. Brussels: International Diabetes Federation; 2015.
2. Geiss LS, Wang J, Cheng YJ, Thompson TJ, Barker L, Li Y, et al. Prevalence and incidence trends for diagnosed diabetes among adults aged 20 to 79 years, United States, 1980–2012. JAMA. 2014;312:1218–26.
3. Gregg EW, Li Y, Wang J, Burrows NR, Ali MK, Rolka D, et al. Changes in diabetes-related complications in the United States, 1990–2010. N Engl J Med. 2014;370:1514–23.
4. World Health Organization. Global status report on noncommunicable diseases 2014. Geneva: WHO Press; 2014.
5. Shaw JE, Sicree RA, Zimmet PZ. Global estimates of the prevalence of diabetes for 2010 and 2030. Diabetes Res Clin Pract. 2010;87:4–14.
6. Hu F. Globalization of diabetes: the role of diet, lifestyle, and genes. Diabetes Care. 2011;34:1249–57.
7. Egede LE, Dagogo-Jack S. Epidemiology of type 2 diabetes: focus on ethnic minorities. Med Clin N Am. 2005;89:949–75.
8. Tanizawa Y, Riggs AC, Dagogo-Jack S, Vaxillaire M, Froguel P, Liu L, et al. Isolation of the human LIM/homeodomain gene islet-1 and identification of a simple sequence repeat polymorphism. Diabetes. 2004;43:935–41.
9. Ehm MG, Karnoub MC, Sakul H, Gottschalk K, Holt DC, Weber JL, American Diabetes Association GENNID Study Group. Genetics of NIDDM, et al. Genome wide search for type 2 diabetes susceptibility genes in four American populations. Am J Hum Genet. 2000;66:1871–81.
10. McCarthy M, Zeggini E. Genome-wide association studies in type 2 diabetes. Curr Diab Rep. 2009;9: 164–71.
11. Hivert MF, Jablonski KA, Perreault L, Saxena R, McAteer JB, Franks PW, et al. Updated genetic score based on 34 confirmed type 2 diabetes Loci is associated with diabetes incidence and regression to normoglycemia in the diabetes prevention program. Diabetes. 2011;60:1340–8.
12. Dagogo-Jack S. Predicting diabetes: our relentless quest for genomic nuggets. Diabetes Care. 2012; 35:193–5.
13. American Diabetes Association. Standards of medical care in diabetes—2016. Diabetes Care. 2016; 39:S1–112.
14. Fujimoto WY, Leonetti DL, Kinyoun JL, Newell-Morris L, Shuman WP, Stolov WC, et al. Prevalence of diabetes mellitus and impaired glucose tolerance among second-generation Japanese-American men. Diabetes. 1987;36:721–9.
15. Dagogo-Jack S, Santiago JV. Pathophysiology of type 2 diabetes and modes of action of therapeutic interventions. Arch Intern Med. 1997;157: 1802–17.
16. Defronzo RA. Banting lecture. From the triumvirate to the ominous octet: a new paradigm for the treatment of type 2 diabetes mellitus. Diabetes. 2009;58:773–95.
17. DeFronzo RA. Insulin resistance, lipotoxicity, type 2 diabetes and atherosclerosis: the missing links. The Claude Bernard Lecture 2009. Diabetologia. 2010; 53:1270–87.
18. Rasmussen BB, Holmbäck UC, Volpi E, Morio-Liondore B, Paddon-Jones D, Wolfe RR. Malonyl coenzyme A and the regulation of functional carnitine palmitoyltransferase-1 activity and fat oxidation in human skeletal muscle. J Clin Invest. 2002; 110:1687–93.
19. Kitabchi AE, Temprosa M, Knowler WC, Kahn SE, Fowler SE, Haffner SM, et al. Role of insulin secretion and sensitivity in the evolution of type 2 diabetes in the diabetes prevention program: effects of lifestyle intervention and metformin. Diabetes. 2005;54:2404–14.
20. Larson-Meyer DE, Heilbronn LK, Redman LM, Newcomer BR, Frisard MI, Anton S, et al. Effect of calorie restriction with or without exercise on insulin sensitivity, β-cell function, fat cell size, and ectopic lipid in overweight subjects. Diabetes Care. 2006; 29:1337–44.
21. Kelley DE. Effects of weight loss on glucose homeostasis in NIDDM. Diabetes Rev. 1995;3:366–77.
22. Schneider SH, Morgado A. Effects of fitness and physical training on carbohydrate metabolism and associated cardiovascular risk factors in patients with diabetes. Diabetes Rev. 1995;3:378–407.
23. Rogers MA, Yamamoto C, King DS, Harberg JM, Ensani AA, Holloszy JO. Improvement in glucose tolerance after one week of exercise in patients with mild NIDDM. Diabetes Care. 1988;11:613–8.
24. Eriksson KF, Lindgarde F. Prevention of type 2 diabetes mellitus by diet and physical exercise. Diabetologia. 1991;34:891–8.
25. Mikines KJ, Sonne B, Farrell PA, Tronier B, Galbo H. Effect of physical exercise on sensitivity and responsiveness to insulin in humans. Am J Physiol. 1988;254:E248–59.
26. Goodyear LJ, Kahn BB. Exercise, glucose transport, and insulin sensitivity. Annu Rev Med. 1998; 49:235–61.
27. Steven S, Hollingsworth KG, Al-Mrabeh A, Avery L, Aribisala B, Caslake M, et al. Very-low-calorie diet and 6 months of weight stability in type 2 diabetes: pathophysiologic changes in responders and nonresponders. Diabetes Care. 2016. pii: dc151942. [Epub ahead of print].
28. Dagogo-Jack S, Edeoga C. Understanding and identifying pre-diabetes – can we halt the diabetes epidemic? Eur Endocrinol. 2008;4:16–8.
29. Pour OR, Dagogo-Jack S. Prediabetes as a therapeutic target. Clin Chem. 2011;57:215–20.

30. Maschirow L, Khalaf K, Al-Aubaidy HA, Jelinek HF. Inflammation, coagulation, endothelial dysfunction and oxidative stress in prediabetes — biomarkers as a possible tool for early disease detection for rural screening. Clin Biochem. 2015;48:581–5.
31. Nyenwe EA, Dagogo-Jack S. Metabolic syndrome, prediabetes and the science of primary prevention. Minerva Endocrinol. 2011;36:129–45.
32. Tabák A, Herder C, Rathmann W, Brunner E, Kivimäki M. Prediabetes: a high-risk state for diabetes development. Lancet. 2012;379:2279–90.
33. Weir G, Bonner-Weir S. Five stages of evolving progression to diabetes. Diabetes. 2004;53:S16–21.
34. Weyer C, Bogardus C, Mott DM, Pratley R. The natural history of insulin secretory dysfunction and insulin resistance in the pathogenesis of type 2 diabetes mellitus. J Clin Invest. 1999;104:787–94.
35. Toft-Nielsen MB, Damholt MB, Madsbad S, Hilsted LM, Hughes TE, Michelsen BK, et al. Determinants of the impaired secretion of glucagon-like peptide-1 in type 2 diabetic patients. J Clin Endocrinol Metab. 2001;86:3717–23.
36. Papaetis G. Incretin-based therapies in prediabetes: current evidence and future perspectives. World J Diabetes. 2014;5:817–34.
37. Lopategi A, López-Vicario C, Alcaraz-Quiles J, García-Alonso V, Titos E, Clària J, et al. Role of bioactive lipid mediators in obese adipose tissue inflammation and endocrine dysfunction. Mol Cell Endocrinol. 2016;419:44–59.
38. Cerasi E, Luft R. The prediabetic state, its nature and consequences – a look toward the future. Diabetes. 1972;21 Suppl 2:685–94.
39. Centers for Disease Control and Prevention. National diabetes statistics report: estimates of diabetes and its burden in the United States, 2014. Atlanta: US Department of Health and Human Services; 2014.
40. Edelstein SL, Knowler WC, Bain RP, et al. Predictors of progression from impaired glucose tolerance to NIDDM: an analysis of six prospective studies. Diabetes. 1997;46:701–10.
41. Knowler WC, Bennett PH, Hamman RF, Miller M. Diabetes incidence and prevalence in Pima Indians: a 19-fold greater incidence than in Rochester, Minnesota. Am J Epidemiol. 1978;108:497–505.
42. Brancati FL, Kao WH, Folsom AR, Watson RL, Szklo M. Incident type 2 diabetes mellitus in African American and white adults: the Atherosclerosis Risk in Communities Study. JAMA. 2000;283:2253–9.
43. Weyer C, Tataranni PA, Bogardus C, Pratley R. Diabetes Care. 2000;24:89–94.
44. Meigs JB, Muller DC, Nathan DM, Blake DR, Andres R. Diabetes. 2003;52:1475–84.
45. Dagogo-Jack S, Edeoga C, Ebenibo S, Nyenwe E, Wan J. Lack of racial disparity in incident prediabetes and glycemic progression among black and white offspring of parents with type 2 diabetes: the pathobiology of prediabetes in a biracial cohort (POP-ABC) study. J Clin Endocrinol Metab. 2014;99: E1078–87.
46. Boucher AB, Adesanya EAO, Owei I, Gilles AK, Ebenibo S, Wan J, Edeoga C, Dagogo-Jack S. Dietary habits and leisure-time physical activity in relation to adiposity, dyslipidemia, and incident dysglycemia in the Pathobiology of Prediabetes in A Biracial Cohort Study. Metabolism. 2015;64: 1060–7.
47. Jiang Y, Owei I, Wan J, Ebenibo S, Dagogo-Jack S. Adiponectin levels predict prediabetes risk: the pathobiology of prediabetes in a biracial cohort (POP-ABC) study. BMJ Open Diabetes Res Care. 2016;4:e000194. doi:10.1136/bmjdrc-2016.
48. Pan XR, Li GW, Hu YH, Wang JX, Yang WY, An ZX, et al. Effects of diet and exercise in preventing NIDDM in people with impaired glucose tolerance: the Da Qing IGT and Diabetes Study. Diabetes Care. 1997;20:537–44.
49. Tuomilehto J, Lindstrom J, Eriksson J, Valle T, Hamalainen H. Prevention of type 2 diabetes mellitus by changes in lifestyle among subjects with impaired glucose tolerance. N Engl J Med. 2001;344: 1343–50.
50. DPP Research Group. Reduction in the incidence of type 2 diabetes with lifestyle intervention or metformin. N Engl J Med. 2002;346:393–403.
51. Ramachandran A, Snehalatha C, Mary S, Mukesh B, Bhaskar AD, Vijay V, Indian Diabetes Prevention Programme (IDPP). The Indian Diabetes Prevention Programme shows that lifestyle modification and metformin prevent type 2 diabetes in Asian Indian subjects with impaired glucose tolerance (IDPP-1). Diabetologia. 2006;49:289–97.
52. American Diabetes Association. Economic costs of diabetes in the U.S. in 2012. Diabetes Care. 2013;36: 1033–46.
53. Zhang P, Zhang X, Brown J, Vistisen D, Sicree R, Shaw J, Nichols G. Global healthcare expenditure on diabetes for 2010 and 2030. Diabetes Res Clin Pract. 2010;87:293–301.
54. Barceló A, Aedo C, Rajpathak S, Robles S. The cost of diabetes in Latin America and the Caribbean. Bull World Health Organ. 2003;81:19–27.
55. Deeb LC, Tan MH, Alberti KGMM. Insulin availability among International Diabetes Federation member associations. Diabetes Care. 1994;17:220–3.
56. Dagogo-Jack S. DCCT results and diabetes care in developing countries. Diabetes Care. 1995;18:416–7.
57. Beran D, Yudkin JS. Diabetes care in sub-Saharan Africa. Lancet. 2006;368:1689–95.
58. Dagogo-Jack S. Pattern of foot ulcer in diabetic Nigerians. Pract Diabetes Dig. 1991;2:75–8.
59. Dagogo-Jack S. Diabetic in-patient mortality in Nigeria. Pract Diabetes Dig. 1991;2:117–9.
60. Dagogo-Jack S. Primary prevention of cardiovascular disease in diabetic patients. Cardiol Q. 2006;12: 20–5.
61. Nathan DM, Bayless M, Cleary P, Genuth S, Gubitosi-Klug R, Lachin JM, DCCT/EDIC Research Group, et al. Diabetes control and complications trial/epidemiology of diabetes interventions and

complications study at 30 years: advances and contributions. Diabetes. 2013;62:3976–86.
62. UK Prospective Diabetes Study (UKPDS) Group. Intensive blood-glucose control with sulphonylureas or insulin compared with conventional treatment and risk of complications in patients with type 2 diabetes (UKPDS 33). Lancet. 1998;352:837–53.
63. Hayward RA, Reaven PD, Wiitala WL, Bahn GD, Reda DJ, Duckworth, VADT Investigators, et al. Follow-up of glycemic control and cardiovascular outcomes in type 2 diabetes. N Engl J Med. 2015; 372:2197–206.
64. Gaede P, Lund-Andersen H, Parving HH, Pedersen O. Effect of a multifactorial intervention on mortality in type 2 diabetes. N Engl J Med. 2008;358:580–91.
65. Banegas JR, López-García E, Dallongeville J, Guallar E, Halcox JP, Borghi C, et al. Achievement of treatment goals for primary prevention of cardiovascular disease in clinical practice across Europe: the EURIKA study. Eur Heart J. 2011;32:2143–53.
66. Ali MK, Bullard KM, Saaddine JB, Cowie CC, Imperatore G, Gregg EW. Achievement of goals in U.S. diabetes care, 1999–2010. New Engl J Med. 2013;368:1613–24.
67. Dagogo-Jack S. Preventing diabetes-related morbidity and mortality in the primary care setting. J Natl Med Assoc. 2002;94:549–60.
68. Dagogo-Jack S. Primary prevention of type 2 diabetes in developing countries. J Natl Med Assoc. 2006;98:415–9.
69. Echouffo-Tcheugui JB, Dagogo-Jack S. Preventing diabetes mellitus in developing countries. Nat Rev Endocrinol. 2012;8:557–62.
70. Dabelea D, Knowler WC, Pettitt DJ. Effect of diabetes in pregnancy on offspring: follow-up research in the Pima Indians. J Matern Fetal Med. 2000; 9:83–8.
71. Francis-Emmanuel PM, Thompson DS, Barnett AT, Osmond C, Byrne CD, Hanson MA, et al. Glucose metabolism in adult survivors of severe acute malnutrition. J Clin Endocrinol Metab. 2014;99:2233–40.
72. Dagogo-Jack S. HIV therapy and diabetes risk (Editorial). Diabetes Care. 2008;31:1267–8.
73. Yarasheski K, Tebas P, Sigmund CM, Dagogo-Jack S, Bohrer A, Turk J, Cryer PE, Powderly WG. Insulin resistance in HIV-protease inhibitor-associated diabetes. J Acquir Immune Defic Syndr. 1999;21:209–16.
74. Perreault L, Pan Q, Mather KJ, Watson KE, Hamman RF, Kahn SE, Diabetes Prevention Program Research Group. Effect of regression from prediabetes to normal glucose regulation on long-term reduction in diabetes risk: results from the Diabetes Prevention Program Outcomes Study. Lancet. 2012;379:2243–51.
75. Diabetes Prevention Program Research Group. 10-year follow-up of diabetes incidence and weight loss in the Diabetes Prevention Program Outcomes Study. Lancet. 2009;374:1677–86.
76. Lindström J, Ilanne-Parikka P, Peltonen M, Aunola S, Eriksson JG, Hemiö K. Sustained reduction in the incidence of type 2 diabetes by lifestyle intervention: follow-up of the Finnish Diabetes Prevention Study. Lancet. 2006;368:1673–9.
77. Li G, Zhang P, Wang J, An Y, Gong Q, Gregg EW, et al. Cardiovascular mortality, all-cause mortality, and diabetes incidence after lifestyle intervention for people with impaired glucose tolerance in the Da Qing Diabetes Prevention Study: a 23-year follow-up study. Lancet Diabetes Endocrinol. 2014;2:474–80.
78. Simmons D, Rush E, Crook N. Development and piloting of a community health worker-based intervention for the prevention of diabetes among New Zealand Maori in Te Wai o Rona: diabetes prevention strategy. Public Health Nutr. 2008;11:1318–25.
79. Ackermann RT, Marrero DG. Adapting the Diabetes Prevention Program lifestyle intervention for delivery in the community: the YMCA model. Diabetes Educ. 2007;33(69):74–5, 77–8.
80. Albright AL, Gregg EW. Preventing type 2 diabetes in communities across the U.S.: the National Diabetes Prevention Program. Am J Prev Med. 2013;44(4 Suppl 4):S346–51.
81. Albright A. The National Diabetes Prevention Program: from research to reality. Diabetes Care Educ Newsl. 2012;33(4):4–7.
82. Hays LM, Finch EA, Saha C, Marrero DG, Ackermann RT. Effect of self-efficacy on weight loss: a psychosocial analysis of a community-based adaptation of the diabetes prevention program lifestyle intervention. Diabetes Spectr. 2014;27:270–5.
83. Velicer WF, Brick LA, Fava JL, Prochaska JO. Testing 40 predictions from the transtheoretical model again. With confidence. Multivar Behav Res. 2013;48:220–40.
84. Norcross JC, Krebs PM, Prochaska JO. Stages of change. J Clin Psychol. 2011;67:143–54.
85. Pan WH, Flegal KM, Chang HY, Yeh WT, Yeh CJ, Lee WC. Body mass index and obesity-related metabolic disorders in Taiwanese and US whites and blacks: implications for definitions of overweight and obesity for Asians. Am J Clin Nutr. 2004;79: 31–9.
86. Yang W, Lu J, Weng J, Jia W, Ji L, Xiao J. Prevalence of diabetes among men and women in China. N Engl J Med. 2010;362:1090–101.
87. Pohl JH, Greer JA, Hasan KS. Type 2 diabetes mellitus in children. Endocr Pract. 1998;4:413–6.
88. Kaufman FR. Type 2 diabetes mellitus in children and youth: a new epidemic. J Pediatr Endocrinol Metab. 2002;15 Suppl 2:737–44.
89. Alberti G, Zimmet P, Shaw J, Bloomgarden Z, Kaufman F, Silink M, Consensus Workshop Group. Type 2 diabetes in the young: the evolving epidemic: the international diabetes federation consensus workshop. Diabetes Care. 2004;27:1798–811.
90. Wiegand S, Maikowski U, Blankenstein O, Biebermann H, Tarnow P, Gruters A. Type 2 diabetes and impaired glucose tolerance in European children and adolescents with obesity - a problem that is no longer restricted to minority groups. Eur J Endocrinol. 2004;151:199–20.

91. Caprio S. Development of type 2 diabetes mellitus in the obese adolescent: a growing challenge. Endocr Pract. 2012;18:791–5.
92. TODAY Study Group. Rapid rise in hypertension and nephropathy in youth with type 2 diabetes: the TODAY clinical trial. Diabetes Care. 2013;36:1735–41.
93. HEALTHY Study Group. A school-based intervention for diabetes risk reduction. N Engl J Med. 2010;363:443–5.
94. The Diabetes Prevention Program Research Group. The Diabetes Prevention Program (DPP): description of lifestyle intervention. Diabetes Care. 2002;25: 2165–71.
95. Eriksson KF, Lindgarde F. Prevention of type 2 (noninsulin-dependent) diabetes mellitus by diet and physical exercise: the 6-year Malmo feasibility study. Diabetologia. 1991;4:891–8.
96. Pate RR, Pratt M, Blair SN, Haskell WL, Macera CA, Bouchard C, et al. Physical activity and public health: recommendation from the Centers for Disease Control and Prevention and the American College of Sports Medicine. JAMA. 1995;273:402–7.
97. Kimm SY, Glynn NW, Kriska AM, Barton BA, Kronsberg SS, Daniels SR, et al. Decline in physical activity in black and white girls during adolescence. N Engl J Med. 2002;347:709–15.
98. Hood MS, Little JP, Tarnopolsky MA, Myslik F, Gibala MJ. Low-volume interval training improves muscle oxidative capacity in sedentary adults. Med Sci Sports Exerc. 2011;43:1849–56.
99. Tate DF, Wing RR, Winett RA. Using Internet technology to deliver a behavioral weight loss program. JAMA. 2001;285:1172–7.
100. Neve M, Morgan PJ, Jones PR, Collins CE. Effectiveness of web-based interventions in achieving weight loss and weight loss maintenance in overweight and obese adults: a systematic review with meta-analysis. Obes Rev. 2010;11:306–21.
101. Kodama S, Saito K, Tanaka S, Horikawa C, Fujiwara K, Hirasawa R, et al. Effect of Web-based lifestyle modification on weight control: a meta-analysis. Int J Obes (Lond). 2012;36:675–85.
102. Kohl LF, Crutzen R, de Vries NK. Online prevention aimed at lifestyle behaviors: a systematic review of reviews. J Med Internet Res. 2013;15:e146. doi:10.2196/jmir.2665.
103. Watson S, Woodside JV, Ware LJ, Hunter SJ, McGrath A, Cardwell CR, et al. Effect of a web-based behavior change program on weight loss and cardiovascular risk factors in overweight and obese adults at high risk of developing cardiovascular disease: randomized controlled trial. J Med Internet Res. 2015;17(7):e177. doi:10.2196/jmir.3828.
104. US Department of Agriculture Center for Nutrition Policy and Promotion. Dietary guidelines for Americans. http://www.cnpp.usda.gov/dietaryguidelines.htm. Accessed 5 Apr 2016.
105. Camelon KM, Hådell K, Jämsén PT, Ketonen KJ, Kohtamäki HM, Mäkimatilla S, et al. The Plate Model: a visual method of teaching meal planning. DAIS Project Group. Diabetes Atherosclerosis Intervention Study. J Am Diet Assoc. 1998;98:1155–8.
106. Wing RR, Phelan S. Long-term weight loss maintenance. Am J Clin Nutr. 2005;82(Suppl):222S–5.
107. Hamman RF, Wing RR, Edelstein SL, Lachin JM, Bray GA, Delahanty L, Hoskin M, Kriska AM, Mayer-Davis EJ, Pi-Sunyer X, Regensteiner J, Venditti B, Wylie-Rosett J, Diabetes Prevention Program Research Group. Effect of weight loss with lifestyle intervention on risk of diabetes. Diabetes Care. 2006;29:2102–7.
108. Chiasson JL, Josse RG, Gomis R, Hanefeld M, Karasik A, Laakso M, STOP-NIDDM Trial Research Group. Acarbose for prevention of type 2 diabetes mellitus: the STOP-NIDDM randomised trial. Lancet. 2002;359:2072–7.
109. Orgerson JS, Hauptman J, Boldrin MN, Sjöström L. XENical in the prevention of Diabetes in Obese Subjects (XENDOS) study: a randomized study of orlistat as an adjunct to lifestyle changes for the prevention of type 2 diabetes in obese patients. Diabetes Care. 2004;27:155–61.
110. DREAM (Diabetes REduction Assessment with ramipril and rosiglitazone Medication) Trial Investigators. Effect of rosiglitazone on the frequency of diabetes in patients with impaired glucose tolerance or impaired fasting glucose: a randomised controlled trial. Lancet. 2006;368:1096–105.
111. DeFronzo RA, Tripathy D, Schwenke DC, Banerji M, Bray GA, Buchanan TA, ACT NOW Study, et al. Pioglitazone for diabetes prevention in impaired glucose tolerance. N Engl J Med. 2011;364:1104–15 (Erratum in: N Engl J Med. 2011;365:189).
112. Zinman B, Harris SB, Neuman J, Gerstein HC, Retnakaran RR, Raboud J, et al. Low-dose combination therapy with rosiglitazone and metformin to prevent type 2 diabetes mellitus (CANOE trial): a double-blind randomised controlled study. Lancet. 2010;376:103–11.
113. NAVIGATOR Study Group. Effect of valsartan on the incidence of diabetes and cardiovascular events. N Engl J Med. 2010;362:1477–90 (Erratum in: N Engl J Med. 2010;362:1748).
114. DPP Research Group. Effects of withdrawal from metformin on the development of diabetes in the diabetes prevention program. Diabetes Care. 2003;26: 977–80.
115. DREAM Trial Investigators. Incidence of diabetes following ramipril or rosiglitazone withdrawal. Diabetes Care. 2011;34:1265–9.
116. Tripathy D, Schwenke DC, Banerji M, Bray GA, Buchanan TA, Clement SC, et al. Diabetes incidence and glucose tolerance after termination of pioglitazone therapy: results from ACT NOW. J Clin Endocrinol Metab. 2016:jc20154202. [Epub ahead of print].
117. Ramachandran A, Snehalatha C, Mary S, Selvam S, Kumar CK, Seeli AC, Shetty AS. Pioglitazone does

not enhance the effectiveness of lifestyle modification in preventing conversion of impaired glucose tolerance to diabetes in Asian Indians: results of the Indian Diabetes Prevention Programme-2 (IDPP-2). Diabetologia. 2009;52:1019–26.
118. Greenway FL. Physiological adaptations to weight loss and factors favouring weight regain. Int J Obes (Lond). 2015. doi:10.1038/ijo.2015.59.
119. Nathan DM, Davidson MB, DeFronzo RA, Heine RJ, Henry RR, Pratley R, Zinman B. Impaired fasting glucose and impaired glucose tolerance. Diabetes Care. 2007;30:753–9.
120. Twigg SM, Kamp MC, Davis TM, Neylon EK, Flack JR. Australian Diabetes Society and Australian Diabetes Educators Association. Prediabetes: a position statement from the Australian Diabetes Society and Australian Diabetes Educators Association. Med J Aust. 2007;186:461–5.
121. Indian Health Services. 2008 IHS guidelines for care of adults with prediabetes and/or the metabolic syndrome in clinical settings. http://aianp.ucdenver.edu/sdpi/common/initiative/DP_Appendices/DPIAN6%20IHS%20Guidelines%20PreDiabetes%20Metsyn%20Sept%202008.pdf. Accessed 3 Apr 2016.
122. Dagogo-Jack S, Askari H, Tykodi G. Glucoregulatory physiology in subjects with low-normal, high-normal, or impaired fasting glucose. J Clin Endocrinol Metab. 2009;94:2031–6.
123. Kanat M, Mari A, Norton L, Winnier D, DeFronzo RA, Jenkinson C, Abdul-Ghani MA. Distinct β-cell defects in impaired fasting glucose and impaired glucose tolerance. Diabetes. 2012;61:447–53.
124. Rhee MK, Herrick K, Ziemer DC, Vaccarino V, Weintraub WS, Narayan KM, et al. Many Americans have pre-diabetes and should be considered for metformin therapy. Diabetes Care. 2010;33:49–54.
125. Diabetes Prevention Program (DPP) Research Group. Cost associated with the primary prevention of type 2 diabetes mellitus in the Diabetes Prevention Program. Diabetes Care. 2003;26:36–47.
126. Diabetes Prevention Program Research Group. Within-trial cost-effectiveness of lifestyle intervention or metformin for the primary prevention of type 2 diabetes. Diabetes Care. 2003;26:2518–23.
127. Herman WH, Hoerger TJ, Brandle M, Hicks K, Sorensen S, Zhang P, Diabetes Prevention Program Research Group, et al. The cost-effectiveness of lifestyle modification or metformin in preventing type 2 diabetes in adults with impaired glucose tolerance. Ann Intern Med. 2005;142:323–32.
128. Diabetes Prevention Program Research Group. The 10-year cost-effectiveness of lifestyle intervention or metformin for diabetes prevention: an intent-to-treat analysis of the DPP/DPPOS. Diabetes Care. 2012; 35:723–30.
129. Ramachandran A, Snehalatha C, Yamuna A, Mary S, Ping Z. Cost-effectiveness of the interventions in the primary prevention of diabetes among Asian Indians: within-trial results of the Indian Diabetes Prevention Programme (IDPP). Diabetes Care. 2007;30:2548–52.
130. Ackermann RT, Marrero DG, Hicks KA, Hoerger TJ, Sorensen S, Zhang P, et al. An evaluation of cost sharing to finance a diet and physical activity intervention to prevent diabetes. Diabetes Care. 2006;29: 1237–41.
131. Dagogo-Jack S. 2015 Presidential address: 75 years of battling diabetes-our global challenge. Diabetes Care. 2016;39:3–9.

Diabetes in Sub-Saharan Africa

3

Felix Assah and Jean Claude Mbanya

Overview

Type 2 diabetes[1] is a global problem with major public health and socioeconomic challenges. From recent estimates of the International Diabetes Federation (IDF) [1], the number of adults with diabetes in the world currently stands at 415 million with a projected rise to 642 million by 2040. An estimated 14.2 (9.5–29.4‡) million people aged 20–79 have diabetes in the sub-Saharan Africa (SSA) region, representing a regional prevalence of 2.1–6.7 %‡. SSA has the highest proportion of undiagnosed cases of diabetes; over two-thirds (66.7 %) of people with diabetes are unaware of their status. The majority of people with diabetes (58.8 %) live in cities, even though the population in the region (61.3 %) is predominantly rural. With increasing urbanisation and population ageing, diabetes will pose an even greater threat. It is expected that by 2040 there will be 34.2 million adults in the region living with diabetes, more than double the number in 2015 [1].

[1]This chapter will focus on type 2 diabetes and will be referred to as diabetes throughout.

F. Assah, MD, PhD (✉) • J.C. Mbanya, MD, PhD, FRCP
Faculty of Medicine and Biomedical Sciences,
University of Yaoundé I, Yaoundé, Cameroon
e-mail: kembeassah@yahoo.com;
jcmbanya@yahoo.co.uk

Diabetes prevalence in adults is in general much higher on islands in sub-Saharan Africa, compared to the mainland. The highest prevalence is found in the Seychelles (17.4 % age-adjusted comparative prevalence, 17.4 % raw prevalence), followed by the island of Reunion (15.8 % age-adjusted, 18.2 % raw) and Comoros (9.9 % age-adjusted, 7.5 % raw). Some of Africa's most populous countries have the highest numbers of people with diabetes, including South Africa (2.3 [1.2–4.6‡] million), Democratic Republic of Congo (1.8 [1.5–2.2‡] million), Nigeria (1.6 [1.2–3.8‡] million) and Ethiopia (1.3 [0.8–3.5‡] million). Nearly half of all adults with diabetes in the region live in these four countries [1].

Despite the paucity of data from Africa, over the past few decades, diabetes, which was previously considered to be rare or unknown in rural Africa, has emerged as an important non-communicable disease (NCD) in the region [2–4]. Global estimates and projections [1, 5–7] confirm the diabetes epidemic, through the increasing numbers of people with diabetes and impaired glucose tolerance (IGT). These reports not only show that diabetes in adults is a global problem but also that populations of developing countries, minority groups and disadvantaged communities in industrialised countries face the greatest risk. The large increase that is expected to occur in developing regions of the world has principally been attributed to population ageing and urbanisation [1, 5, 7].

S. Dagogo-Jack (ed.), *Diabetes Mellitus in Developing Countries and Underserved Communities*,
DOI 10.1007/978-3-319-41559-8_3

Epidemiology of Diabetes in Africa

Historical Perspective

In 1901, Doctor Cook, a medical missionary working in Uganda, reported that diabetes was rather uncommon, but very fatal in sub-Saharan Africa [8]. For over half a century after that, diabetes continued to be regarded as a disease of affluent societies. Almost no data was available as very few studies were carried out on diabetes in sub-Saharan Africa until the latter half of the twentieth century. The limited number of early studies completed between the 1960s and early 1980s reported prevalence rates of mostly <1 %, except for South Africa with 0.6–3.6 % and Ivory Coast with 5.7 % [2]. Doctor Cook's initial report is no longer accurate today as it is known that most of the people living with diabetes are in developing countries. The burden of diabetes in sub-Saharan Africa is already substantial and continues to increase at a very rapid rate. Current predictions estimate that the number of people living with the chronic condition on the continent will almost double over the next 20 years [1].

Current Trends

Sub-Saharan Africa is currently facing a multiple disease burden characterised by simultaneous health challenges from chronic non-communicable diseases (NCDS), HIV/AIDS, other infectious diseases and malnutrition [9]. The emerging and increasing burden of obesity, diabetes and other NCDs is not accompanied by any marked improvements in control of infections or undernutrition. Studies have reported high rates of coexistence of obesity and undernutrition in the same communities and even same households [10, 11]. The current epidemiologic transition in sub-Saharan Africa is unique and not the same as most Western countries. The transition in Africa follows a delayed model [12] which is characterised by high fertility and high but reducing mortality, resulting in a double demographic disease pattern.

The burden of diabetes in sub-Saharan Africa is already substantial and continues to increase at a very rapid rate. A recent review paper reported that diabetes in sub-Saharan African countries has reached epic proportions. The overall pooled prevalence was estimated at 5.7 % for diabetes, 4.5 % for impaired fasting glycaemia and 7.9 % for impaired glucose tolerance [13]. Diabetes prevalence in sub-Saharan African countries varies by two factors: the first is the level of urbanisation, from 1 % in rural Uganda to 12 % in urban Kenya, and the second is by ethnicity, from 8 % in Zimbabwe to 18 % in sub-Saharan African countries with advanced economies or with significant numbers of Indian subpopulations such as South Africa, Kenya and Seychelles [10, 14]. Data from several point prevalence studies in Cameroon show a more than tenfold increase in diabetes prevalence over a period of one decade [15]; Fig. 3.1.

Current predictions estimate that the number of people living with diabetes on the continent will almost double over the coming 20 years [1, 51, 110]. This, together with the growing incidence of type 2 diabetes in younger age groups (including in some obese children even before puberty), constitutes a serious cause for concern. In developed countries, most people with diabetes are above the age of retirement (>60 years), whilst in developing countries, those most frequently affected are in the middle, productive years of their lives, aged between 35 and 64 [16]. All types of diabetes are on the increase, particularly type 2 diabetes, and the number of people with diabetes will increase by 55 % by 2035 [1] (Fig. 3.2) (IDF 2015). This underlines the fact that the economic burden of diabetes in developing countries will be amplified by its effect on the working age group.

Risk Factors for Diabetes in Africa [9]

Age, Gender and Family History

Similar to data from other parts of the world, studies from sub-Saharan Africa (SSA) show that diabetes prevalence increases with age (Fig. 3.3) [18–21]. Therefore, as living standards improve in SSA with a resulting increase in life expectancy,

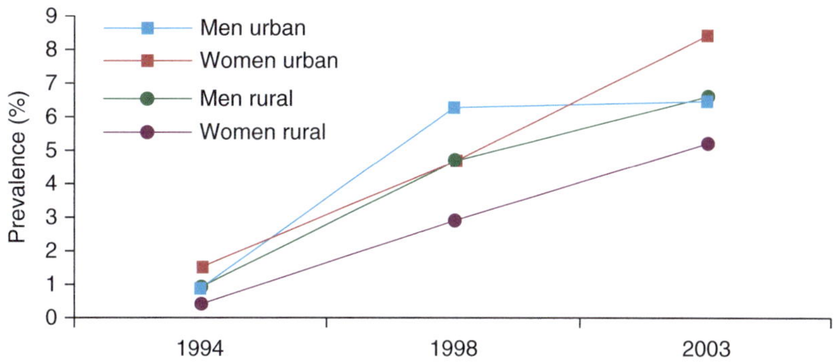

Fig. 3.1 Prevalence of type 2 diabetes in Cameroon, 1994–2003 (prevalence standardised to new world population distribution)

IDF region	2013 Millions	2035 Millions	Increase %
Africa	19.8	41.4	109 %
Middle East and North Africa	34.6	67.9	96 %
South-East Asia	72.1	123	71 %
South and Central America	24.1	38.5	60 %
Western Pacific	138.2	201.8	46 %
North America and Caribbean	36.7	50.4	37 %
Europe	56.3	68.9	22 %
World	**381.8**	**591.9**	**55 %**

Fig. 3.2 The number of people living with diabetes in 2013 and projections for 2035 (in millions of cases), with projected percent changes (Source of data: IDF Diabetes Atlas [17]. *AFR* Africa, *MENA* Middle East and North Africa, *EUR* Europe, *NAC* North America and Caribbean, *SACA* South and Central America, *SEA* South-East Asia, *WP* Western Pacific)

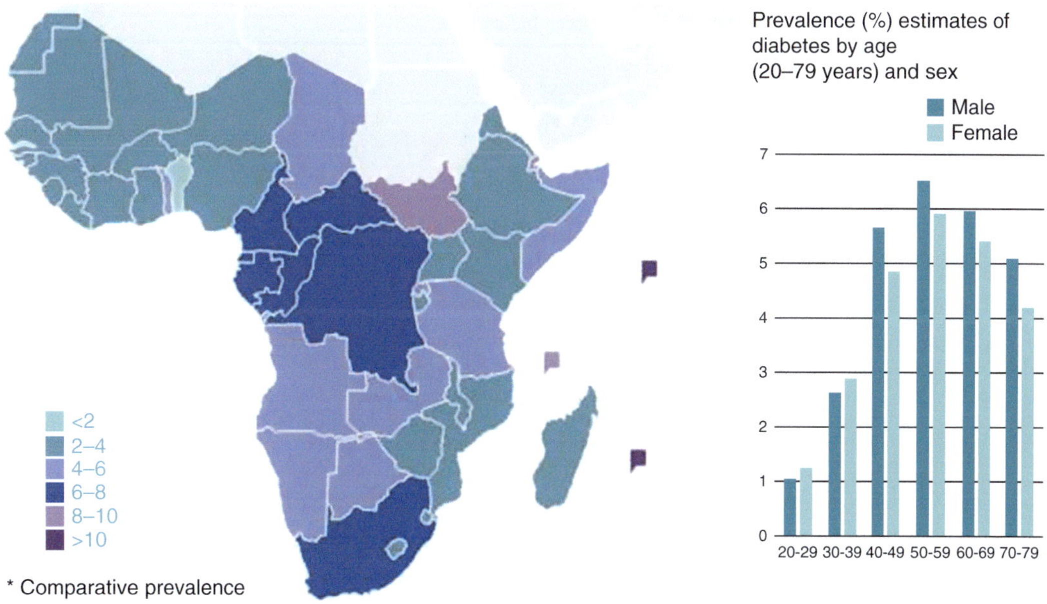

Fig. 3.3 An estimated number of adults with diabetes in sub-Saharan Africa by age group and sex (Source of data: IDF [1])

the prevalence of diabetes is expected to increase accordingly. In addition, the age at onset of diabetes may shift more towards younger adults due to the effects of urbanisation and westernisation – increasing obesity, sedentary lifestyle and other diabetes risk factors in younger age groups.

There is no discernable gender difference in either the prevalence or distribution of diabetes in SSA [22]. This is consistent with observations from other parts of the world as well as with global estimates [23]. It must also be noted that a positive family history of diabetes is an independent diabetes risk factor [18, 19, 24].

Ethnicity, Urbanisation, Migration and Diabetes

Studies from Tanzania and South Africa have shown that diabetes prevalence is lower in the indigenous African community [20, 25, 26] than in migrant Asian Indians [27–29] and when compared with a population of mixed ancestry (Khoi-East Indian-Europid) [30] (Table 3.1). The prevalence rates in Caucasians in SSA have been quite similar to those in Europe (6–10 %), also relatively high [31].

SSA is experiencing the fastest rate of urbanisation worldwide, with an average annual rate of change of the urban population of more than 3 % [34]. Currently, more than one-third of the population in SSA live in urban areas. It is estimated that this could increase to 45 % by 2025, with a demographic inflection point to be attained by 2035 – more urban than rural residents [35]. This increase in the urban population is influenced by both the inherent growth of the urban population due to persistent high fertility and longer life expectancy, and also a massive rural-urban migration [34]. This rapid urbanisation in SSA has been identified as a major determinant of the rising burden of diabetes and other cardiovascular diseases [12, 23, 36, 37].

Table 3.1 Ethnic differences in the prevalence of diabetes mellitus (D) and impaired glucose tolerance (IGT) and the effect of migration in Africa

Country	Author year	Ethnic group	Prevalence (%)[a]	
Locality	(Reference)		D	IGT
Tanzania	McLarty (1989) [26]	Native African	1.1	8.4
	Ramaiya (1991) [27]	Asian Indian	9.1	16.2
	Swai (1990) [28]	Asian Indian	7.1	21.5
South Africa				
KwaZulu Natal	Omar (1993) [25]	Native African	5.3	7.7
	Omar (1994) [29]	Asian Indian	13.0	6.9
Cape Province	Levitt (1993) [20]	Native African	8.0	7.0
	Levitt (1999) [30]	Mixed ancestry (Khoi-East Indian-Europid)	10.8	10.2
Sudan	Elbagir (1996) [19]	Native African	3.4[b]	2.9[b]
	Elbagir (1998) [18]	Mixed Egyptian ancestry	10.4	9.8
Nigeria	Cooper (1997) [32]	Native African	2.0	–
Caribbean		African – origin	7.2	–
United States		African – origin	10.8	–
United Kingdom		African – origin	10.6	–
Cameroon Rural	Mbanya (1999) [33]	Native African	0.8	6.4/3.1[c]
Cameroon Urban		Native African	2.0	1.6/4.6[c]
Caribbean		African – origin	8.5	16.3/19.6[c]
United Kingdom		African – origin	14.6	11.1/14.4[c]

[a]Age-adjusted prevalence except where indicated
[b]For crude prevalence
[c]Male/female

Many studies have clearly demonstrated a positive rural-urban gradient in the prevalence of diabetes and its risk factors, particularly obesity. Urban residence is associated with a two- to five-fold increased risk of prevalent diabetes or impaired fasting glycaemia (Fig. 3.4) [18, 21, 33, 36, 38–42]. Most of these studies considered only the current residence and so may be confounded by the effects of recent rural-urban migration or vice versa. A study from Cameroon [43] that examined both current urban residence as well as total lifetime exposure to an urban environment found that both lifetime exposure to an urban environment and current residence were independently associated with diabetes. Lifetime exposure to an urban environment was strongly associated with fasting blood glucose ($r=0{\cdot}23$; $P<0{\cdot}001$), with the prevalence of diabetes or IFG being higher for individuals with a longer exposure to the urban environment.

Most of these studies from SSA are cross-sectional studies, requiring that inferences about causality or direction be made with caution. Longitudinal studies to provide more robust data on direction and magnitude of change are almost inexistent. In a prospective study of recent rural-to-urban migrants in Tanzania [42], during the first 6 months of urban residence, there was no significant change in their HbA1c level compared to an age, sex and village-matched nonmigrant cohort. However, there was an increase in mean body mass index (BMI) in the recent migrants compared to the nonmigrants. More data is needed to provide answers about societal changes and their influence on human behaviour and cardiovascular risk factors such as diabetes.

A limitation to the discussion on urban and rural differences is the lack of a universally accepted definition for an urban area. Studies of rural-urban differences in diabetes have used local or national norms to define urbanised regions, which may not be similar across studies. The existence of geographically separate residential areas by social class within urban areas may further confound observed differences between studies. Apart from heterogeneity in the definition and attributes of 'urban area' across studies, the degree of urbanisation may influence the magnitude of differences in estimates of diabetes or its risk factors. A study in Benin [44] that recruited participants from rural, semiurban and urban areas observed a positive rural and semiurban to urban gradient in metabolic syndrome and

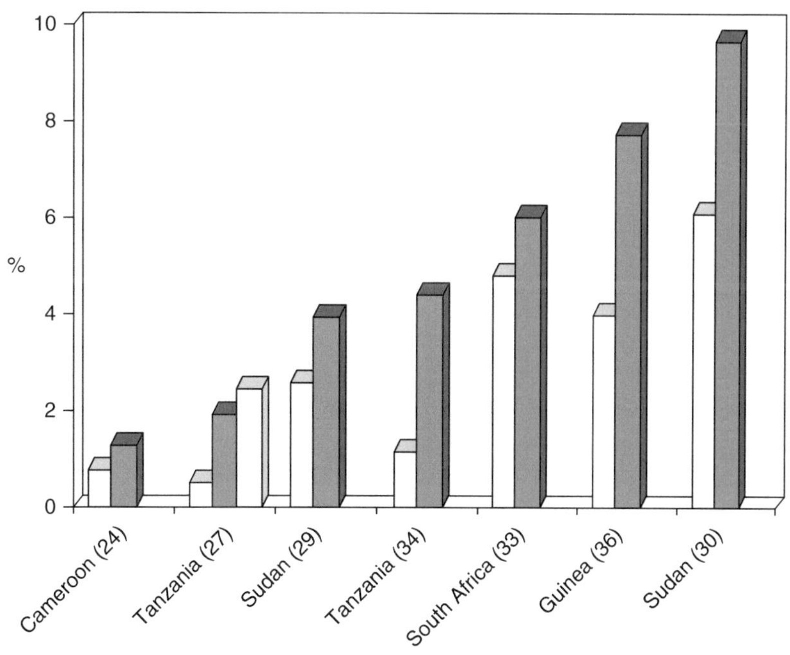

Fig. 3.4 Prevalence of diabetes mellitus (D) in rural [ ] and urban [ ] communities in community studies in Africa, using randomly selected samples

obesity, but not for blood glucose or prevalence of diabetes. The prevalence of high fasting blood glucose was significantly lower in urban dwellers compared to their semiurban or rural counterparts.

The impact of environmental influence (migration) in populations of similar genetic origin has been confirmed in two studies which showed that diabetes prevalence was lower in native West African populations in Nigeria and Cameroon than in West African–origin communities living abroad, in the Caribbean, United Kingdom and United States [32, 33] (Table 3.1). In a study comparing rural and urban Ghanaians in Ghana with Ghanaians in the Netherlands [45] adjusting for age and educational level, the Ghanaians living in the Netherlands were more likely to be obese than those in rural Ghana.

Currently, there are growing concerns about the diabetes burden in indigenous populations because these populations may be experiencing a very rapid lifestyle transition. Active subsistence lifestyle is rapidly giving way to sedentary 'Western' lifestyles. Indigenous populations are generally neglected in terms of healthcare and research, hence the scanty nature of data about them. A study from South Africa reported a diabetes prevalence of about 5 % among the QwaQwa people [46]. There is currently an increasing global awareness of the vulnerability of indigenous peoples as a result of their socioeconomic disadvantage, limited access to care and marginalisation from the majority of the population [17].

From the above data, it appears to be difficult to categorise ethnicity, urbanisation and migration as distinct and separate risk factors for diabetes. Instead, the correlation should be noted and further study undertaken in this area.

Diabetes and Obesity

Published studies indicate a simultaneous rise in overweight/obesity and diabetes prevalence in most SSA countries [47] (Fig. 3.5). Most people with diabetes are obese at the time of diagnosis [48]. Studies conducted in African countries (Ghana [49, 50], Togo [51], Rwanda [52], South Africa [53] and Nigeria [69]) have reported significant associations between type 2 diabetes and

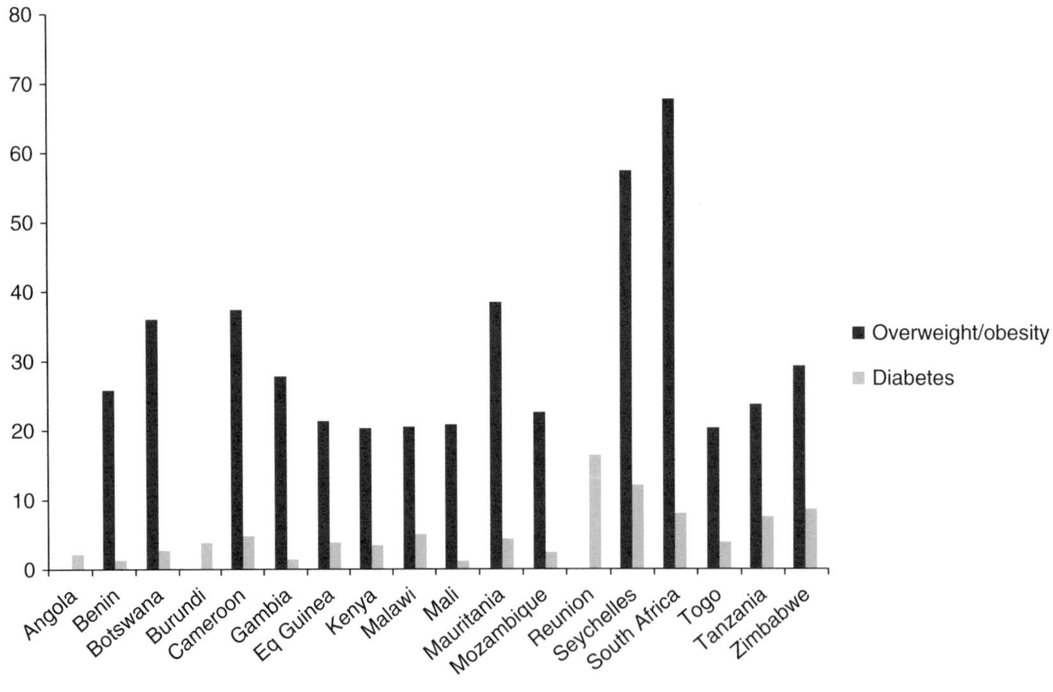

Fig. 3.5 Comparison of overweight/obesity and diabetes prevalence in sub-Saharan Africa (SSA)

obesity. Many studies of people living with diabetes in Africa have consistently reported excess body weight in >50 % of studied samples. However, there is lack of agreement regarding which of the anthropometric variables used to measure obesity can best predict the development of diabetes. One case-control study conducted in a Ghanaian sample [50] suggests that measures of central, rather than general, obesity appear to be significantly related to type 2 diabetes in Africans. There is little or no data from longitudinal studies with hard endpoints that can shed more light on the predictive value of these different measures of obesity in Africans. This means that there are no African-specific cut-off points for estimating obesity risk, hence the continued use of Caucasian cut-off points for Africans. Further research is needed to establish cut-off points based on African data [55].

Adiposity

In most studies in sub-Saharan Africa (SSA), adiposity has generally been found to be associated with diabetes. These studies have shown that diabetes prevalence is higher with increased BMI (BMI-specific rates) [24, 26, 32, 56], waist-hip ratio (WHR-specific rates) [20, 24, 57] and waist circumference (WC-specific rates) [24]. This means that overall obesity (BMI) as well as central obesity (WC and WHR) are associated with an increased risk for diabetes.

Some researchers have been proposing theories suggesting that some alternate distributions of body fat (such as in the hips, thighs or legs) could confer lower risk for diabetes. The protective role of hip circumference as observed in rural South Africans, confirming recent findings in Australians, requires further evaluation in Africa [24].

Emerging evidence is demonstrating that present day lifestyle habits are not the only contributing factor to adiposity. The developmental origins of adult disease suggest that intrauterine growth retardation and the resulting low birth weight predispose individuals to metabolic disorders in their adulthood [58–60]; the high prevalence of stunting and malnutrition [61, 62] in SSA might escalate the development of these disorders. This combination of childhood stunting and adulthood obesity has led to the proposition that such individuals in their early years acquire the contentious 'thrifty phenotype' such that when they rapidly adapt to sedentary lifestyles and high-calorie diets later in their lives, they will be highly prone to obesity-related disorders [59, 63]. The thrifty phenotype hypothesis seems to apply better for the sub-Saharan African populations rather than the thrifty gene hypothesis (theorises that genes derived from times of deprivation may result in adaptations that have adverse effects in times of plenty) [59, 64]. This is because the prevalence rates of T2DM and obesity have been on the increase since the advent of dramatic nutritional/lifestyle changes.

Physical Activity, Diet and Diabetes

Available data strongly links the current epidemiological transition in SSA with rapid urbanisation and westernisation of lifestyle. This changing lifestyle is characterised by decreased levels of physical activity and increased consumption of energy dense or high-fat diets. Although the suggestion of lower physical activity in urban areas compared to rural areas is intuitively plausible, most of the studies on physical activity levels have used self-reported information, mainly using physical activity questionnaires which have not been validated in the population [30, 43, 65–69]. Few studies have used locally validated physical activity questionnaires to demonstrate an urbanisation gradient [42, 70] and the increased risk of diabetes associated with reduced physical activity levels [30].

Studies documenting temporal trends of physical activity levels in SSA using comparable methods are lacking. The adoption and use of the WHO STEPS Global Physical Activity Questionnaire for surveillance of habitual physical activity by many SSA countries [71] will hopefully provide some answers in the near future about trends in population levels of physical activity over time – despite the limitations of self-reported physical activity [68, 69].

Most of the studies which have used objective methods to measure physical activity or energy expenditure are small etiologic studies in specific populations or questionnaire validation studies [65–67, 70, 72–74] and may not be representative of the general population. However, a study in Cameroon [65] using the doubly labelled water method to measure physical activity in free-living adults found physical activity energy expenditure to be inversely associated with 2-h glucose levels independent of age, sex, adiposity or aerobic fitness. Larger studies in Cameroon and Kenya have used a combined heart rate and motion sensor to objectively measure physical activity in free-living individuals [39, 75, 76]. These studies demonstrate a significantly higher physical activity level in rural compared to urban dwellers, and a beneficial association between physical activity and abnormal glucose tolerance.

A high-fat, high-calorie diet is associated with the development of obesity and diabetes. The difficulties of assessing diet and nutritional data in free-living individuals in epidemiologic studies pose an even bigger challenge in many resource-limited settings. Consequently, population level dietary data relevant to diabetes and other chronic NCDs in SSA are scanty [77–79]. A study in South African Blacks showed a temporal trend of increasing consumption of fat and decreasing carbohydrates in both urban and rural areas [77]. However, urbanisation may also lead to a better supply of fruits and vegetables which improve the micronutrient and fibre content of the diet in urban compared to rural areas [79]. The notion of increased consumption of fat as a marker of urbanisation and westernisation of the African diet is not supported by the findings of a study by Mennen et al. which reported the highest consumption of fat in rural Cameroonians, compared to urban Cameroonians, Black Jamaicans and Blacks in Manchester, UK [78].

Impact of HIV/AIDS

In SSA, chronic NCDs such as diabetes receive limited attention due in part to misconceptions that the adult population will be decimated by HIV/AIDS and that few will live long enough to develop such diseases. However, a South African study [80], which modelled the impact of HIV/AIDS for the years 1995 and 2010, clearly showed that the total number of people with diabetes and the number of people with diagnosed diabetes (patient load) will increase regardless of the expected impact of HIV/AIDS on population growth rates and any change (no change, increase) in diabetes prevalence. Since this analysis did not take into consideration the potential impact of antiretroviral therapy (ART) on improving survival rates or possible increase in diabetes incidence, it is likely to be a conservative estimate. However, the ART of choice in sub-Saharan Africa, with its limited healthcare resources, has been linked with an increase in the numbers of people developing prediabetes, and its increased use in the treatment of HIV/AIDS is also projected to cause adverse metabolic abnormalities among patients in SSA [81]. Because of the sheer numbers of people with HIV/AIDS, this effect could directly influence the emerging diabetes crisis in sub-Saharan Africa. Long-term studies to examine the effect of ART on the rising burden of diabetes in SSA are needed.

Clinical Manifestations

The presence of atypical forms of diabetes in sub-Saharan Africa makes it sometimes difficult to classify persons living with diabetes based on established clinical criteria. The disease process may involve peripheral resistance to insulin, increased hepatic production of glucose and lack of insulin production from the pancreas. There are also other causes of diabetes such as genetic abnormalities, surgery, drug usage and infectious diseases [82].

Diabetes mellitus is defined as a "metabolic disorder caused by different factors characterized by a chronic high level of blood sugar with disturbances to carbohydrate, fat, and protein metabolism resulting from defects in insulin secretion, insulin action, or both" [83]. Scientists have divided diabetes into three different types: Type 1 diabetes mellitus (formerly insulin-dependent diabetes mellitus – IDDM) or type 1 diabetes is also known as juvenile onset diabetes. Type 2 diabetes mellitus (non-insulin-dependent diabetes mellitus (formerly non-insulin-dependent diabetes, NIDDM) or type 2 diabetes – adult-onset diabetes) is found in individuals who are insulin-resistant and who usually have relative insulin deficiency. Gestational diabetes mellitus (GDM), the third type, is defined as any degree of glucose intolerance with onset or first recognition during pregnancy. Recently, diabetologists have added a fourth category, tropical diabetes, suggested first in 1907, but made popular by Hugh Jones (J-type diabetes) during the mid-1950s by his study of 13 Jamaican patients [84, 85]. However, tropical diabetes is less than 1 % of the diabetes cases in Africa and is thought to be related to malnutrition [31].

The diagnosis of diabetes usually involves symptoms of diabetes plus either casual plasma glucose concentration ≥200 mg/dl (11.1 mmol/l), a fasting plasma glucose ≥126 mg/dl (7.0 mmol/l) or a 2-h post-load glucose ≥200 mg/dl (11.1 mmol/l) during an oral glucose tolerance test (OGTT) conducted as per WHO recommendations using a glucose load containing the equivalent of 75 g anhydrous glucose dissolved in water [48]. In 2010, a WHO expert committee further adopted cut-off points for using glycated haemoglobin (HbA1c) in the diagnosis of diabetes. It concluded that HbA1c can be used as a diagnostic test for diabetes providing that stringent quality assurance tests are in place and assays are standardised to criteria aligned to the international reference values, and there are no conditions present which preclude its accurate measurement. An HbA1c of 6.5 % was therefore recommended as the cut-off point for diagnosing diabetes, though a value less than 6.5 % does not exclude diabetes diagnosed using glucose tests [86]. The practicality of using HbA1c for diabetes diagnosis in Africa still faces challenges, particularly the high cost of the test relative to blood glucose measurements and also the high prevalence of haemoglobinopathies such as sickle cell anaemia. As the OGTT is much more demanding in terms of time and logistics, HbA1c offers real hope for widespread use in both clinical and research settings even in remote parts of the continent.

Beran et al. surveyed the availability of diagnostic testing tools in a sample of healthcare settings in three countries and found that in Mozambique, urine glucose strips were available in only 18 % of health facilities surveyed, ketone testing strips in 8 % and blood glucose metres in 21 %, whilst availability in Mali was 54, 43 and 13 % and in Zambia 61, 54 and 49 %, respectively [87, 88]. Low levels of adequate glucose control in those diagnosed with diabetes were reported in several prevalence studies [89, 90]. Only 27 % of people diagnosed with type 2 diabetes receiving treatment in a study conducted in Cameroon had adequately controlled glucose levels [89]. Of the 99 people with type 1 diabetes in a Tanzanian survey, only one person achieved suggested glucose targets [90]. None of the 99 people with type 1 diabetes had the ability to monitor their glucose levels at home, and hospitals were unable to routinely do this [68]. A regular supply of insulin was unaffordable for many people with diabetes, with 1 month's insulin supply costing 19.6 days wages in Malawi [91] and 25 % of the minimum wage in Tanzania [92]. One Sudanese study found that 65 % of a family's annual household expenditure on health was spent on caring for a diabetic child [93].

Beran and Yudkin found that state interventions affected insulin price, reporting that an annual supply of insulin cost 5 % of GDP in Mozambique, where it was subsidised by the government, whereas it cost 25 % of GDP in Mali without subsidies [88]. One study investigated insulin availability and reported that one in five hospitals and none out of six health centres surveyed had a regular insulin supply [87].

Economic Cost of Diabetes

Healthcare in most of SSA is almost entirely privately purchased, even though the majority of the poorest people on earth live in SSA. A recent study by Kirigia et al. [94] clearly demonstrates that the cost of diabetes care is going to be overwhelming for the poorest countries of the region. This study shows that whilst the direct cost of diabetes per person with diabetes is only a fraction (<25 %) of the GNI per capita for the 12 richest countries, the direct cost for the 34 poorest countries of the region is 125 % of their GNI per capita (Fig. 3.6). For these poorest countries, the total cost (direct and indirect costs) of diabetes per person with diabetes is more than double the GNI per capita.

The few studies which have examined the cost of diabetes care (usually in small samples) in the region confirm the above estimates. Akoussou-Zinsou and Amedegnato reported in 2001 that the direct cost of diabetes care at a teaching hospital in Togo was USD 342 and USD 110 per person for 'complicated' and 'uncomplicated' diabetes patients, respectively. The estimated GNI per capita for Togo at the time was approximately USD 385. Chale et al. [95] reported an average annual direct cost of diabetes care in Tanzania in 1989–1990 of USD 287 for a patient requiring insulin and USD 103 for a patient not requiring insulin. In a study on type 1 diabetes patients in Sudan, Elrayah et al. [93] reported a partial direct cost of care for each child with type 1 diabetes of USD 283, in a country with a GDP per capita of USD 300 and a per capita government expenditure on health of USD 300.

These data indicate undeniably that the cost of diabetes care constitutes a huge burden for SSA. In the absence of a publicly funded healthcare system, these costs are borne almost entirely by individuals – individuals who are among the poorest people in the world. In this context, poor disease prognosis, with high morbidity and mortality seem to be the unavoidable outcome.

Healthcare Access for Diabetes and its Complications

Many SSA countries have made significant efforts in initiating and improving care for diabetes and other chronic diseases. However, two-

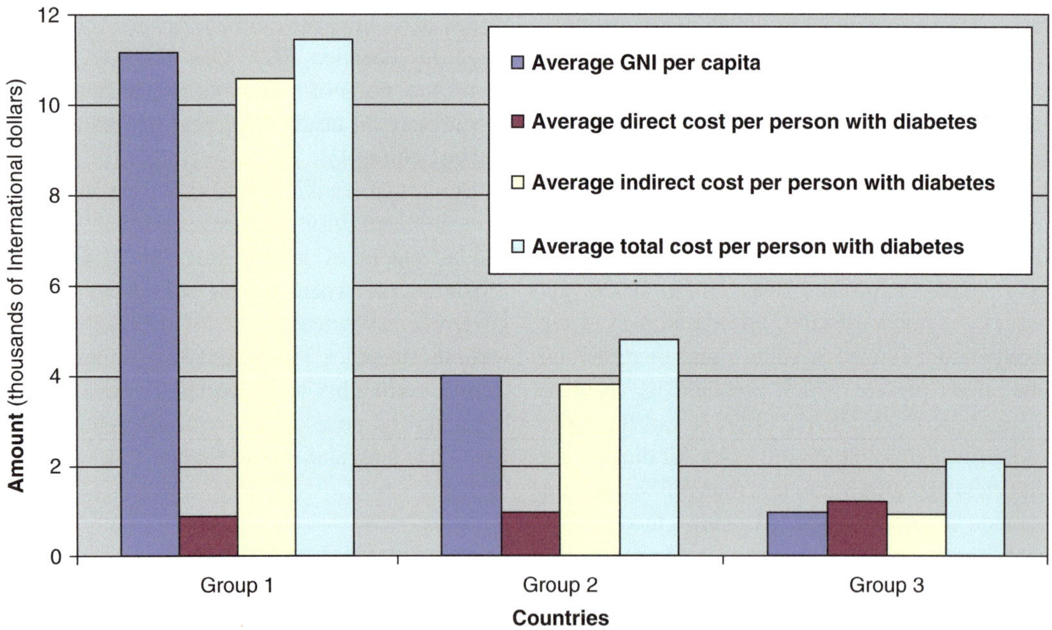

Fig. 3.6 Direct, indirect and total cost of diabetes per person with diabetes compared to the average GNI per capita in countries of WHO Africa region grouped according to the average GNI per capita of the countries (Adapted from Kirigia et al. [94])

thirds of people with diabetes in low- and middle-income countries have poor diabetes control because of inadequate access to care – oral antidiabetic agents and insulin are not available at all times in many parts of the developing world [96]. A few countries have now established successful National Diabetes Programmes and guidelines for the management of diabetes [97–99]. For most countries, there is still much improvement required. Limited financial resources are a major handicap even with the availability of scientific information and political will – both of which are still largely lacking in many SSA countries.

It is possible to set up effective diabetes care at the peripheral level using basic resources in terms of personnel and equipment. Nurse-led care including education has been shown to be successful in resource-limited settings over an 18-month period [100]. It would however be a real challenge to translate such experiments over a larger scale and a much longer period. Work carried out by the International Insulin Foundation [101] identified key areas to be addressed in the fight against diabetes in SSA, encompassing policy improvement, better organisation and delivery of care and patient education. Whiting et al. [102] reviewed challenges to the delivery of diabetes care in a few countries which had reported data on diabetes healthcare delivery, and could still identify the following barriers to adequate diabetes care:

- Patient attendance is poor (there are many reasons for this and more work is required to explore them).
- Consultation times are very short, leaving little or no time for patient education.
- Staff levels are inadequate and more use could be made of trained nurses and other health workers.
- Staff training is limited, and continuing education or in-service training, especially of lower cadres, is needed.
- Complications are not monitored or evaluated in a systematic manner.
- Control of blood glucose and blood pressure is very poor.
- Referral systems are inadequate.
- Patient education is almost nonexistent.
- Organisation of services is generally poor.
- Better record keeping will assist improvements in care.

Therefore, even when diabetes care programmes are introduced, a lot will still need to be done to enable them meet their objective of reducing morbidity and mortality linked to diabetes and its complications. A few of the drawbacks above relate to inadequate healthcare staff levels as well as patient-related factors. Patient education and empowerment in the form of a peer support system could offer some hope of better diabetes control by improving compliance and optimising self-care practices.

Advocacy and Policy for Diabetes Control and Prevention

The adoption of a World Diabetes Day Resolution by the United Nations General Assembly [103] is acknowledgement of the fact that diabetes is a real and imminent threat to social and economic development globally. The UN resolution calls for member states 'to develop national policies for the prevention, treatment and care of diabetes in line with the sustainable development of their healthcare systems, taking into account the internationally agreed development goals, including the Millennium Development Goals'. In SSA specifically, the IDF Africa Region, the World Health Organization (WHO)-AFRO and the African Union have jointly issued a Diabetes Declaration and Strategy for Africa [104]. The declaration is a call to action for governments of African countries and all partners and stakeholders in diabetes to prevent diabetes and related non-communicable diseases and to improve quality of life and reduce morbidity and premature mortality from diabetes (*Panel*).

The IDF-Africa, the WHO-AFRO and the Africa Union call on governments of African countries, non-government organisations, international donor agencies, industry, health care providers and all partners in diabetes to ensure:

- Adequate, appropriate and affordable medications and supplies for people living with diabetes
- Earlier detection and optimal quality of care for diabetes
- Effective efforts to create healthier environments and prevent diabetes
- The identification and dissemination of information, education and communication to empower people with diabetes to access appropriate diabetes services and improve self-care
- Equitable access to care and prevention services for people with or at risk of diabetes
- Awareness of diabetes in the community and among health care providers
- A truly integrated approach which utilises the whole health workforce to address infectious and non-communicable diseases simultaneously
- Government commitment to reducing the personal and public health burden of diabetes
- Partnership and collaboration within and between government sectors, private sectors, non-government organisations and communities to create community and workplace environments that promote better health.

The advocacy for diabetes prevention and control in SSA is largely based on general principles that are generally accepted. There is very little evidence available from local data to substantiate the implementation of prevention or control interventions.

Future Perspectives of Diabetes Prevention and Control

Diabetes is perhaps the index case of the general problem of non-communicable disease healthcare delivery in developing countries. There have been scattered reports [100, 105–109] of successful attempts to improve diabetes care delivery and outcome, but sadly these have largely been initiated either by local hospitals or by external funding and support. The lessons appear to be that real improvements in diabetes care and outcome in Africa are achievable. However, although external support, local health facilities, support groups and diabetes associations all have a role to play, national government health departments need to take the responsibility of instigating widespread permanent change and improvement. The costs need not be great, as patient education (one of the least expensive of diabetes treatments) has been shown to be a major and effective part of all the currently described care delivery packages [100, 105–109]. The integration of traditional healers should also be considered as part of these reforms, since, to the everyday African, they are very much a part of illness management.

References

1. International Diabetes Federation. IDF diabetes atlas. Brussels, Belgium: International Diabetes Federation; 7th ed. 2015.
2. McLarty DG, Pollitt C, Swai AB. Diabetes in Africa. Diabet Med. 1990;7(8):670–84.
3. Motala AA, Omar MA, Pirie FJ. Diabetes in Africa. Epidemiology of type 1 and type 2 diabetes in Africa. J Cardiovasc Risk. 2003;10(2):77–83.
4. Levitt NS. Diabetes in Africa: epidemiology, management and healthcare challenges. Heart. 2008; 94(11):1376–82.
5. International Diabetes Federation. IDF diabetes atlas. Brussels, Belgium: International Diabetes Federation; 3rd ed. 2008.
6. King H, Aubert RE, Herman WH. Global burden of diabetes, 1995–2025: prevalence, numerical estimates, and projections. Diabetes Care. 1998;21(9): 1414–31.
7. Wild S, Roglic G, Green A, Sicree R, King H. Global prevalence of diabetes: estimates for the

year 2000 and projections for 2030. Diabetes Care. 2004;27:1047–53.
8. Cook A. Notes on the diseases met with in Uganda, Central Africa. J Trop Med. 1901;4:175–8.
9. Mbanya JC, Motala AA, Sobngwi E, Assah FK, Enoru ST. Diabetes in sub-Saharan Africa. Lancet. 2010;375(9733):2254–66.
10. Hall V, Thomsen RW, Henriksen O, Lohse N. Diabetes in Sub-Saharan Africa 1999–2011: epidemiology and public health implications. A systematic review. BMC Public Health. 2011;11:564.
11. Kimani-Murage EW, Muthuri SK, Oti SO, Mutua MK, Van de V, Kyobutungi C. Evidence of a double burden of malnutrition in urban poor settings in Nairobi, Kenya. PLoS One. 2015;10(6):e0129943.
12. Omran AR. The epidemiologic transition: a theory of the epidemiology of population change. 1971. Milbank Q. 2005;83:731–57.
13. Hilawe EH, Yatsuya H, Kawaguchi L, Aoyama A. Differences by sex in the prevalence of diabetes mellitus, impaired fasting glycaemia and impaired glucose tolerance in sub-Saharan Africa: a systematic review and meta-analysis. Bull World Health Organ. 2013;91(9):671–682D.
14. Bovet P, Gabriel A, Shamlaye C, Paccaud F. Diabetes in Africa: the situation in the Seychelles. Heart. 2009;95(6): 506–7.
15. Mbanya JC, Kengne AP, Assah F. Diabetes care in Africa. Lancet. 2006;368(9548):1628–9.
16. Tabish SA. Is diabetes becoming the biggest epidemic of the twenty-first century? Int J Health Sci (Qassim). 2007;1(2):V–VIII.
17. International Diabetes Federation. IDF diabetes atlas. Brussels, Belgium: International Diabetes Federation; 6th ed. 2013.
18. Elbagir MN, Eltom MA, Elmahadi EM, Kadam IM, Berne C. A high prevalence of diabetes mellitus and impaired glucose tolerance in the Danagla community in northern Sudan. Diabet Med. 1998;15(2): 164–9.
19. Elbagir MN, Eltom MA, Elmahadi EM, Kadam IM, Berne C. A population-based study of the prevalence of diabetes and impaired glucose tolerance in adults in Northern Sudan. Diabetes Care. 1996;19(10): 1126–8.
20. Levitt NS, Katzenellenbogen JM, Bradshaw D, Hoffman MN, Bonnici F. The prevalence and identification of risk factors for NIDDM in urban Africans in Cape Town, South Africa. Diabetes Care. 1993; 16(4):601–7.
21. Balde NM, Diallo I, Balde MD, Barry IS, Kaba L, Diallo MM, et al. Diabetes and impaired fasting glucose in rural and urban populations in Futa Jallon (Guinea): prevalence and associated risk factors. Diabetes Metab. 2007;33(2):114–20.
22. Motala AA, Omar MAK, Pirie FJ. Epidemiology of diabetes in Africa. In: Ekoe J-M, Rewers M, Williams R, Zimmet P, eds. The epidemiology of diabetes mellitus (2nd edn). Chichester: Wiley, 2008; 133–46.
23. International Diabetes Federation. IDF diabetes atlas. Brussels, Belgium: International Diabetes Federation; 4th ed. 2009.
24. Motala AA, Esterhuizen T, Gouws E, Pirie FJ, Omar MA. Diabetes and other disorders of glycemia in a rural South African community: prevalence and associated risk factors. Diabetes Care. 2008;31(9): 1783–8.
25. Omar MA, Seedat MA, Motala AA, Dyer RB, Becker P. The prevalence of diabetes mellitus and impaired glucose tolerance in a group of urban South African blacks. S Afr Med J. 1993;83(9):641–3.
26. McLarty DG, Swai AB, Kitange HM, Masuki G, Mtinangi BL, Kilima PM, et al. Prevalence of diabetes and impaired glucose tolerance in rural Tanzania. Lancet. 1989;1(8643):871–5.
27. Ramaiya KL, Swai AB, McLarty DG, Alberti KG. Impaired glucose tolerance and diabetes mellitus in Hindu Indian immigrants in Dar es Salaam. Diabet Med. 1991;8(8):738–44.
28. Swai AB, McLarty DG, Sherrif F, Chuwa LM, Maro E, Lukmanji Z, et al. Diabetes and impaired glucose tolerance in an Asian community in Tanzania. Diabetes Res Clin Pract. 1990;8(3):227–34.
29. Omar MA, Seedat MA, Dyer RB, Motala AA, Knight LT, Becker PJ. South African Indians show a high prevalence of NIDDM and bimodality in plasma glucose distribution patterns. Diabetes Care. 1994; 17(1):70–3.
30. Levitt NS, Steyn K, Lambert EV, Reagon G, Lombard CJ, Fourie JM, et al. Modifiable risk factors for type 2 diabetes mellitus in a peri-urban community in South Africa. Diabet Med. 1999;16: 946–50.
31. Sobngwi E, Mauvais-Jarvis F, Vexiau P, Mbanya JC, Gautier JF. Diabetes in Africans – part 1: epidemiology and clinical specificities. Diabetes Metab. 2001;27:628–34.
32. Cooper RS, Rotimi CN, Kaufman JS, Owoaje EE, Fraser H, Forrester T, et al. Prevalence of NIDDM among populations of the African diaspora. Diabetes Care. 1997;20:343–8.
33. Mbanya JCN, Cruickshank JK, Forrester T, Balkau B, Ngogang JY, Riste L, et al. Standardised comparison of glucose intolerance in West African-origin populations of rural and urban Cameroon, Jamaica, and Caribbean migrants to Britain. Diabetes Care. 1999;22: 434–40.
34. United Nations Population Fund. State of world population 2007: unleashing the potential of urban growth.
35. Population Division of the Department of Economic and Social Affairs of the United Nations Secretariat. World urbanization prospects: the 2007 revision. 2008
36. Mayosi BM, Flisher AJ, Lalloo UG, Sitas F, Tollman SM, Bradshaw D. The burden of non-communicable diseases in South Africa. Lancet. 2009;374:934–47.
37. Popkin BM, Gordon-Larsen P. The nutrition transition: worldwide obesity dynamics and their determinants. Int J Obes Relat Metab Disord. 2004;28 Suppl 3:S2–9.

38. Aspray TJ, Mugusi F, Rashid S, Whiting D, Edwards R, Alberti KG, et al. Rural and urban differences in diabetes prevalence in Tanzania: the role of obesity, physical inactivity and urban living. Trans R Soc Trop Med Hyg. 2000;94:637–44.
39. Christensen DL, Friis H, Mwaniki DL, Kilonzo B, Tetens I, Boit MK, et al. Prevalence of glucose intolerance and associated risk factors in rural and urban populations of different ethnic groups in Kenya. Diabetes Res Clin Pract. 2009;84:303–10.
40. Mbanya JC, Ngogang J, Salah JN, Minkoulou E, Balkau B. Prevalence of NIDDM and impaired glucose tolerance in a rural and an urban population in Cameroon. Diabetologia. 1997;40:824–9.
41. Mollentze WF, Moore AJ, Steyn AF, Joubert G, Steyn K, Oosthuizen GM, et al. Coronary heart disease risk factors in a rural and urban orange free state black population. S Afr Med J. 1995;85:90–6.
42. Unwin N, McLarty D, Machibya H, Aspray T, Tamin B, Carlin L, et al. Changes in blood pressure and lipids associated with rural to urban migration in Tanzania. J Hum Hypertens. 2006;20:704–6.
43. Sobngwi E, Mbanya JC, Unwin NC, Porcher R, Kengne AP, Fezeu L, et al. Exposure over the life course to an urban environment and its relation with obesity, diabetes, and hypertension in rural and urban Cameroon. Int J Epidemiol. 2004;33:769–76.
44. Ntandou G, Delisle H, Agueh V, Fayomi B. Abdominal obesity explains the positive rural-urban gradient in the prevalence of the metabolic syndrome in Benin, West Africa. Nutr Res. 2009;29:180–9.
45. Agyemang C, Owusu-Dabo E, de Jonge A, Martins D, Ogedegbe G, Stronks K. Overweight and obesity among Ghanaian residents in The Netherlands: how do they weigh against their urban and rural counterparts in Ghana? Public Health Nutr. 2009;12:909–16.
46. Mollentze WF, Osthuizen GM, et al. The prevalence of diabetes mellitus in two South African black populations. Diabetologia. 1992;5:511. 1992.
47. World Health Organization. Global status report on noncommunicable diseases 2010. Geneva: World Health Organization; 2011. 2011.
48. American Diabetes Association. Position statement: diagnosis and classification of diabetes mellitus. Diabetes Care. 2004;27(1):s5–10.
49. Danquah I, Bedu-Addo G, Terpe KJ, Micah F, Amoako YA, Awuku YA, et al. Diabetes mellitus type 2 in urban Ghana: characteristics and associated factors. BMC Public Health. 2012;12:210.
50. Frank LK, Heraclides A, Danquah I, Bedu-Addo G, Mockenhaupt FP, Schulze MB. Measures of general and central obesity and risk of type 2 diabetes in a Ghanaian population. Trop Med Int Health. 2013;18(2):141–51.
51. Barruet R, Gbadoe AD. Type 2 diabetes mellitus in children in black Africa: description of first five cases in Togo. Med Trop (Mars). 2006;66(5):481–3.
52. Buresi D. Clinical study of diabetes mellitus in hospital practice in Northern Rwanda (apropos of 86 case reports). Med Trop (Mars). 1988;48(3):229–35.
53. Erasmus RT, Blanco BE, Okesina AB, Gqweta Z, Matsha T. Assessment of glycaemic control in stable type 2 black South African diabetics attending a peri-urban clinic. Postgrad Med J. 1999;75(888):603–6.
54. Oguntibeju OO, Odunaiya N, Oladipo B, Truter EJ. Health behaviour and quality of life of patients with type 2 diabetes attending selected hospitals in South Western Nigeria. West Indian Med J. 2012; 61(6):619–26.
55. Mbanya JC, Assah FK, Saji J, Atanga EN. Obesity and type 2 diabetes in Sub-Saharan Africa. Curr Diab Rep. 2014;14(7):501.
56. Fisch A, Pichard E, Prazuck T, Leblanc H, Sidibe Y, Brucker G. Prevalence and risk factors of diabetes mellitus in the rural region of Mali (West Africa): a practical approach. Diabetologia. 1987;30(11):859–62.
57. Fisch A, Pichard E, Prazuck T, Leblanc H, Cisse H. Suitability of reflectometry in epidemiology of diabetes mellitus in Africans. Lancet. 1990;335(8690): 661–2.
58. Prentice AM, Moore SE. Early programming of adult diseases in resource poor countries. Arch Dis Child. 2005;90(4):429–32.
59. Joffe B, Zimmet P. The thrifty genotype in type 2 diabetes: an unfinished symphony moving to its finale? Endocrine. 1998;9(2):139–41.
60. Pettitt DJ, Aleck KA, Baird HR, Carraher MJ, Bennett PH, Knowler WC. Congenital susceptibility to NIDDM. Role of intrauterine environment. Diabetes. 1988;37(5):622–8.
61. Martorell R, Kettel Khan L, Hughes ML, Grummer-Strawn LM. Overweight and obesity in preschool children from developing countries. Int J Obes Relat Metab Disord. 2000;24:959–67. (8): 959–967.
62. de Onis M, Blossner M. Prevalence and trends of overweight among preschool children in developing countries. Am J Clin Nutr. 2000;72(4):1032–9.
63. Hossain P, Kawar B, El NM. Obesity and diabetes in the developing world – a growing challenge. N Engl J Med. 2007;356:213–5.
64. Levitt NS, Lambert EV. The foetal origins of the metabolic syndrome – a South African perspective. Cardiovasc J S Afr. 2002;13(4):179–80.
65. Assah FK, Ekelund U, Brage S, Mbanya JC, Wareham NJ. Free-living physical activity energy expenditure is strongly related to glucose intolerance in Cameroonian adults independently of obesity. Diabetes Care. 2009;32(2):367–9.
66. Cole AH, Ogbe JO. Energy intake, expenditure and pattern of daily activity of Nigerian male students. Br J Nutr. 1987;58:357–67.
67. Luke A, Dugas LR, Ebersole K, Durazo-Arvizu RA, Cao G, Schoeller DA, et al. Energy expenditure does not predict weight change in either Nigerian or African-American women. Am J Clin Nutr. 2009;89: 169–76.
68. Neilson HK, Robson PJ, Friedenreich CM, Csizmadi I. Estimating activity energy expenditure: how valid are physical activity questionnaires? Am J Clin Nutr. 2008;87:279–91.

69. Wareham NJ, Rennie KL. The assessment of physical activity in individuals and populations: why try to be more precise about how physical activity is assessed? Int J Obes Relat Metab Disord. 1998;22 Suppl 2: S30–8.
70. Singh J, Prentice AM, Diaz E, Coward WA, Ashford J, Sawyer M, et al. Energy expenditure of Gambian women during peak agricultural activity measured by the doubly-labelled water method. Br J Nutr. 1989;62: 315–29.
71. World Health Organization. STEPwise approach to chronic disease risk factor surveillance. Geneva: World Health Organization; 2009.
72. Heini AF, Minghelli G, Diaz E, Prentice AM, Schutz Y. Free-living energy expenditure assessed by two different methods in rural Gambian men. Eur J Clin Nutr. 1996;50:284–9.
73. Huss-Ashmore R, Goodman JL, Sibiya TE, Stein TP. Energy expenditure of young Swazi women as measured by the doubly-labelled water method. Eur J Clin Nutr. 1989;43:737–48.
74. Kolbe-Alexander TL, Lambert EV, Harkins JB, Ekelund U. Comparison of two methods of measuring physical activity in South African older adults. J Aging Phys Act. 2006;14:98–114.
75. Dirk Lund Christensen. Glucose intolerance in relation to body composition, physical activity and other predictors among the Luo, Kamba and Maasai of Kenya. PhD Thesis, University of Copenhagen. 2008.
76. Assah FK. Physical activity, cardiorespiratory fitness and metabolic health in Cameroon. PhD Thesis, University of Cambridge. 2009.
77. Bourne LT, Lambert EV, Steyn K. Where does the black population of South Africa stand on the nutrition transition? Public Health Nutr. 2002;5:157–62.
78. Mennen LI, Jackson M, Sharma S, Mbanya JCN, Cade J, Walker S, et al. Habitual diet in four populations of African origin: a descriptive paper on nutrient intakes in rural and urban Cameroon, Jamaica and Caribbean migrants in Britain. Public Health Nutr. 2001;4:765–72.
79. Vorster HH, Venter CS, Wissing MP, Margetts BM. The nutrition and health transition in the North West Province of South Africa: a review of the THUSA (Transition and Health during Urbanisation of South Africans) study. Public Health Nutr. 2005;8: 480–90.
80. Levitt NS, Bradshaw D. The impact of HIV/AIDS on type 2 diabetes prevalence and diabetes healthcare needs in South Africa: projections for 2010. Diabet Med. 2006;23(1):103–4.
81. Young F, Critchley JA, Johnstone LK, Unwin NC. A review of co-morbidity between infectious and chronic disease in Sub-Saharan Africa: TB and diabetes mellitus, HIV and metabolic syndrome, and the impact of globalization. Glob Health. 2009;5:9.
82. Idemyor V. Diabetes in sub-Saharan Africa: health-care perspectives, challenges, and the economic burden of disease. J Natl Med Assoc. 2010;102(7): 650–3.
83. World Health Organisation. Definition, diagnosis and classification of diabetes mellitus and its complications. WHO/NCD/NCS/99.2. Geneva: World Health Organization; 1999.
84. McMillan DE. Tropical malnutrition diabetes. Diabetologia. 1986;29(2):127–8.
85. Ducorps M, Ndong W, Jupkwo B, Belmejdoub G, Poirier JM, Mayaudon H, et al. Epidemiological aspects of diabetes in Cameroon: what is the role of tropical diabetes? Diabetes Metab. 1997;23(1):61–7.
86. World Health Organization. Use of glycated hemoglobin (HbA1c) in the diagnosis of diabetes mellitus. Geneva: World Health Organization; 2010.
87. Beran D, Yudkin JS, de Court. Access to care for patients with insulin-requiring diabetes in developing countries: case studies of Mozambique and Zambia. Diabetes Care. 2005;28(9):2136–40.
88. Beran D, Yudkin JS. Looking beyond the issue of access to insulin: what is needed for proper diabetes care in resource poor settings. Diabetes Res Clin Pract. 2010;88(3):217–21.
89. HoPiT Research Group. Cameroon burden of diabetes project (Cambod): baseline survey report. Yaoundé: HoPiT Research Group; 2004.
90. Majaliwa ES, Munubhi E, Ramaiya K, Mpembeni R, Sanyiwa A, Mohn A, et al. Survey on acute and chronic complications in children and adolescents with type 1 diabetes at Muhimbili National Hospital in Dar es Salaam, Tanzania. Diabetes Care. 2007;30(9):2187–92.
91. Mendis S, Fukino K, Cameron A, Laing R, Filipe Jr A, Khatib O, et al. The availability and affordability of selected essential medicines for chronic diseases in six low- and middle-income countries. Bull World Health Organ. 2007;85(4):279–88.
92. Neuhann HF, Warter-Neuhann C, Lyaruu I, Msuya L. Diabetes care in Kilimanjaro region: clinical presentation and problems of patients of the diabetes clinic at the regional referral hospital - an inventory before structured intervention. Diabet Med. 2002;19(6):509–13.
93. Elrayah H, Eltom M, Bedri A, Belal A, Rosling H, Ostenson CG. Economic burden on families of childhood type 1 diabetes in urban Sudan. Diabetes Res Clin Pract. 2005;70(2):159–65.
94. Kirigia JM, Sambo HB, Sambo LG, Barry SP. Economic burden of diabetes mellitus in the WHO African region. BMC Int Health Hum Rights. 2009;9:6.
95. Chale SS, Swai AB, Mujinja PG, McLarty DG. Must diabetes be a fatal disease in Africa? Study of costs of treatment. BMJ Clin Res Ed. 1992;304(6836): 1215–8.
96. Deeb LC, Tan MH, Alberti KG. Insulin availability among International Diabetes Federation member associations. Report of the Task Force on Insulin Distribution. Diabetes Care. 1994;17(3):220–3.
97. Njamnshi A, Hiag AB, Mbanya J-C. From research to policy: the development of a national diabetes programme in Cameroon. Diabetes Voice. 2006;51(3): 18–21.

98. Ramaiya K. Tanzania and diabetes – a model for developing countries? BMJ. 2005;330(7492):679.
99. Daniels A, Biesma R, Otten J, Levitt NS, Steyn K, Martell R, et al. Ambivalence of primary healthcare professionals towards the South African guidelines for hypertension and diabetes. S Afr Med J. 2000; 90(12):1206–11.
100. Gill GV, Price C, Shandu D, Dedicoat M, Wilkinson D. An effective system of nurse-led diabetes care in rural Africa. Diabet Med. 2008;25(5):606–11.
101. Beran D, Yudkin JS. Diabetes care in sub-Saharan Africa. Lancet. 2006;368(9548):1689–95.
102. Whiting DR, Hayes L, Unwin NC. Diabetes in Africa. Challenges to health care for diabetes in Africa. J Cardiovasc Risk. 2003;10(2):103–10.
103. United Nations. World diabetes day. A/RES/61/225. 12-20-2006.
104. IDF Africa. Diabetes declaration and strategy for Africa. International Diabetes Federation; 2006.
105. Huddle KR, Gill GV. Reducing acute hyperglycaemic mortality in African diabetic patients. Diabet Med. 1989;6(1):64–6.
106. Acheampong JW, Boateng KA, Eghan BA, Story P, Parry EHO, Tomlinson S. The impact of diabetes nurses in the Komfo Anokye Teaching Hospital, Ghana. Diabetes Int. 2000;10:81–93.
107. Mamo Y, Seid E, Adams S, Gardiner A, Parry E. A primary healthcare approach to the management of chronic disease in Ethiopia: an example for other countries. Clin Med (Lond). 2007;7(3):228–31.
108. Coleman R, Gill G, Wilkinson D. Noncommunicable disease management in resource-poor settings: a primary care model from rural South Africa. Bull World Health Organ. 1998;76(6):633–40.
109. Windus DW, Ladenson JH, Merrins CK, Seyoum M, Windus D, Morin S, et al. Impact of a multidisciplinary intervention for diabetes in Eritrea. Clin Chem. 2007;53(11):1954–9.
110. Otaigbe BE, Imafidon EE. Type 2 diabetes mellitus in a Nigerian child: a case report. Afr Health Sci. 2011;11(3):454–6.

4 Type 2 Diabetes in the Middle East and North Africa (MENA)

Yasmin Khan and Osama Hamdy

Introduction

The Middle East and North Africa (MENA) region encompasses approximately 22 countries and comprises 6 % of the world's population. It is a geographic area with rich history and linguistic, ethnic, and cultural diversity. According to WHO statistics from 2010, Egyptians account for more than one-third of the population in this region, followed by North Africans and Arabs from the Gulf (Fig. 4.1). The MENA region has one of the highest prevalence rates of diabetes in the world (11 %) (Fig. 4.2).

Diabetes is a global pandemic affecting more than 415 million adults worldwide. This number is expected to surge to 642 million by 2040 [1]. According to the International Diabetes Federation (IDF), over 35 million people in MENA have diabetes. Saudi Arabia leads the MENA region with the highest prevalence of diabetes (23.9 %), and Egypt is the country with the largest number of diabetes patients (7.5 million) [1]. The rapid rise is due to a multitude of factors, including economic and demographic changes over the last few decades that have led to a decrease in physical activity and rise in obesity. The MENA region has among the highest obesity rates in the world (Fig. 4.3).

Diabetes is associated with early mortality and increased risk for microvascular and macrovascular complications. Approximately 40 % of patients with diabetes have chronic kidney disease, and almost 60–70 % of patients with diabetes have mild to severe forms of nervous system damage. In addition, patients with diabetes are two to four times more likely to have fatal or nonfatal coronary events or stroke. Almost 70–80 % of patients with diabetes die from one of these two conditions. The American Heart Association considers diabetes to be one of the six major controllable risk factors for cardiovascular disease. Researchers also consider diabetes as a risk equivalent to having a prior heart attack.

In addition to being a major public health problem, diabetes is also associated with significant healthcare costs. Worldwide, the global cost of diabetes continues to soar and is now estimated to be 825 billion dollars per year [2]. The IDF estimates that in 2015, countries in the Middle East spent over 17 billion dollars on diabetes care. This figure accounts for only 2.5 % of global spending on the disease [1]. Healthcare expenditure

Y. Khan, MD, MPH (✉)
Adult Diabetes Section, Joslin Diabetes Center, Boston, MA, USA
e-mail: Yasmin.Khan@joslin.harvard.edu

O. Hamdy, MD, PhD, FACE
Joslin Diabetes Center, Harvard Medical School, Boston, MA, USA
e-mail: osama.hamdy@joslin.harvard.edu

S. Dagogo-Jack (ed.), *Diabetes Mellitus in Developing Countries and Underserved Communities*,
DOI 10.1007/978-3-319-41559-8_4

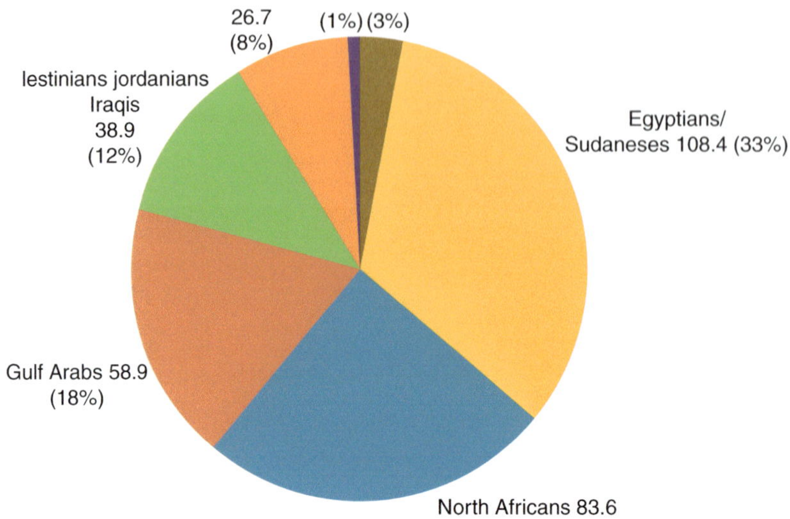

Fig. 4.1 Ethnicity of the MENA region (Source: 2010 WHO statistics)

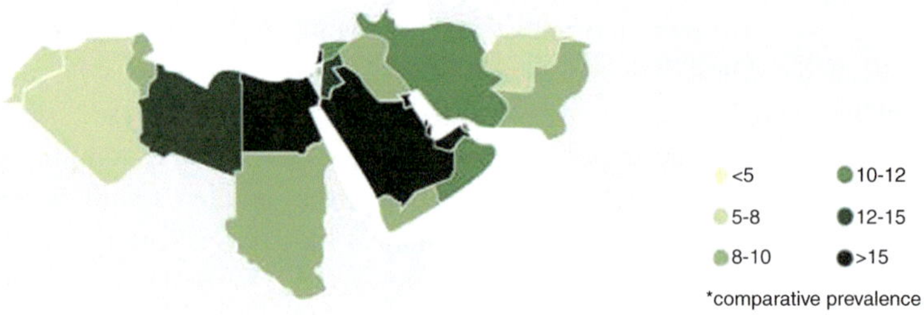

Fig. 4.2 Comparative prevalence of diabetes in MENA (Source: IDF Diabetes Atlas)

varies greatly across the region due to economic inequalities. In Egypt, a cost analysis from 2010 estimated the economic impact of diabetes to be $1.29 billion. This number excluded the cost associated with prediabetes and also the cost related to loss of productivity. This figure, adjusted for inflation, can be expected to double by the year 2030. According to the IDF, in Egypt the current spending on diabetes is among the lowest in the MENA at $116 per patient per year (16% of total healthcare expenditure). Countries with the highest spending per person with diabetes are Qatar, Kuwait, UAE, and Bahrain, with a range of $1,000–2,000 per year. This is still lower than spending for developed countries, which usually ranges from $2,000 to 7,000 per patient per year [1]. The rising epidemic will continue to strain the economies of the MENA region, and health authorities should urgently address the problem of diabetes to avoid major spending on healthcare in the coming years.

Epidemiology of Diabetes in MENA

The MENA region can be described as a global hotspot for diabetes. According to the IDF, approximately 37 million adults aged 20–79 are living with diabetes across the region. By 2040, this number is expected to rise to 72 million. Of particular concern is that over 40% of individuals with diabetes are undiagnosed and are at increased risk for developing complications from diabetes. Moreover, in 2015 there were 342,000 deaths related to diabetes. A further 30.2 million people in the region, or 7.8% of the adult population, are estimated to have impaired glucose tolerance and are therefore at high risk of developing diabetes in the future [1].

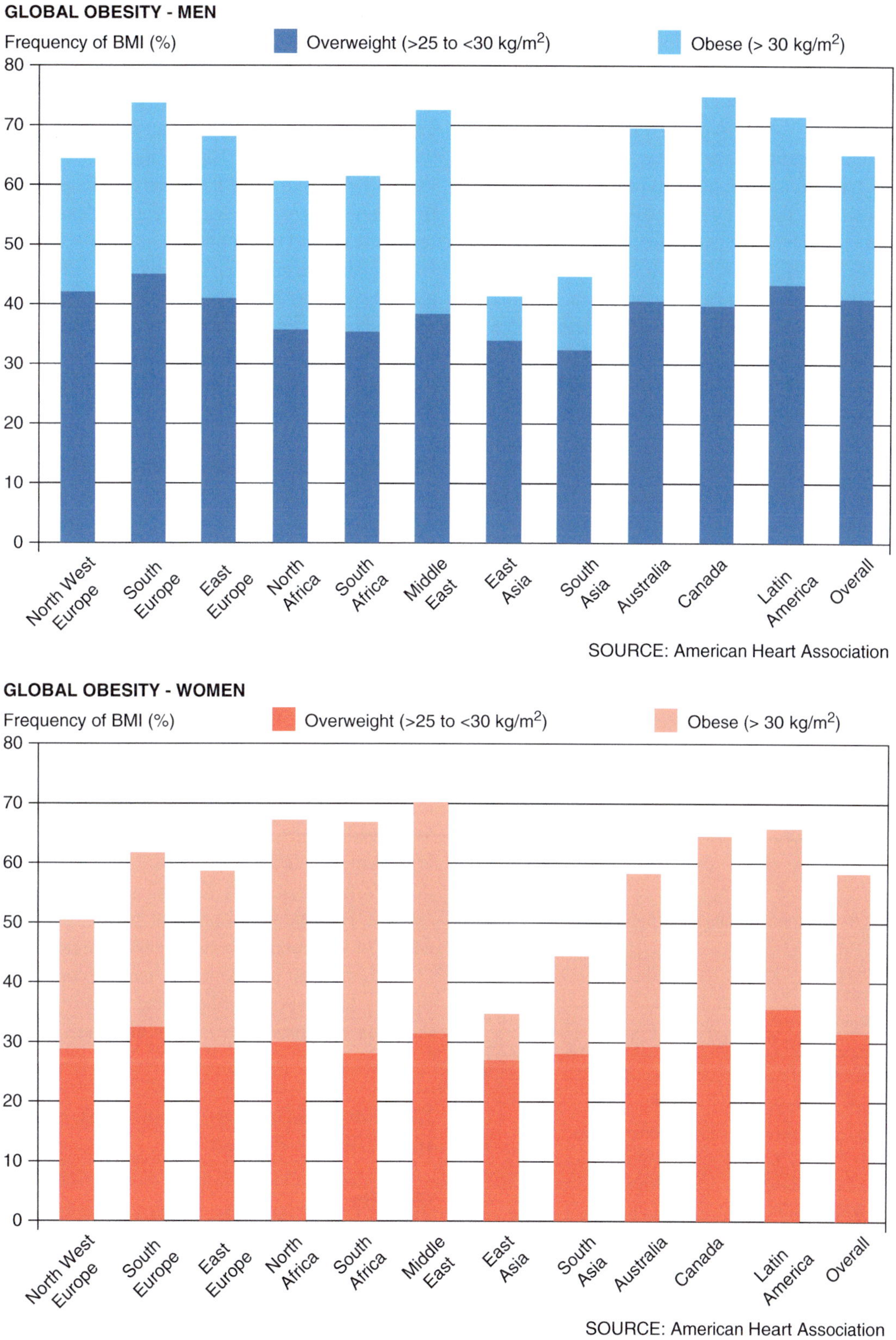

Fig. 4.3 Global prevalence of obesity (Source: AHA)

Prevalence of Diabetes

Diabetes prevalence varies greatly across the region. The highest prevalence is seen in the Gulf countries, with Saudi Arabia, Kuwait, and Bahrain leading the way (Fig. 4.4). The high rates of diabetes are due in large part to the economic growth of the last few decades and the subsequent change in diet and lifestyle of these populations. Saudi Arabia has a diabetes prevalence of 23.9 % among adults. The prevalence is higher among Saudis residing in urban areas (25.5 %) when compared to rural areas (19.5 %) [3]. There is little gender difference with respect to diabetes prevalence in the region. As expected, type 2 diabetes (T2D) cases predominate and constitute approximately 90–95 % of all patients with diabetes. However, it is worth mentioning that Saudi Arabia has one of the world's highest annual incidence rates of type 1 diabetes in children, with 31.4 new cases per 100,000 individuals per year [4]. This is the highest incidence of type 1 diabetes of any country outside of Europe.

The countries with the largest number of people affected by diabetes are Egypt (7.5 million), Pakistan (7 million), and Iran (4.5 million) (Fig. 4.4). These figures reflect the large populations of these countries. In Egypt, the prevalence of diabetes is around 15.6 % among adults between 20 and 79 years of age. The International Diabetes Federation (IDF) estimates that 7.5 million individuals in Egypt have diabetes and another 2.2 million have prediabetes. Furthermore, reports indicate that 43 % of patients with diabetes and most patients with prediabetes in Egypt are likely undiagnosed. It is estimated that 42 % of patients with diabetes in Egypt have retinopathy, 5 % are legally blind, and 22 % have peripheral neuropathy. Diabetes is also the leading cause of end-stage renal disease and leg amputation in Egypt [5–7]. It is especially alarming that the prevalence of diabetes in Egypt has increased rapidly within a relatively short period of time from approximately 4.4 million in 2007 to 7.5 million in 2013. This number is projected to rise to 13.1 million by 2035 (Fig. 4.5).

Top 5 countries for number of pepole with diabetes (20-79 years), 2014

Countries/territories	Millions
Egypt	7.593
Pakistan	6.944
Iran (Islamic Republic of)	4.582
Saudi Arabia	3.806
Sudan	3.007

Top 5 countries for diabetes comparative prevalence (%) (20-79 years), 2014

Countries/territories	%
Saudi Arabia	23.9
Kuwait	23.1*
Bahrain	21.9*
Qatar	19.8
United Arab Emirates	19

Fig. 4.4 Diabetes in the MENA region, 2014 (Source: IDF Atlas, sixth edition)

Prevalence of Diabetes Complications

Among patients with diabetes, the prevalence of microvascular and macrovascular complications is relatively high in Arab populations. A recent cross-sectional study from Saudi Arabia showed that the prevalence of peripheral neuropathy among patients with diabetes was 19.9 % [8]. Among Saudi patients with T2D for at least 10 years, the prevalence of retinopathy was 31 % [9]. In Jordan, data from a national diabetes center showed that 45 % of patients had retinopathy, 33 % had nephropathy, and 5 % had a history of amputation [10]. Diabetes is also frequently associated with psychological distress. A study from UAE demonstrated that up to 33.8 % of patients with diabetes had depression or anxiety or both [11]. Diabetic patients with depression are less likely to adhere to medical treatment and engage in self-care. Overall, the high prevalence of diabetic complications in this region highlights the need for early detection and prompt treatment of this disease.

Risk Factors for Type 2 Diabetes in the MENA Region

Obesity

Obesity and physical inactivity are the two major risk factors for diabetes in the MENA region. The countries with the highest prevalence of obesity are Saudi Arabia, United Arab Emirates, and Egypt (Fig. 4.6). Over the last few decades, there

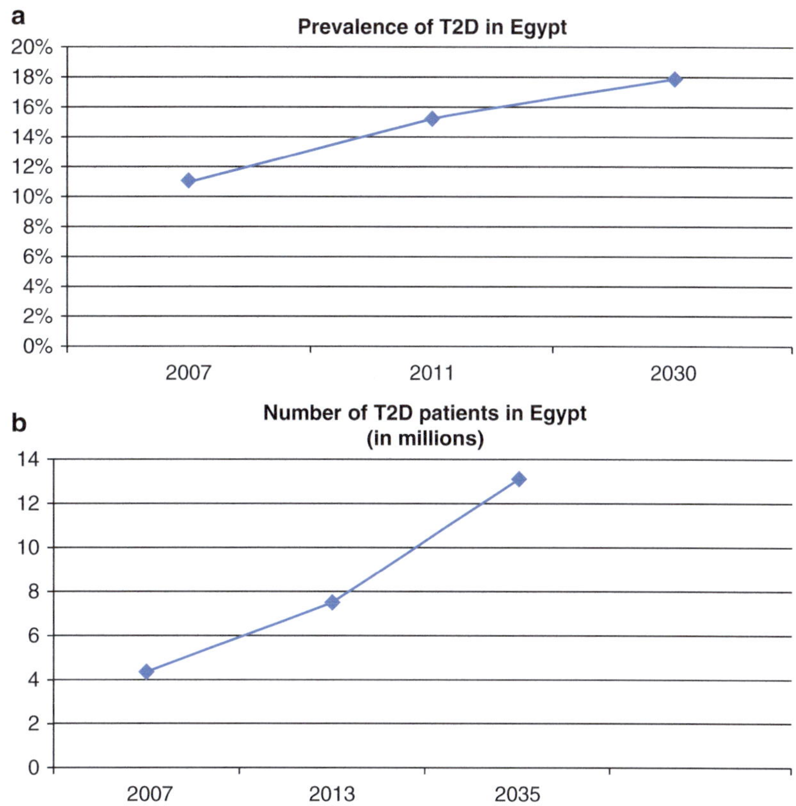

Fig. 4.5 The rising prevalence of type 2 diabetes in Egypt. (**a**) Projected trends of the prevalence rate of T2D in Egypt. (**b**) The projected trend of the total number of patients with T2D in Egypt

has been a dramatic increase in obesity, particularly among Arab women. Results from a national survey conducted in Saudi Arabia showed the prevalence of obesity was 44 % among women and 26 % among men [12]. Similar results were seen in the 2008 Egypt Demographic and Health Survey, which assessed the nutritional status of adults aged 15–59 years old, and found that approximately 50 % of men and 65–80 % of women were overweight or obese [13]. The Egyptian National Hypertension Survey program, which was conducted in six Egyptian governorates and included 2,313 adults older than 25 years of age, showed that 50 % of surveyed individuals had central obesity. This was shown to be strongly associated with increased risk of diabetes and cardiovascular disease [14–16].

An alarming trend is the increased rates of obesity among children and adolescents. Obesity during childhood is a risk factor for obesity and related chronic diseases during adulthood, such as cardiovascular disease, diabetes mellitus, and hypertension. The highest prevalence of obesity among children has been reported in Bahrain (38.5 %), while the lowest was reported in Iran (3 %) [17]. Cross-sectional data from Saudi Arabia showed that a very high proportion of Saudi adolescents (84 % of males and 91.2 % of females) spent more than 2 h on TV or video screen daily and almost half of the males and three-quarters of the females did not meet daily physical activity guidelines [18]. In Egypt, data from the most recent Demographic and Health Survey show that 35 % of males and 36 % of females aged 5–19 are overweight [13]. These trends are largely the result of an unhealthy eating pattern and decreased physical activity that has emerged over the last few decades.

Genetics of Diabetes

Central adiposity is common among Arab populations and genetic factors are likely to play a role in the development of obesity and diabetes. The genetics underlying T2D is multifactorial and complex in

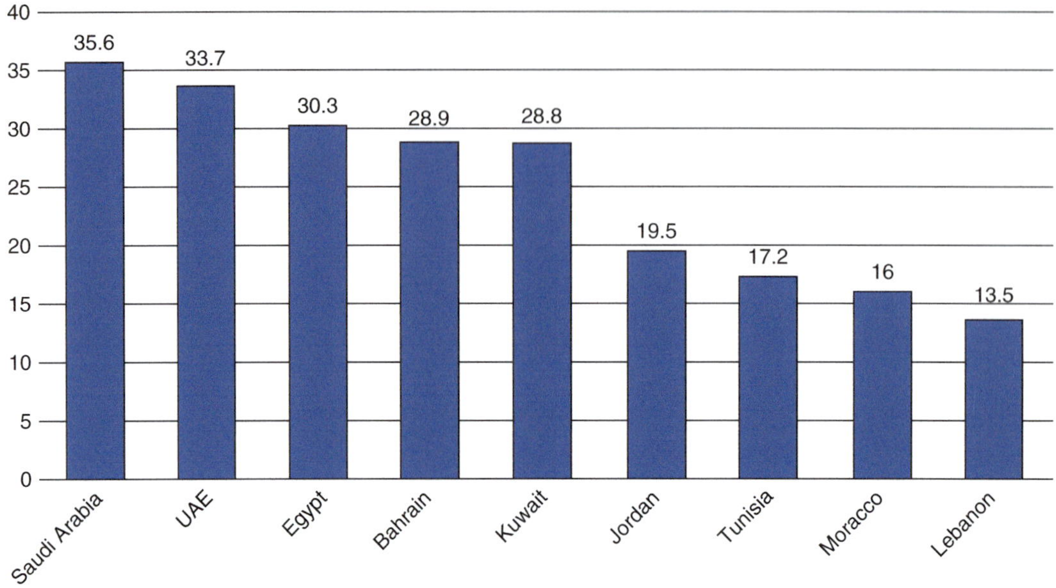

Fig. 4.6 Prevalence (%) of obesity in Arab countries (Source: 2010 WHO statistics)

nature. Although genetic studies from the region are limited, there is evidence that variations in the *ADIPOQ* gene, which encodes adiponectin, are associated with increased BMI and waist circumference [19]. Adiponectin is released by adipocytes and is found in lower levels among obese subjects. Recent studies from Jordan and Tunisia have also shown that variants in the *ADIPOQ* gene strongly correlate with risk of T2D [20, 21]. In the Lebanese population, mutations in both *CDKAL1* and *IGF2BP2* genes have been shown to be associated with T2D [22, 23]. Interestingly, variants of the *TCF7L2* gene, which have been associated with T2D across multiple ethnic groups, have only a weak association with diabetes in Arab populations. Another consideration is that the genetic risk is increased among populations that have traditions of consanguineous marriages. Certainly more research is needed to further our understanding of the genetic basis of diabetes in this region.

Physical Inactivity

Physical inactivity is the other major risk factor for the development of T2D in MENA. Rapid economic development, increased availability of cars, access to migrant labor, and widespread use of computers and television have all contributed to a sedentary lifestyle. Low levels of physical activity are prevalent throughout the region. In a cross-sectional study of adults in Saudi Arabia aged 30–70, the prevalence of inactivity was very high at 96.1 % [24]. In Cairo, absence of weekly physical activity was reported among 81 % of the 4,918 households surveyed in 1995 [13]. The majority of individuals did not engage in any physical activity or walk regularly. Physical activity levels were especially low among women [24]. The major reasons for decreased physical activity, particularly among Egyptian women, include the general lack of exercise facilities, overcrowded urban cities, and poor physical education in schools [13]. Furthermore, urban planning in many cities does not encourage or support an active lifestyle. The lack of regular physical activity represents a major public health concern that needs to be addressed by each individual country in a culturally appropriate way.

Chronic Hepatitis C Infection

The burden of hepatitis C virus (HCV) is growing in the MENA region. If untreated, HCV can lead to liver cirrhosis, hepatocellular cancer, and death. Egypt has the highest prevalence of chronic hepatitis C infection in the world. This is attributed to the mass intravenous treatment campaign of bilharziasis between 1960 and 1980 with the use of poorly sterilized needles. The Egypt Demographic and Health Survey showed that 15 % of Egyptians are serologically positive for HCV antibodies and 10 % have active infection [13]. Meanwhile in the Gulf region, infection rates are relatively low. In Qatar, 1.1 % of the population carries the virus.

The prevalence of T2D among patients with HCV is 13–33 %. A meta-analysis of the association of HCV and T2D showed that patients with HCV are more likely to develop T2D. The odds ratio was particularly high among male patients (OR, 1.26; 95 % CI, 1.03–1.54) and those older than 40 years of age (OR, 7.39; 95 % CI, 5.82–9.38). Not only does HCV increase the risk of diabetes, it is also associated with poor glycemic control and increased prevalence of diabetes complications. A study of 438 patients with T2D (113 Egyptians and 325 Kuwaitis) showed that poor glycemic control was mostly seen in patients positive for HCV. In another cross-sectional study of 489 patients with T2D who attended an outpatient clinic and dialysis unit in Egypt, the prevalence of HCV infection was 12.9 % among patients attending the outpatient clinic and 18.7 % among patients on dialysis [25–28].

Early treatment of HCV can help delay or prevent T2D. It has been shown that effective elimination of HCV in patients with prediabetes improved glycemic tolerance and significantly reduced A1C levels. Prospectively, 34.8 % of patients who were treated became normoglycemic and only 5.5 % developed diabetes. The sustained response to antiviral therapy was the only independent predictor of improved glycemic control [29]. With the development of newer and effective medications for HCV, the risk for T2D may significantly reduce in Egypt.

Pesticide Exposure

There is growing evidence that pesticide use is associated with T2D. Exposure to pesticides may occur either directly among farmers and applicators or indirectly due to chronic exposure to low levels of pesticides through contaminated food. Pesticides can affect multiple pathways involved in glucose regulation. Organophosphorus and organochlorine pesticides in particular lead to a deleterious effect on glucose metabolism and insulin secretion. It is hypothesized that the involved mechanisms include oxidative stress, pancreatitis, and inhibition of cholinesterase [30, 31].

Pesticides are widely used in the MENA region, as 43 % of the population lives in rural areas and depends on farming for livelihood. Pesticide usage is high in Lebanon, Kuwait, and Egypt. Egypt ranks fifth among African nations with respect to pesticide consumption. The most commonly used pesticides in Egypt are dichlorodiphenyltrichloroethane (DDT), which is an organochlorine compound, and chlorpyrifos and malathion, which are organophosphorus compounds [32–35]. Growing evidence suggests a strong association between exposure to these pesticides and increased risk for insulin resistance and T2D. Raafat et al. found a positive association between chronic exposure to malathion and insulin resistance [36]. Another study showed a U-shaped dose-response association between features of metabolic syndrome, such as high body mass index, dyslipidemia (increased serum triglycerides, increased LDL cholesterol, decreased HDL cholesterol), and insulin resistance with exposure to various pesticides [37]. Currently, pesticide regulations are inadequate and a greater commitment to food safety is needed to protect the health of consumers.

Cultural Factors Affecting Type 2 Diabetes in the MENA Region

Dietary Pattern

Over the last three decades, the MENA region has experienced a major shift in its traditional eating patterns, referred to as the "nutrition transition," due to urbanization and rapid economic development. The traditional diet was rich in vegetables, legumes, fruits, whole wheat bread, and fish, with low to moderate in amount of animal protein. Presently, a dietary pattern with high consumption of saturated fat, refined carbohydrates, processed meat, and sugar-sweetened beverages has emerged throughout the region. This pattern has been associated with an increased risk of T2D. Meanwhile, diets characterized by high intakes of vegetables, fruits, and whole grains have been shown to be protective against T2D [38].

Recent meta-analyses of observational and prospective cohort studies have shown a strong association between high consumption of white rice and an increased risk of T2D [39]. High consumption of trans fat has also been shown to be a risk factor for cardiovascular disease. Egypt and Pakistan are the world's highest consumers of this unhealthy type of fat. Partially hydrogenated oil, which contains trans fat, is also used frequently for daily cooking and for preparing fried foods throughout the region.

Sociocultural factors also play an important role in the pattern of food consumption. With longer working hours and more women entering the workforce, there has been a gradual shift toward larger and later dinner. Dining out is also on significant rise, especially among youth. Western fast-food restaurants have also proliferated throughout the MENA region. Together with a strong culture of hospitality and frequent family gatherings around food, these trends have nudged society toward consumption of bigger portions and no doubt are contributing to the increased prevalence of obesity and T2D in the MENA region.

Sedentary Lifestyle

Low levels of physical activity are further exacerbating the problem of obesity and diabetes. The increased number of cars, vast expansion of cities, and hot climate contribute to decreased physical daily activity. In addition, there are various cultural and social norms that may discourage exercise. In Egypt, there is a tendency to avoid exercise in public areas, while few are able to afford membership in private athletic facilities. Overall, exercise facilities are limited and community sports facilities are scarce. Even in schools, reduced time for physical activity and limited availability of spaces for sports reinforces a sedentary lifestyle for Egyptian youth. It is also worth mentioning that in Egypt and Gulf countries, reduced exposure to sunlight with traditional clothing among women contributes to vitamin D deficiency, which has been linked to increased rates of obesity and T2D [40].

Women are facing more obstacles to physical activity compared to men. In Bahrain, for example, the main barriers to exercise perceived by women were home commitments (49 %), care of children (36 %), and negative attitudes by family members toward women practicing exercise/sports (24 %) [41, 42]. Of the women studied, the majority believed that there is gender discrimination when it comes to sports, since sports and other recreational facilities are provided mostly for men [42]. Furthermore, in the Middle East, women athletes continue to struggle for women's participation in sports at the national and international level. In 2012, Sarah Attar and Wojdan Shaherkani made history when they became the first women to compete for Saudi Arabia in the London Olympics.

Smoking

Smoking represents a major public health crisis in the MENA region. Smoking is directly linked to increased incidence of microvascular and macrovascular diseases in patients with diabetes. In Jordan, 43.4 % of men smoke, which represents the highest prevalence in the region. Among women, Lebanon leads the way with a smoking prevalence of 21.2 %. Egypt represents one of the largest tobacco markets in the world, with over 20 billion cigarettes smoked annually and a smoking prevalence of 39.7 % among adult men. Smoking is still rare among Egyptian women. Despite high taxes on cigarettes and increasing public health education, smoking remains a common unhealthy habit in the MENA region [43].

Health Illiteracy

Health literacy may be defined as the degree to which an individual has the capacity to obtain and understand basic health information to make appropriate health decisions. Health illiteracy is common in the MENA region. Obesity is frequently regarded as a cosmetic problem and rarely viewed as a disease. Most patients with T2D believe that diabetes should only be treated by oral medications and often resist insulin injections when indicated. Routine daily glucose monitoring is essentially nonexistent or limited due to cost or fear of frequent finger sticks. Furthermore, it has been demonstrated that patients rarely change their diet or exercise habits following a diagnosis of diabetes. A recent survey of 575 patients from a diabetes outpatient clinic in the UAE showed that the majority (72 %) of patients had negative attitudes toward having the disease, and 31 % of patients had poor knowledge of diabetes [44].

In a study from Egypt, the majority of 560 patients with T2D surveyed believed that T2D is an infectious disease originally caused by stress. Moreover, only 38.4 % of patients had a positive attitude toward self-management. Interestingly, these study patients believed that the efficacy of herbal medicine in treating T2D was sufficiently high and neglected the positive role of regular exercise in diabetes management. Most of patients also believed that patients suffering from polyuria should reduce their volume of drinking water [45]. All of these factors result in poor glycemic control, late diagnosis, and increased prevalence of diabetes complications.

Poor Adherence

In the MENA region, as elsewhere, nonadherence with diabetes management is common and is one of the main factors for poor glycemic control. Daily testing of blood glucose is very rare and frequent omission of insulin injections is common, even in patients with type 1 diabetes. Even among educated patients, poor adherence with healthy eating and physical activity is common. Furthermore, fear of hypoglycemia among patients treated with insulin leads to suboptimal control and frequent reduction in insulin dosing either intentionally or upon recommendation of treating physicians. Frequently, diagnosis of diabetes complications, especially retinopathy and nephropathy, is too late and does not allow for effective prevention. Unfortunately, many patients consider their disease and its complications as inevitable and feel powerless to alter the course of the disease. A recent study from Egypt showed that improvement with medication adherence can be achieved through improving patient education about the disease, simplifying the drug regimen, and reducing medication cost [46].

Healthcare Quality

The high prevalence of diabetes and other chronic diseases has placed a great burden on the region's health systems. Many patients with diabetes are either treated in the limited number of public hospitals, in the private healthcare sector through out-of-pocket fee for service, or in the scarce diabetes centers in major cities. Furthermore, patients with diabetes face many barriers to care including cost, access to physicians and diabetes educators, and access to medicines such as insulin.

Human resources for diabetes care are often inadequate. Overall, there is a shortage of physicians, nurses, and health educators in the region. For example, a study in Saudi Arabia found that less than 10 % of health centers were staffed with diabetes educators, and only 40 % of patients with retinopathy were referred to eye clinics [47]. Another study examined the delivery of health education to T2D patients in four healthcare centers (two rural and two urban) in Alexandria, Egypt. Although diabetes knowledge was satisfactory among the 88 physicians surveyed in this study, 95.5 % of physicians from rural areas and 89.8 % of those from urban health centers neglected the fundamental role of patient education and regular exercise in managing T2D [45]. All of these factors contribute to suboptimal quality of care for patients with diabetes.

Prevention of T2D

Type 2 diabetes is a largely preventable disease. Research has shown that lifestyle modification can significantly reduce the incidence of type 2 diabetes by up to 58 % [48]. Early diagnosis and prevention of diabetes is a key priority for countries of the MENA region. The Arab Taskforce for Obesity was created in 2010 to limit the rise of obesity among Arab countries. This represented a collaboration of 14 Arab countries. The goals of the taskforce are to promote healthy eating, increase physical activity, raise awareness about obesity and its complications, and develop national guidelines for controlling the rise in obesity, especially in children.

Effective screening is one of the most important factors in diabetes prevention and control. The Weqaya program in Abu Dhabi is an example of a successful screening program. The program was launched in 2008, and to date over 94 % of the national population has been screened for cardiovascular risk factors, including diabetes, using A1c criteria [49]. Approximately 45 % of the screened population was found to have diabetes or prediabetes. In Oman, a diabetes risk score was developed that used age, waist circumference, body mass index, family history of diabetes, and hypertension status to correctly identify individuals at high risk of type 2 diabetes in a community setting. Interestingly, testing with Dutch, Thai, and Finnish diabetes risk scores showed poor performance in this population [50]. This suggests that customized screening tools may be of benefit in Arab populations. Ideally, screening for diabetes should be part of a larger national prevention program. Abu Dhabi, Qatar, UAE, and Kuwait are examples of countries that are leading the way with national strategies for diabetes prevention.

Future Directions

Although the prevalence of diabetes is increasing throughout the MENA region, data on obesity and diabetes in many countries are lacking. Healthcare research is not seen as a priority in many countries of the region. Gaps exist in our knowledge of epidemiological variation of diabetes, as Arab populations are widely distributed across both Asia and Africa. Research on social and cultural barriers to diabetes care can add further insight into the prevention and treatment of this disease.

To curb the diabetes epidemic, public health strategies that focus on primary prevention through promotion of a healthy diet and lifestyle should be prioritized. Primary care is now seen as having a key role in prevention and early detection of diabetes. Traditionally, diabetes has been managed by specialist centers, but the majority of people with diabetes can be effectively managed by multidisciplinary teams of physicians, diabetes educators, nurses, and pharmacists. Countries should develop and organize their health systems to provide integrated and continuous care for patients from prediabetes to severe diabetes with complications.

Strategies to Improve Diabetes Care in the MENA Region

As outlined in this chapter, the diabetes epidemic is driven by a complex multitude of factors. As awareness of diabetes in the region rises, a targeted multi-sector response is necessary to address this global crisis. Fundamental changes in public policies and health systems are required. The following points should be urgently considered:

1. Screen for diabetes.
   Health authorities should implement efficient screening programs for high-risk individuals, especially adults who are overweight and obese with a positive family history of diabetes. Focusing on primary care and preventive services will avoid costly complications of diabetes down the road.
2. Create a National Diabetes Prevention Program.
   Develop a comprehensive and accessible lifestyle program with simple methods to facilitate implementation on large scale. Increase public awareness of diabetes and emphasize that early diagnosis can reduce the risk of diabetes and its complications. Addressing childhood obesity and obesity among women should be a priority of such programs.

3. Improve diabetes education.
   Diabetes education remains the cornerstone of diabetes management. General diabetes and nutrition education should be conducted at schools, community centers, and healthcare facilities. Public and private media can also play vital role in disseminating accurate information about diabetes to the public. The goal is to encourage citizens to be engaged in a healthy lifestyle and also to reduce consumption of processed food, refined carbohydrates, and trans fat.
4. Strengthen clinical care for diabetes.
   Improve human resources for healthcare. The concept of a diabetes management team should be introduced that includes a certified diabetes educator (CDE) and registered dietitian (RD). Health authorities should develop or encourage training programs that aim to prepare enough CDEs and RDs to treat the growing number of patients with diabetes. Education programs should emphasize self-management and dispel fears about finger sticks and insulin injections. Physicians and patients alike should be encouraged to be involved in this process. In addition, mobile technology in the form of apps, reminders, and education material can also be used to enhance a comprehensive diabetes management plan.
5. Treat hepatitis C infection.
   The risk of hepatitis C infection should be reduced to minimize the health and economic burden of diabetes. Early management with a focus toward elimination of HCV in infected patients can also reduce T2D risk. Newer and effective medications should be available at reduced price or provided through the national insurance service.
6. Regulate pesticide use.
   Implementation of an effective pesticide regulatory program, with regular surveying of pesticide residues in drinking water and food, should be mandated. Health education is also warranted to reduce uncontrolled exposure to pesticides by minimizing the misuse and improper handling of pesticides and providing protective personal equipment. Special attention should be made to avoid the involvement of women and children in pesticide application.
7. Develop clinical guidelines.
   Guidelines should be published for diabetes management that are culturally suitable for patients. Such guidelines should consider the unique risk factors highlighted in this chapter. Guidelines can help standardize clinical practice to improve patient care. There is a great opportunity for local diabetes associations and scientific bodies to champion the development of these guidelines and audit their implementation.

Summary and Conclusions

Diabetes is a growing public health problem in the MENA region. Its high prevalence continues to rise due to the increased prevalence of central obesity, sedentary lifestyle, change in diet patterns, increased prevalence of hepatitis C, and possibly the increased use of uncontrolled pesticides. Smoking among men, health illiteracy, and poor adherence increase the frequency of diabetes complications. Health authorities, through a limited healthcare budget, are striving to improve diabetes care, but many strategies and guidelines for standard of care are still needed to augment this effort.

References

1. International Diabetes Federation. IDF diabetes. 7th ed. Brussels: International Diabetes Federation; 2015. http://www.diabetesatlas.org.
2. NCD Risk Factor Collaboration. Worldwide trends in diabetes since 1980: a pooled analysis of 751 population-based studies with 4.4 million participants. Lancet. 2016;387(10027):1513–30.
3. Al-Nozha MM, Al-Maatouq MA, Al-Mazrou YY, Al-Harthi SS. Diabetes mellitus in saudi arabia. Saudi Med J. 2004;25:1603–10.
4. Habeb AM, Al-Magamsi MS, Halabi S, Eid IM, Shalaby S, Bakoush O. High incidence of childhood type 1 diabetes in Al-Madinah, North West Saudi Arabia (2004–2009). Pediatr Diabetes. 2011;12(8): 676–81.
5. Al-rubeaan K. International journal of diabetes mellitus type 2 diabetes mellitus red zone. Int J Diabetes Mellitus. 2010;2:1–2.
6. Jain S, Saraf S. Type 2 diabetes mellitus—its global prevalence and therapeutic strategies. Diabetes Metab Syndr: Clin Res Rev. 2010;4:48–56.

7. Whiting DR, Guariguata L, Weil C, et al. IDF diabetes atlas: global estimates of the prevalence of diabetes for 2011 and 2030. Diabetes Res Clin Pract. 2011;94: 311–21.
8. Wang DD, Bakhotmah BA, Hu FB, Alzahrani HA. Prevalence and correlates of diabetic peripheral neuropathy in a saudi arabic population: a cross-sectional study. PLoS One. 2014;9(9):e106935.
9. El-Asrar AMA, Al-Rubeaan KA, Al-Amro SA, Kangave D, Moharram OA. Risk factors for diabetic retinopathy among Saudi diabetics. Int Ophthalmol. 1998;22(3):155–61.
10. Jbour AS, Jarrah NS, Radaideh AM, Shegem NS, Bader IM, Batieha AM, Ajlouni KM. Prevalence and predictors of diabetic foot syndrome in type 2 diabetes mellitus in Jordan. Saudi Med J. 2003;24(7): 761–4.
11. El-Rufaie OE, Bener A, Ali TA, Abuzeid M. Psychiatric morbidity among type II diabetic patients: a controlled primary care survey. Prim Care Psychiatry. 1997;3:189–94.
12. AlQuaiz AM, Siddiqui AR, Qureshi RH, Fouda MA, AlMuneef MA, Habib FA, Turkistani IM. Women health in Saudi Arabia: a review of non-communicable diseases and their risk factors. Pak J Med Sci. 2014;30(2):422.
13. EL-Zanaty F, Way A. Egypt demographic and health survey 2008. Cairo: Ministry of Health, El-Zanaty and Associates, and Macro International; 2009. p. 431.
14. Population Council. http://www.popcouncil.org/uploads/pdfs/2010PGY_SYPEFinalReport_FrontMatter.pdf.
15. Ibrahim MM, Elamragy AA, Girgis H, et al. Cut off values of waist circumference & associated cardiovascular risk in Egyptians. BMC Cardiovasc Disord. 2011;11:53.
16. Herman WH, Ali MA, Aubert RE, et al. Diabetes mellitus in Egypt: risk factors and prevalence. Diabet Med. 1995;12(12):1126–31.
17. Mirmiran P, Sherafat-Kazemzadeh R, Jalali-Farahani S, Azizi F. Childhood obesity in the Middle East: a review/Revue sur l'obésité de l'enfant au Moyen-Orient. East Mediterr Health J. 2010;16(9):1009.
18. Al-Hazzaa HM, Abahussain NA, Al-Sobayel HI, Qahwaji DM, Musaiger AO. Physical activity, sedentary behaviors and dietary habits among Saudi adolescents relative to age, gender and region. Int J Behav Nutr Phys Act. 2011;8(1):140.
19. Zadjali F, Al-Yahyaee S, Hassan MO, Albarwani S, Bayoumi RA. Association of adiponectin promoter variants with traits and clusters of metabolic syndrome in Arabs: family-based study. Gene. 2013;527(2): 663–9.
20. Alkhateeb A, Al-Azzam S, Zyadine R, Abuarqoub D. Genetic association of adiponectin with type 2 diabetes in Jordanian Arab population. Gene. 2013; 512(1):61–3.
21. Mtiraoui N, Ezzidi I, Turki A, Chaieb A, Mahjoub T, Almawi WY. Single-nucleotide polymorphisms and haplotypes in the adiponectin gene contribute to the genetic risk for type 2 diabetes in Tunisian Arabs. Diabetes Res Clin Pract. 2012;97(2):290–7.
22. Nemr R, Almawi AW, Echtay A, Sater MS, Daher HS, Almawi WY. Replication study of common variants in CDKAL1 and CDKN2A/2B genes associated with type 2 diabetes in Lebanese Arab population. Diabetes Res Clin Pract. 2012;95(2):e37–40.
23. Nemr R, Echtay A, Dashti EA, Almawi AW, Al-Busaidi AS, Keleshian SH, Irani-Hakime N, Almawi WY. Strong association of common variants in the IGF2BP2 gene with type 2 diabetes in Lebanese Arabs. Diabetes Res Clin Pract. 2012;96(2):225–9.
24. Al-Nozha MM, Al-Hazzaa HM, Arafah MR, Al-Khadra A, Al-Mazrou YY, Al-Maatouq MA, Khan NB, Al-Marzouki K, Al-Harthi SS, Abdullah M, Al-Shahid MS. Prevalence of physical activity and inactivity among Saudis aged 30–70 years. A population-based cross-sectional study. Saudi Med J. 2007;28(4):559–68.
25. Miller FD, Abu-Raddad LJ. Evidence of intense ongoing endemic transmission of hepatitis C virus in Egypt. Proc Natl Acad Sci U S A. 2010;107: 14757–62.
26. Chehadeh W, Abdella N, Ben-Nakhi A, et al. Risk factors for the development of diabetes mellitus in chronic hepatitis C virus genotype 4 infection. J Gastroenterol Hepatol. 2009;24:42–8.
27. Chehadeh W, Kurien SS, Abdella N, et al. Hepatitis C virus infection in a population with high incidence of type 2 diabetes: impact on diabetes complications. J Infect Public Health. 2011;4:200–6.
28. Greca LF, Pinto LC, Rados DR, et al. Clinical features of patients with type 2 diabetes mellitus and hepatitis C infection. Braz J Med Biol Res Rev Bras Pesqui Méd Biol Soc Bras Biofís … [et al]. 2012;45:284–90.
29. Huang JF, Yu ML, Huang CF, et al. The outcomes of glucose abnormalities in pre-diabetic chronic hepatitis C patients receiving peginterferon plus ribavirin therapy. Liver Int. 2012;32:962–9.
30. FAO/RNEA. Report of the workshop on implementation of the International Code of Conduct on the distribution and use of pesticides in the Near East, 16–21 Sept 1995, Cairo; 1995.
31. WRI. Pesticides and the immune system: the public health risks. Washington, DC: World Resources Institute; 1996.
32. Ambio O. Pesticide use, habits and health awareness among Egyptian farmers. Ann Occup Hyg. 1996; 40(5):499–509.
33. Wessels D, Barr DB, Mendola P. Use of biomarkers to indicate exposure of children to organophosphate pesticides: implications for a longitudinal study of children's environmental health. Environ Health Perspect. 2003;111(16):1939–46.
34. Mansour SA. Pesticide exposure—Egyptian scene. Toxicology. 2004;198(1–3):91–115.
35. El-Sebae AH, Zeid MA, Saleh MA. Status and environmental impact of toxaphene in the third world—a

case study of African agriculture. Chemosphere. 1993;27(10):2063–72.
36. Raafat N, Abass MA, Salem HM. Malathion exposure and insulin resistance among a group of farmers in Al-Sharkia governorate. Clin Biochem. 2012; 45:1591–5.
37. Lee DH, Steffes MW, Sjödin A, et al. Low dose organochlorine pesticides and polychlorinated biphenyls predict obesity, dyslipidemia, and insulin resistance among people free of diabetes. PLoS One. 2011;6(1), e15977.
38. Brunner EJ, Mosdøl A, Witte DR, Martikainen P, Stafford M, Shipley MJ, Marmot MG. Dietary patterns and 15-y risks of major coronary events, diabetes, and mortality. Am J Clin Nutr. 2008;87(5):1414–21.
39. Hu EA, Pan A, Malik V, Sun Q. White rice consumption and risk of type 2 diabetes: meta-analysis and systematic review. BMJ. 2012;344:e1454.
40. Fields J, Trivedi NJ, Horton E, et al. Vitamin D in the Persian Gulf: integrative physiology and socioeconomic factors. Curr Osteoporos Rep. 2011;9:243–50.
41. Musaiger AO. Overweight and obesity in the Arab countries: the need for action. Arab Cent Nutr. 2007;1:1–8.
42. Musaiger AO, Al-Ansari MS. Barriers to practicing physical activity in the Arab countries, in nutrition and physical activity in the arab countries of the near east. Musaiger AO and Meladi SS, (eds). FAO/Cairo Regional Office, Cairo, Egypt. 2000.
43. Khattab A, Javaid A, Iraqi G, Alzaabi A, Kheder AB, Koniski ML, Shahrour N, Taright S, Idrees M, Polatli M, Rashid N, El Hasnaoui A, BREATHE Study Group. Smoking habits in the Middle East and North Africa: results of the BREATHE study. Respir Med. 2012;106:S16–24.
44. Al-Maskari F, El-Sadig M, Al-Kaabi JM, Afandi B, Nagelkerke N, Yeatts KB. Knowledge, attitude and practices of diabetic patients in the United Arab Emirates. PLoS One. 2013;8(1):e52857.
45. Koura MR, Khairy AE, Abdel-Aal NM, et al. The role of primary health care in patient education for diabetes control. J Egypt Public Health Assoc. 2001; 76(0013-2446 (Print)):241–64.
46. Shams ME, Barakat EA. Measuring the rate of therapeutic adherence among outpatients with T2DM in Egypt. Saudi Pharm J. 2010;18(4):225–32.
47. Al-Ahmadi H, Roland M. Quality of primary health care in Saudi Arabia: a comprehensive review. International J Qual Health Care. 2005;17(4):331.
48. Diabetes Prevention Program Research Group. Reduction in the incidence of type 2 diabetes with lifestyle intervention or metformin. N Engl J Med. 2002;346(6):393.
49. Hajat C, Harrison O, Al Siksek Z. Diagnostic testing for diabetes using HbA1c in the Abu Dhabi population Weqaya: the Abu Dhabi cardiovascular screening program. Diabetes Care. 2011;34(11):2400–2.
50. Al-Lawati JA, Tuomilehto J. Diabetes risk score in Oman: a tool to identify prevalent type 2 diabetes among Arabs of the Middle East. Diabetes Res Clin Pract. 2007;77(3):438–44.

Diabetes in China and the Western Pacific Region

5

Juliana C.N. Chan, Elaine Y.K. Chow, and Andrea O.Y. Luk

Introduction

According to the International Diabetes Federation (IDF) Atlas, 382 million people have diabetes in 2013, and by 2035, this will rise to 582 million, with China, India and the United States of America (USA) as the top three countries contributing to half of the global population of diabetes. The Western Pacific (WP) Region is the world's most populous region with 39 countries and territories and home to 35 % of the world population. It has the largest country, China, with one billion people and the smallest Pacific Island nations with less than 1000 people. It is also a region of transition with enormous diversity in terms of ethnicity, demographics, cultures, politics, religions, technological and socioeconomic development as well as health-care systems, all of which are implicated in the causality and consequences of diabetes [1].

According to the latest estimates by the IDF, 8.6 % of adults in the WP Region, i.e. 138.2 million people, have diabetes which is expected to increase to 201.8 million in the next 20 years. While China has the biggest diabetic population with 98 million people affected, the WP Region also has areas with the highest prevalence, such as some Pacific Islands with a diabetes prevalence of 30 %. A major concern is the high prevalence of undiagnosed diabetes and prediabetes which can lead to late presentation with expensive and difficult-to-treat complications. Figure 5.1 summarises the IDF estimates regarding the prevalence, disease burden and distribution of type 1 and type 2 diabetes in different age and gender groups as well as countries within the WP Region in 2013 (Table 5.1) [1].

Adding to this health-care challenge are the rapid societal transition and changing demographics occurring within an unprepared health-care system designed for provision for acute and episodic rather than chronic care. In many emerging economies, the lack of societal, environmental and financial protection has led to the widening social disparity which has exposed the genetically vulnerable and socially disadvantaged to develop this silent killer often due to lack of information, awareness and intervention [2, 3]. In this chapter, we will review the epidemiology, aetiology, morbidity, diagnosis, treatment and care delivery for diabetes focusing in China and WP Region. We will also discuss the current unmet needs and possible solutions for the prevention and control of diabetes in this populous region.

J.C.N. Chan, MD, FRCP (✉) • E.Y.K. Chow, MB, ChB, PhD • A.O.Y. Luk, MBBS, MRCP
Department of Medicine and Therapeutics, Hong Kong Institute of Diabetes and Obesity and Li Ka Shing Institute of Health Sciences, The Chinese University of Hong Kong, Prince of Wales Hospital, Shatin, Hong Kong, SAR, China
e-mail: jchan@cuhk.edu.hk

S. Dagogo-Jack (ed.), *Diabetes Mellitus in Developing Countries and Underserved Communities*, DOI 10.1007/978-3-319-41559-8_5

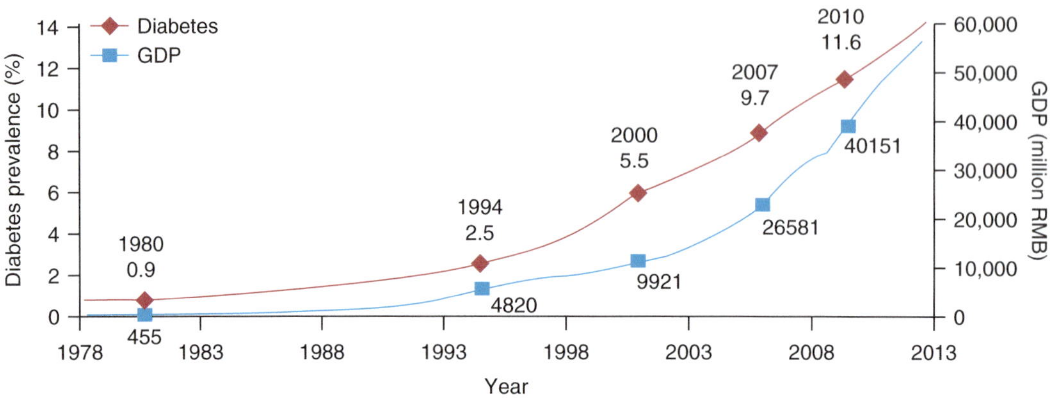

Fig. 5.1 The growth of gross domestic product (*GDP*) and prevalence of diabetes increased in a parallel manner in China during the last three decades [3]

Rapid Transition and the Obesity Epidemic

The impact of rapid urbanisation on the diabetes epidemic is exemplified by the parallel increase in gross domestic product (GDP) and diabetes prevalence in China (Fig. 5.1). In less than three decades, while the GDP has increased by 100-fold, the prevalence of diabetes has also increased by tenfold. In the 2010 National Survey of 98,658 adults and using both 75 g oral glucose tolerance test (OGTT) and glycated haemoglobin (A1c) as diagnostic criteria, one in nine Chinese had diabetes, one in three had obesity (general or central) closely associated with hypertension and dyslipidemia and one in two had prediabetes. Amongst those with diabetes, only 30 % were diagnosed and amongst the diagnosed, only 30 % were treated and amongst the treated, only 40 % were controlled, defined as A1c less than 7 % [4].

Table 5.1 Key facts and figures about diabetes in the Western Pacific Region [1]

At a glance	2013	2035
Total population (millions)	2278	2476
Adult population (20–79 years, millions)	1613	1818
Diabetes (20–79 years)		
Regional prevalence (%)	8.6	11.1
Comparative prevalence (%)*	8.1	8.4
Number of people with diabetes (millions)	138.2	201.8
IGT (20–79 years)		
Regional prevalence (%)	6.8	9.0
Comparative prevalence (%)*	6.6	7.8
Number of people with IGT (millions)	110.1	164.5
Type 1 diabetes (0–14 years)		
Number of children with type 1 diabetes (thousands)	32.5	–
Number of newly diagnosed cases per year (thousands)	5.3	–
Health expenditure due to diabetes (20–79 years, USD)		
Total health expenditure, $R=2^{\#}$, (billions)	88.4	98.4

*Age-adjusted
#R=2 (the diabetes cost ratio assumes that healthcare costs for people with diabetes are on average two fold higher than people without diabetes).

According to the Diabetes Epidemiology Collaborative Analysis of Diagnostic Criteria in Asia (DECODA) data, 30–50 % of subjects in the WP Region had metabolic syndrome, characterised by central obesity and clustering of cardiometabolic risk factors, and a strong predictor for future development of diabetes [5]. In 2008, 60–70 % of people in Tonga, Nauru and Cook Islands were considered obese [6]. In 2004, the sex-standardised diabetes prevalence was reported to be 13.0 % in men and 14.4 % in women in Nauru. The age-specific prevalence rose from 4.5 % in the 15–24 age group to 42.7 % in the 55–64 age group [7]. Tables 5.2 and 5.3 summarise the prevalence and number of people with diabetes in the WP countries based on the IDF figures published in 2013 [8].

Rapid quantitative and qualitative changes in nutritional intake, notably a shift from a traditional high-fibre, low-fat diet to an energy-

Table 5.2 Top ten countries in the Western Pacific Region in terms of number of subjects affected by diabetes [8]

Country/territory	Number of subjects (in 1000s), 2013
1. China	98,407.379
2. Indonesia	8554.165
3. Japan	7203.776
4. Republic of Korea	3323.903
5. Vietnam	3299.113
6. Philippines	3256.215
7. Thailand	3150.670
8. Myanmar	1988.846
9. Malaysia	1913.236
10. Taiwan	1721.062

Table 5.3 Top ten countries in the Western Pacific Region in terms of prevalence of diabetes [8]

Country/territory	Prevalence (%), 2013
1. Tokelau	37.49
2. Federated States of Micronesia	35.03
3. Marshall Islands	34.89
4. Kiribati	28.77
5. Cook Islands	25.66
6. Vanuatu	23.97
7. Nauru	23.29
8. French Polynesia	22.41
9. New Caledonia	19.49
10. Guam	19.48

dense diet with increased meat and fat consumption as well as reduced physical activity due to mechanisation and increased use of mobile vehicles, are important drivers for this global epidemic [9]. In the islands of Vanuatu, researchers reported close associations of economic development with increased consumption of animal proteins and simple carbohydrates, as well as increased tobacco and alcohol consumption in men in areas with high tourism [10]. In China, during the last two decades, changes in food technology with production of high-calorie foods together with reduced physical activity have contributed to the rising burden of obesity in both adults and children [11].

Unique Aspects of Pathophysiology: Beta-Cell Function Versus Visceral Obesity

Age, family history and obesity are the main risk factors for diabetes [4] although inadequate beta-cell response to overcome insulin resistance due to factors such as ageing, obesity and inflammation remains the primary culprit [12]. In an analysis of 74 study cohorts comprising 3813 individuals (19 African, 31 Caucasian and 24 East Asian cohorts), the authors examined the hyperbolic relationship between insulin sensitivity index (IS) and acute insulin response to glucose (AIRg) in healthy cohorts. Amongst these three subpopulations, Asians had a steep and non-linear relationship with small changes in one variable having large effect sizes on the other. Besides, Asians had the lowest body mass index (BMI) and AIRg and developed diabetes only with a small increase in BMI compared to the Caucasians and Africans [13].

Compared to their Europid counterparts, people of Asian ethnicity are more prone to develop diabetes for the same level of BMI or waist circumference due to their propensity to store excessive body or visceral fat [14]. Even amongst lean subjects and given the same amount of visceral fat, Asians were more insulin resistant than Europids due to increased concentration of free fatty acids and inflammatory markers [15]. Using insulin clamp studies, researchers from Thailand reported insulin deficiency as the predominant feature in lean subjects and insulin resistance and in the overweight and obese subjects [16].

In autopsy studies, Korean researchers have reported close correlations between BMI and relative percentage of beta cells in both diabetic ($r=0.55$) and nondiabetic specimens ($r=0.35$). However, diabetic subjects had a lower percentage of beta cells than nondiabetic subjects for the same BMI [17]. In healthy subjects, both Chinese and South Asian subjects with normal glucose tolerance exhibit higher glucose excursion during an OGTT with reduced rate of glucose disposal than their Caucasian counterparts [18]. This inherently low beta-cell function together with propensity to develop obesity which will impose metabolic stress has provided a highly plausible explanation for the high risk of diabetes in Asian populations undergoing rapid transition (Fig. 5.2).

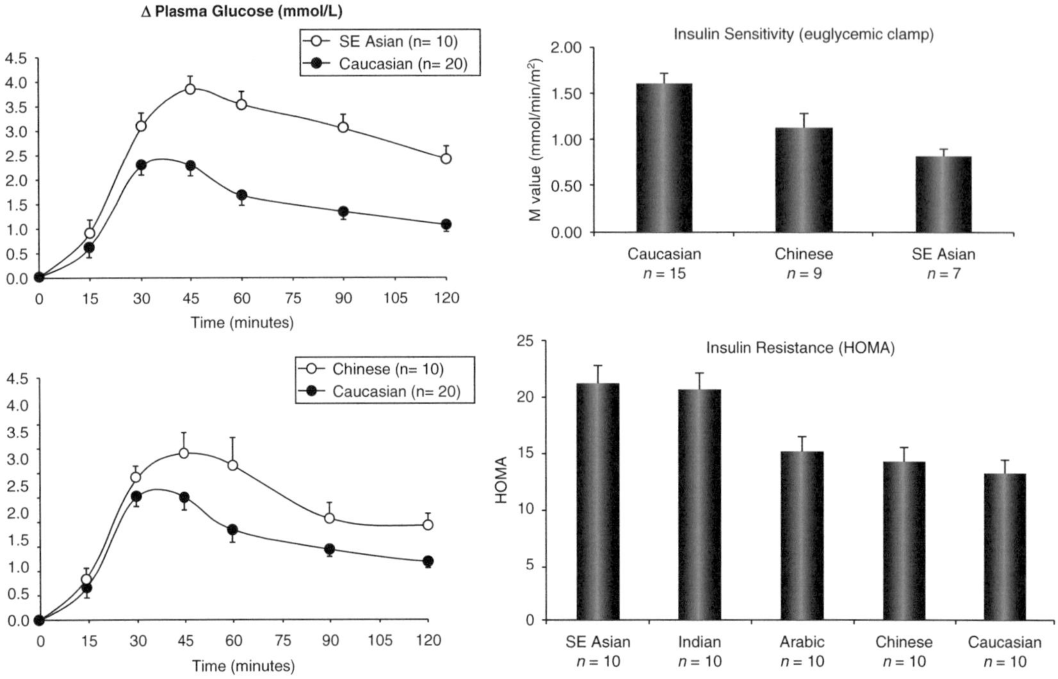

Fig. 5.2 Lean Chinese and Southeast Asians (*open circle*) with normal glucose tolerance exhibited higher glucose excursion during a 75 g oral glucose tolerance test and reduced insulin sensitivity during euglycaemic clamp studies compared to their Europid counterparts (*black circle*), supporting their biological vulnerability to develop diabetes under conditions of metabolic stress [18]

Genomic Landscape of Diabetes in the Region

Most of the genetic variants discovered in the genome-wide association studies (GWAS) in Caucasians have been replicated in Asian populations, albeit often with subtle differences in locations and frequency of genetic variants given the same locus [19] and larger effect size on beta-cell function in Asians for the same variant [20]. Besides, GWAS performed in Japanese, Chinese and Caucasian populations have revealed significant interethnic differences in genomic architecture as well as novel genetic variants in Asian populations which are implicated in protein synthesis and developmental and beta-cell biology [19, 21, 22]. Some of these novel variants were first discovered in patients with familial young-onset diabetes, suggesting that more variants may be discovered in these populations [23, 24]. These findings also support the notion that insufficient beta-cell response to rapid weight gain with progressive personal affluence through multiple generations [19] may contribute to this Asian epidemic with increasingly young age of onset. On the other hand, monogenic diabetes and latent autoimmune diabetes in adults [25] are not uncommon in young Asian populations which further increase the genotypic and phenotypic heterogeneity of diabetes in Asian populations [26] (Fig. 5.3).

In a recent epigenome-wide association study of South Asians and Caucasians, the methylation levels of several genetic loci associated with lipid metabolism and beta-cell biology were found to be associated with increased risk of diabetes in a dose-dependent manner [27]. These findings are in line with the preponderance of noncoding variants linked to diabetes in GWAS, suggesting that dysregulation of expression may be more important than protein changes as a genetic cause for the common form of diabetes [28]. In this light, maternal obesity and gestational diabetes may influence the in utero environment to cause dysregulation of expression of interlinking biological networks through DNA methylation and chromatin modification and contribute towards the high prevalence

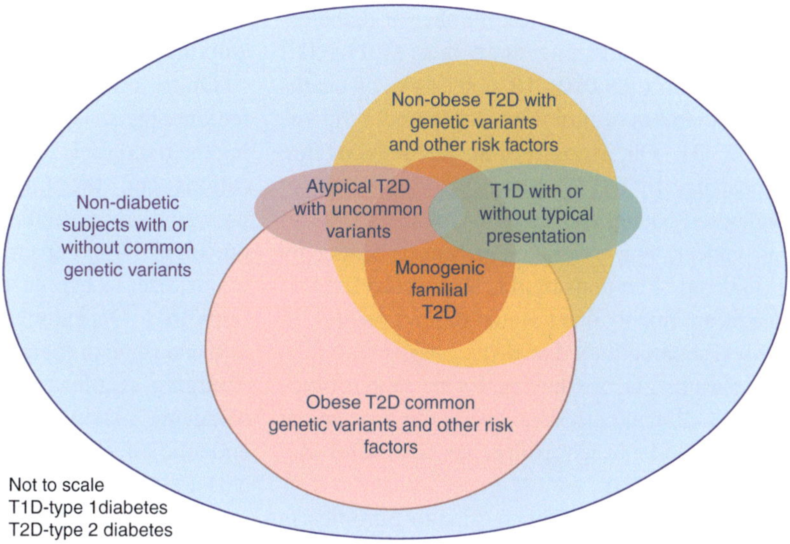

Fig. 5.3 A schematic diagram showing the phenotypic and genotypic heterogeneity of diabetes in Asian populations with complex interactions between genetic, autoimmune and external risk factors

of childhood metabolic syndrome [29] and young-onset diabetes in Asian population [30, 31]. In this context, the 'thrifty genotype or phenotype' theory which states that a trait conducive to survival during energy-scare condition may become maladaptive in an energy-abundant environment may be particularly relevant to emerging economies like China and the WP Region [32]. In support of this notion, early-life exposure to the 1950–1960 famine in China was found to be associated with increased risk of diabetes and metabolic syndrome [33] especially in subjects with low birth weight and adult obesity [34, 35].

Nature Versus Nurture

The combination of low BMI and obesity has put Asians at high risk of diabetes although many of these risk factors are modifiable [36]. First and foremost, health illiteracy and social disparity [37] remain the most important socioeconomic determinant for diabetes and obesity [38, 39]. In these subjects, lack of awareness, poor education, psychosocial stress [40, 41] and long working hours [42] may amplify the adverse effects of behavioural risk factors such as poor sleep hygiene [43] and the use of tobacco [44], alcohol [45] and sugar-sweetened beverages [46] which can unmask diabetes especially in those with genetic predisposition [47].

Amongst these risk factors, low-grade inflammation [48] associated with endemic infections such as chronic hepatitis B viral infections affecting over 10 % of the Asian population [49, 50] as well as beta-cell dysfunction associated with the use of tobacco, with smoking rates as high as 50 % amongst Asian men from China, Japan, Korea and Indonesia [51], may be particularly relevant to the Asian environment. These external factors may interact with cultural factors such as high consumption of rice with high glycaemic index [52] to cause metabolic stress especially in those with compromised beta-cell function. Adding to this multicausality and complexity, environmental pollutants such as persistent organic pollutants (POPs) [53] and bisphenol A (BPA) [54] are endocrine or mitochondrial disruptors which tend to hit emerging economies and/or subjects with low socioeconomic status hardest. By inducing insulin resistance and/or beta-cell dysfunction, these chemicals may increase the risk of obesity and hyperglycaemia especially in subjects with genetic predisposition [54].

Morbidity and Mortality

According to the estimates by IDF in 2013, 36 % of global deaths in adults are due to diabetes affecting 5.1 million people. The most populous

WP Region had the highest number of diabetes-related deaths affecting more men (1,080,000) than women (789,000). Of note, 44 % of deaths due to diabetes occurred in people under the age of 60 [1]. On average, diabetes reduces life expectancy by 6–12 years, especially in people diagnosed young, and increases the risk of vascular, cancer, nonvascular, non-cancer deaths by 1.3–3-fold. The nonvascular, non-cancer-related deaths are mainly due to renal failure, mental illnesses, hepatobiliary disease and sepsis with fasting plasma glucose having linear relationships with all clinical outcomes, even after adjustment for confounders such as age, sex, BMI and lifestyle factors [55].

In the WP Region, in contrast to Europids in whom cardiovascular disease is a leading cause of mortality and morbidity, diabetic kidney disease is a major complication in Asia [26], affecting 50–60 % of type 2 diabetic patients in different clinic settings [56]. In prospective studies, the annual incidence of diabetic kidney disease in Chinese population was 2–4 %, driven primarily by disease duration, smoking, metabolic syndrome, blood pressure and glycaemic control [57]. Other factors such as the use of over-the-counter medications including herbal medicine [58] and chronic hepatitis B infection [50] might also contribute to this high rate of diabetic kidney disease in the WP Region. While many patients in the WP Region die from end-stage renal disease due to lack of access to renal replacement therapy, this devastating condition can be prevented by intensive control of all risk factors using a protocol-driven and collaborative approach [59].

Countries in the WP Region differ considerably in the ecosystem of health-care provision and health literacy. In low-income areas such as some Pacific Islands where health illiteracy is common and access to care is poor, leg amputation continues to be a major cause of morbidity and mortality. In a recent survey of amputations involving 85 people with diabetes from Solomon Islands, Nauru and Vanuatu, delayed treatment (42 %), the use of traditional treatments (18 %) and insufficient knowledge about foot care (11 %) [60] are the main reasons for amputation.

On the other hand, several local, national and regional registries have provided insights regarding the interethnic differences in diabetic complications and the impact of ageing and care provision on the secular changes of these clinical outcomes. Apart from renal failure, stroke is a major disease burden in Asian diabetic populations [61]. Depending on the demographic pattern and stage of societal transition, cancer is now emerging as a leading cause of death especially in ageing societies and areas with high rate of endemic infections (e.g. hepatitis B for liver cancer) and high survival rates from cardiovascular-renal complications [62]. In the Australian National Diabetes Registry of nearly one million subjects, researchers have reported 1.3-fold increased standardised incidence risk of all-site cancer in both type 1 and type 2 diabetes except for prostate and melanoma [63]. In a national insurance database from Taiwan, diabetes-related death rates have declined over time (men, women: 3.92 %, 3.29 % in 2000; 3.64 %, 3.11 % in 2005; and 3.12 %, 2.71 % in 2009). In 2009, the estimated loss of life due to diabetes was 6.1 years in women and 5.3 years in men amongst people diagnosed at the age of 40. The four major causes of death were diabetes, malignancies, heart disease and cerebrovascular disease [64].

In the Hong Kong Diabetes Registry established as a quality improvement programme since 1995, researchers were able to track the secular changes in clinical outcomes in Chinese adults with diabetes, captured by a territory-wide clinical management system. In the early 1990s when universal health-care coverage was still being developed, stroke and end-stage renal failure were the leading causes of death. With ageing, societal affluence and access to interventions, coronary heart disease, cancer and heart failure became the leading causes of death. In 2005 and after a follow-up period of 5.5 years, amongst the 7534 type 2 diabetic patients enrolled in the registry since 1995, 763 died with the main causes of death being neoplasms (24.5 %) and cardiovascular (23.5 %), respiratory (15.3) and renal disease (15.3 %) [65].

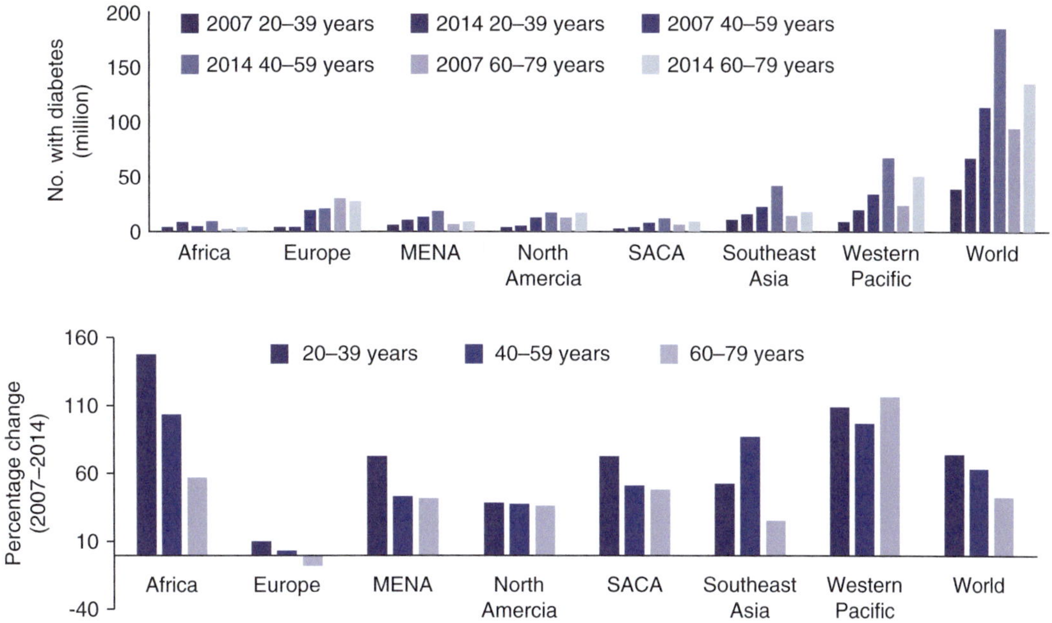

Fig. 5.4 Rates of increase and number of people with diabetes in different age groups showing the growing epidemic of young-onset diabetes especially in Asia (Adapted from IDF Atlas 2015 [1]) (*MENA* Middle East and North Africa, *SACA* South America and Central America)

Emerging Epidemic of Young-Onset Diabetes and Its Comorbidities

In the WP Region, 32,500 children under the age of 15 were estimated to have type 1 diabetes, with the largest number living in the Philippines (7900), followed by China (7700), while Australia has the highest estimated incidence rate of 22.3 cases per 100,000 children. In 2013, 5300 children were diagnosed to have type 1 diabetes in the WP Region [1]. Although type 1 diabetes is often considered a rare disease in non-Caucasian populations, the rising prevalence of young-onset type 2 diabetes is a major health-care challenge. Arbitrarily defined as age of diagnosis less than 40 years, these youths and young adults are high-risk populations for premature noncommunicable disease (NCD) including but not limited to cardiovascular-renal disease and cancer. This growing epidemic of young-onset diabetes is in part driven by the high prevalence of maternal obesity, gestational diabetes and childhood metabolic syndrome which sets up a vicious cycle of 'diabetes begetting diabetes' with enormous implications on the individual, family and society [66]. Between 2007 and 2014, the number of people with diabetes worldwide has increased by 74 % in the 20–39 years age group, from 38 million to 67 million. This compares to a 63 % increase in the 40–59 years age group and a 43 % increase in the 60–79 years age group with an especially sharp increase in the WP Region and Southeast Asia where China and India are located (Fig. 5.4).

In the same registry, the researchers reported the rarity of classical type 1 diabetes which accounted for 3 % in the entire cohort and less than 10 % amongst those diagnosed before the age of 40. Overall, one in five adults with type 2 diabetes had young-onset disease, with 50 % higher risk of cardiovascular-renal disease than their late-onset counterparts at any given age, mainly driven by long disease duration [67]. Amongst these young-onset type 2 diabetic patients, 40 % were lean and 60 % were obese or overweight. Compared to their counterparts with type 1 diabetes, these young-onset type 2 diabetic patients had considerably higher rates of cardiovascular-renal complications, often due to poor control of risk factors, frequent default and treatment non-adherence. By contrast, due to their propensity to develop an acute ketotic presentation, type 1 diabetic patients were less likely to default, and with access to education and insulin, these patients tended to have low incidence of complications despite long disease duration [68].

In a regional database established through the web-based Joint Asia Diabetes Evaluation (JADE) programme which enables care providers to establish registries using a common protocol in a real-world setting, high prevalence of young-onset diabetes (~20 %) and treatment gaps was confirmed in 41,029 adult patients from over ten countries in Asia. These real-world data highlight the heterogeneity in terms of attainment of treatment targets often due to differences in health-care coverage and financial support for essential laboratory investigations and medications as key components for diabetes care. Yet irrespective of these diversities, in all countries, there was a consistent trend that patients with young-onset diabetes were less likely to attain treatment targets for blood glucose and blood lipids and were less likely to be prescribed organ-protective drugs such as statins and renin-angiotensin system (RAS) inhibitor despite having clear indications such as cardiovascular-renal complications [30].

Diagnosis of Diabetes and Prediabetes in Asia

The criteria for diagnosing diabetes and prediabetes in Asia for the most part take references from international guidelines including those of the World Health Organization (WHO) and American Diabetes Association (ADA) [69, 70]. The measurement of fasting plasma glucose for diabetes screening is widely accepted and practised. On the other hand, there are differences in regional recommendations for oral glucose tolerance test (OGTT) and glycated haemoglobin (A1c) in the routine diagnostic process. Approaches to screening are also closely related to health-care access and resources available. For instance, the Chinese Diabetes Society guideline for the prevention and control of type 2 diabetes last updated in 2010 has not yet endorsed the use of HbA1c as an alternative to glucose-based tests for diagnosing diabetes [71]. Similarly, the UNITE FOR Diabetes Philippines in its 2014 practice guideline also recommended against using A1c. They also proposed the use of OGTT for diabetes screening only in individuals with known impaired fasting glucose or metabolic syndrome [72]. In the latest report published in 2010, the Japan Diabetes Society adopted the use of A1c to complement glucose-based tests in diabetes screening but stipulated that an individual meeting the A1c threshold of 6.5 % must concurrently fulfil one other criteria of either fasting plasma glucose ≥7.0 mmol/L or 2-h post-OGTT plasma glucose ≥11.1 mmol/L to establish the diagnosis [73]. This differs from international guidelines which assign similar weights to glucose-based studies and A1c in the diagnostic schema and allows the diagnosis to be made on the basis of A1c measurement alone. The Korean Diabetes Association fully applied the ADA criteria for diagnosing diabetes since 2011 [74].

Glycated haemoglobin has a number of advantages over plasma glucose in that it summarises long-term glucose exposure, has less intra-individual variability and does not require testing during a fasted state [75]. The recommendation to include A1c in diagnostic criteria of diabetes by the international expert committee was based on epidemiological studies which demonstrated a tight association between A1c and diabetic retinopathy in mixed populations [75–77]. Progress in analytic procedures and global movement to certify A1c assay to the National Glycohemoglobin Standardization Program facilitated its wider use as a diagnostic tool as well as in disease monitoring [75, 78]. In developing countries such as China and the Philippines, however, the measurement of A1c has not yet achieved standardisation across the nation, and this remains the key limitation to its application [72].

Notwithstanding logistics of costs and instrumentation, inclusion of A1c in diagnostic criteria will uncover more patients with diabetes than using glucose-based criteria alone. In large population surveys in China and Japan, over half of the participants with newly diagnosed diabetes and prediabetes were detected with A1c. This may be due to the high prevalence of high post-glucose challenge blood glucose levels which may be detected by an integrated value like A1c but missed by using fasting plasma glucose only [4, 79].

Increasingly, it is recognised that ethnicity may modify the relationship between measured A1c and blood glucose levels. Several studies have shown that for similar distribution of blood glucose, A1c levels were consistently higher in Asians compared to Caucasians and that amongst Asians, higher in Indians and Malays relative to Chinese [80, 81]. A few factors may contribute to such racial disparities such as differences in haemoglobin glycation rate and in population prevalence of haemoglobinopathies which interfere with A1c measurement.

Against this background, concerns are raised regarding the optimal A1c threshold for detecting diabetes in Asian groups and whether ethnic-specific standards are required. Studies carried out in Asians have suggested that lower cut-offs of A1c correlated more closely with diabetes as defined using the gold standard of OGTT [82–84]. In a recent population-based study comprising three ethnic groups of Malay, Chinese and Indian which examined the cross-sectional relationship between A1c and moderate retinopathy, it was found that although A1c differed slightly in its sensitivity and specificity in predicting retinopathy amongst different ethnic groups, eye complication was generally rare when A1c fell below 6.5 % [85]. Results from this Asian study concurred with those of a large multinational database which confirmed that an A1c threshold of 6.5 % has similar discriminatory power for the presence or absence of diabetic retinopathy in Caucasians and Asians [77, 85].

Oral glucose tolerance test is the gold standard test for the diagnosis of diabetes and is necessary in making a diagnosis of impaired glucose tolerance (IGT). The requirement of a second blood sample and being more time consuming has greatly limited its practice in many Asian countries. However, the importance of the 2-h plasma glucose has been highlighted in studies conducted in Asia which showed that fasting plasma glucose alone could only identify half of the people with diabetes and that individuals with predominantly post-load hyperglycaemia are phenotypically different from those with fasting hyperglycaemia [86]. As discussed, Asian diabetic patients have lower BMI and less beta-cell reserve than their Caucasian counterparts and thus are more likely to fail glucose stress test. On this premise, a lower threshold to perform OGTT in Asians should be considered. In Chinese, a paired value of A1c ≥6.1 % and fasting plasma glucose ≥6.1 mmol/L had 13–17 times increased likelihood to occur in diabetic subjects compared to nondiabetic subjects [87, 88]. In resource-limited setting, OGTT will have the greatest yield in detecting diabetes when paired A1c and fasting plasma glucose are above these cut-off values.

Translating Primary Prevention of Type 2 Diabetes

The chronic, silent and nonurgent nature of diabetes often leads to late diagnosis and delayed treatment. Once diagnosed, people with diabetes have pluralistic needs including information, social and psychological support, education, medical and surgical treatment, to name but a few. Given these multiple demands, large population size, lack of capacity and resource restraints, prevention and control of diabetes is often challenged with care fragmentation, clinical inertia and treatment non-adherence with insufficient community support [3, 89, 90]. In both randomised disease management programmes and observational cohorts, attaining multiple treatment targets and the use of organ-protective drugs such as statins and RAS inhibitors have been shown to reduce cardiovascular-renal complications and related deaths in the WP Region [91, 92]. Yet large-scale surveys have demonstrated only 30 % of patients with diabetes ever had assessments for risk factors and complications. Amongst those who had assessments, only 30–40 % attained one of the three ABC targets (A1c <7 %, BP <130/80 mmHg, LDL-C <2.6 mmol/L) and 5–10 % attained all three targets [93] with particularly low rates amongst people with young-onset diabetes [30, 94].

Diabetes is a lifelong disease which requires acquisition of knowledge, change of attitudes and formation of new habits in order to reduce disease burden. It is also a biological problem that requires medications, technologies and monitoring which have resource implications. In a survey from Guam involving 125 patients, 40 % were not aware of the type of diabetes they had, 20 % had not received education on self-management and 30–60 % had not received advice on tobacco cessation, immunisation services, nutritional counselling and/or regular eye and foot examinations. Over 50 % of patients expressed their desire to have preventive and education services with enhanced access to specialists and specialised care as well as financial support to cover the costs of chronic care and medications [95].

There is now consensus that a chronic care model involving community mobilisation and engagement supported by an integrated health-care system with country/area appropriate financing and health-care organisation is needed to promote interactions between an informed person with diabetes and a proactive health-care team to achieve positive clinical outcomes [96]. In this information and technology era, there is a growing advocacy to use improvement science, often entailing the use of real-world data, to inform and change clinical practice [97]. In the case of diabetes, changing the workflow and using protocols to collect data systematically for establishing registry can generate personalised report to promote shared decision-making. On a broader perspective, data transparency and comparison of performance indexes may also motivate practice and policy changes through ongoing evaluation and sharing of best care models [98–100].

Western Pacific Diabetes Declaration (WPDD) Plan for Action (2006–2010)

In 2000, at the 51st session of the WHO Regional Committee for the WP, the Committee endorsed the establishment of the WPDD as a regional strategic alliance between the WHO Regional Office for the WP, the Secretariat of the Pacific Community and the IDF-Western Pacific Region as a regional voice to advocate for prevention and control of diabetes. In the WPDD Plan of Action (2005–2010), experts from the region summarised the multidimensional nature of diabetes (Fig. 5.5) and the need to use a multipronged strategy including policies and legislations (Fig. 5.6) to create a health-enabling environment and reform the health-care system to make prevention and control of diabetes accessible, affordable and sustainable [101].

Some Examples of Diabetes Prevention and Control Strategies from China and WP

National Plan for Diabetes and NCD Prevention

In the China National Plan for NCD Prevention and Treatment (2012–2015), the government proposed to use public measures including environmental protection, food safety, clean drinking water, tobacco control and occupational safety to create a health-enabling environment through broad social participation and multisector collaborations. Other proposed practices and policies included universal vaccination, maternal and child health programmes and primary care. Since then, the Chinese government has introduced different health insurance packages at the rural and urban areas and built more than 30,000 community-based clinics to provide basic preventive care programme including regular risk factor surveillance and provision of essential medications for control of blood pressure and blood glucose [102]. Despite these ongoing efforts, given the vastness of the country and size of the population, there remain challenges in communications amongst relevant stakeholders, patient flow between hospitals and primary care clinics, capacity building and public education [103].

Tobacco Control

Several meta-analyses have indicated a dose-dependent risk association of smoking with dia-

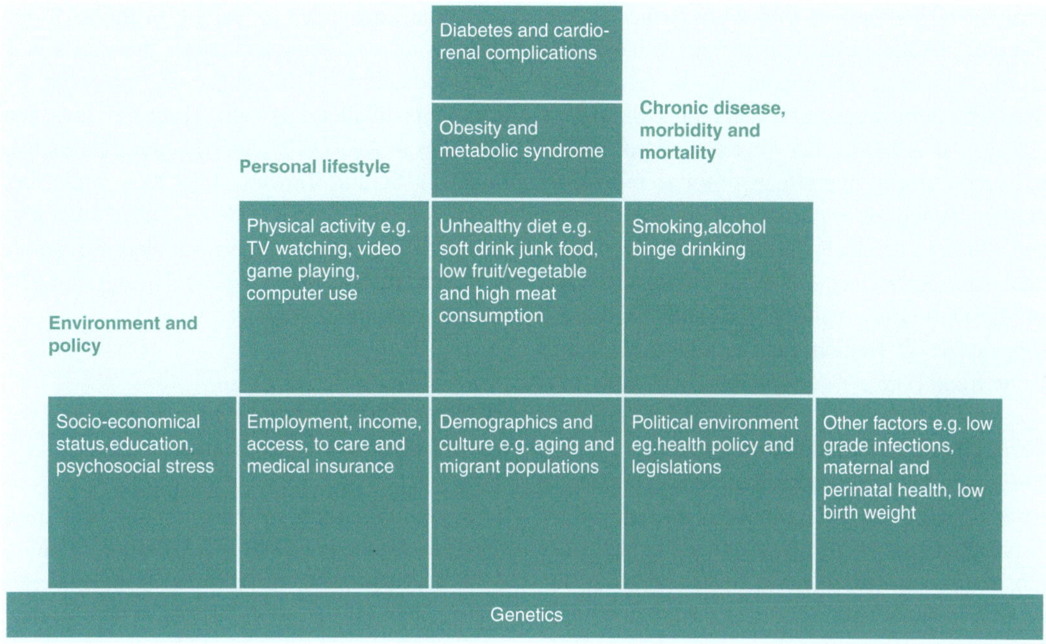

Fig. 5.5 A schematic diagram summarising the interactions amongst predisposing, precipitating and perpetuating factors in the epidemic of diabetes and its comorbidities in the Western Pacific Diabetes Declaration – Plan for Action (2005–2010) [154]

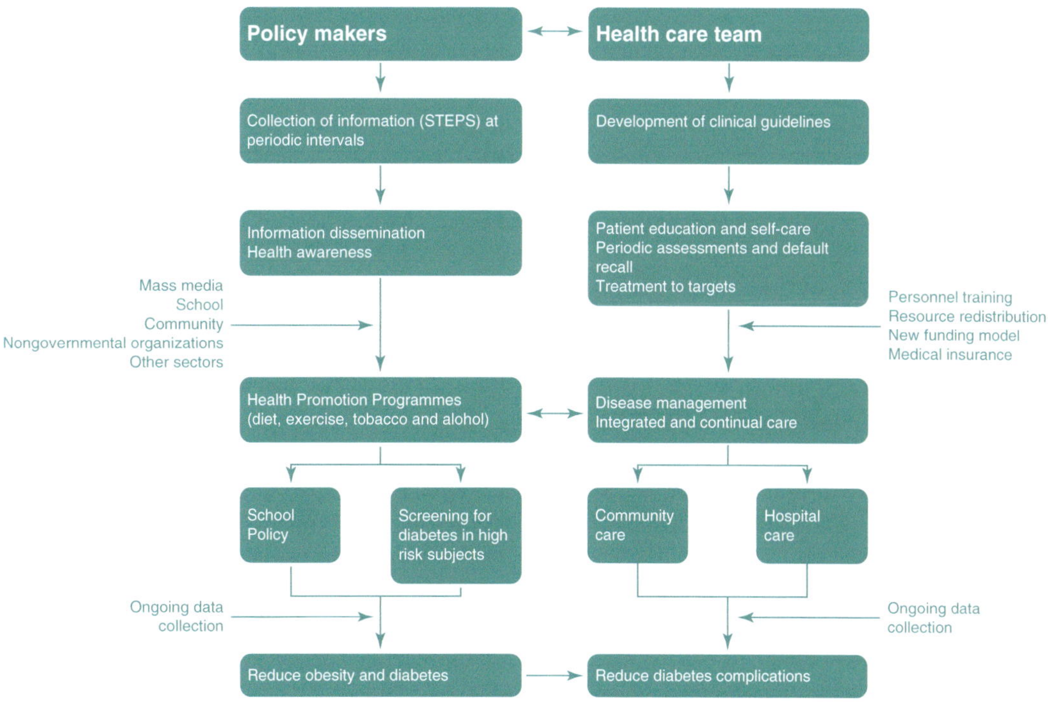

Fig. 5.6 A multipronged strategy using policies, community mobilisation, intersectoral partnerships and clinical leaderships to detect, prevent and control diabetes in the Western Pacific Diabetes Declaration – Plan for Action (2005–2010) [154]

betes [104] as well as that with cardiovascular disease and total mortality in people with diabetes [105]. Although it remains to be confirmed whether smoking cessation will reduce the risk of diabetes, it is likely that tobacco control would reduce the amplifying effects of tobacco on morbidities associated with diabetes, notably, cancer and cardiovascular-renal disease. To this end, there have been successful stories in tobacco control through strong political will and tough measures in the WP Region, such as New Zealand and Hong Kong [106].

Early Detection and Prevention

There is high-level evidence confirming that many cases of diabetes can be prevented or delayed by structured lifestyle modification [107]. That said, most experts and professional bodies proposed targeted or opportunistic screening using known risk factors (e.g. age, sex, family history, obesity (BMI and waist circumference), blood pressure and gestational diabetes) and/or simple risk scores [108] rather than population screening [109]. Given the high prevalence of young-onset diabetes in the WP Region and the importance of disease duration as a determinant for all diabetes-related complications [110], targeted screening in young subjects with family history and/or obesity is likely to be cost-effective due to the high prevalence of diabetes amongst the relatives of affected subjects [111] and the high lifetime risk for complications, once affected [109].

In the early 1990s, China conducted the first randomised 6-year lifestyle modification programme in a workforce who had IGT. These subjects continued to be observed for more than 20 years after completion of the trial which confirmed that early intervention reduced the incidence of diabetes, retinopathy and cardiovascular disease [112, 113]. Similar prevention programmes have also been successfully translated and adapted to meet the special needs in primary care settings in Australia [114] and indigenous populations in Pacific Islands [115].

The negative impact of gestational diabetes on childhood obesity may underlie the growing epidemic of young-onset diabetes and NCD. The WHO has now called for early prevention of diabetes using a life-course strategy that starts with maternal health [116]. However, screening for gestational diabetes is only practised in a few countries in Asia [117]. Several countries such as Japan [118] and Taiwan [119] have embarked upon national urine glucose screening programme, while a few countries such as Singapore have introduced national school programme to control childhood obesity [120].

Rational Selection of Antidiabetes Medications

In previous sections, we have highlighted differences in pathophysiology in Asian populations. Beta-cell dysfunction may be the primary defect in lean individuals, while Asians exhibit greater insulin resistance and visceral adiposity at a lower BMI compared with Caucasian counterparts. Therefore, treatment may be tailored to reflect these ethnic differences. Metformin is widely used as a first-line oral antidiabetic agent. Despite a lower BMI, metformin appears efficacious in Asian populations [121]. Asian diabetic subjects treated with metformin show a similar reduction in insulin resistance and improved glycaemic control as compared with non-Asians [122]. Therefore, metformin, unless contraindicated, is recommended as the first-line therapy according to global guidelines by the IDF [123].

Alpha glucosidase inhibitors (AGI) may have a particular role in early therapy amongst Asians due to high carbohydrate content of Asian diets. The typical Chinese diet has a carbohydrate content of up to 67 % as compared with 40 % amongst Europeans [124]. In one study, treatment with acarbose 50–100 mg three times a day effectively reduced A1c by 0.7 % and improved both fasting and 1 h plasma glucose as compared with placebo in Asians with type 2 diabetes [125]. In the metformin and acarbose in Chinese as the initial hypoglycaemic treatment (MARCH) study, nearly 800 newly diagnosed Chinese patients with type 2 diabetes were randomised to 24 weeks of either acarbose or metformin monotherapy [126].

The reduction in A1c was comparable in the acarbose- and metformin-treated groups (−1.17 % versus −1.19 %), demonstrating noninferiority in overall glucose lowering.

Further, there is a strong evidence that AGI may prevent progression from IGT to type 2 diabetes. In the STOP-NIDDM trial that was conducted in Canada and Europe, the use of acarbose reduced progression to type 2 diabetes by 25 % [127]. These findings have been replicated in the VICTORY study which compared voglibose versus placebo amongst 1780 Japanese individuals with IGT. The use of voglibose was associated with an impressive 40 % lower risk of progression to type 2 diabetes [128]. The control of postprandial glucose excursions may theoretically confer cardioprotection via reduction of oxidative stress. However, the jury is still out as to whether AGI confers any cardiovascular benefit. In an analysis of a large Taiwanese cohort comparing type 2 diabetes patients treated with AGI versus metformin monotherapy, the risk of cardiovascular events was significantly higher amongst those on AGI, adjusted for baseline differences by propensity score [129]. Ongoing trials, such as the Acarbose Cardiovascular Evaluation (ACE) study which evaluates the effect of acarbose on recurrent cardiovascular events and incident diabetes amongst those with history of cardiovascular disease and IGT, may provide much needed answers [130].

Insulin secretagogues including sulfonylureas and glinides are widely used and are generally efficacious in glucose lowering amongst Asians. The glinides target early-phase insulin release, as compared with sulfonylureas which tend to have a longer half-life. Thus, glinides may be particularly effective in Asian Chinese where a defect in early-phase insulin is common [124]. In a trial in Chinese patients which compared repaglinide plus metformin versus repaglinide alone, both arms achieved a similar reduction in A1c (−4.45 % with repaglinide plus metformin versus −4.15 % with repaglinide only) from baseline A1c of 10 %. However, combination treatment with metformin achieved lower fasting plasma glucose as compared with repaglinide alone. There are no head-to-head trials comparing glinides versus other first-line oral antidiabetic drugs; therefore, their role in early therapy remains unclear.

In contrast to Caucasians, the incretin response is preserved in Asians with type 2 diabetes [131]. DPP4 inhibitors may have a larger effect in glucose reduction in Asians as compared with non-Asians. In a systematic review of randomised controlled trials of DPP4 inhibitors, those involving higher proportion of Asian subjects demonstrated greater A1c lowering [132]. Similarly, GLP-1 analogues lowered A1c to a greater extent in Asian-dominant as compared with non-Asian-dominant studies [133]. Although there are no ethnic-specific data of long-term safety of incretin-based therapies, several large-scale cardiovascular end point studies of saxagliptin and sitagliptin have enrolled over 10 % of Asians and demonstrated neutral effects on cardiovascular outcomes [134, 135].

Severe beta-cell dysfunction is common at diagnosis, and there is evidence that early intensive insulin therapy may preserve beta-cell function or even induce remission in Asians. An initial study showed that continuous subcutaneous insulin infusion for 2 weeks in newly diagnosed type 2 diabetes Chinese patients led to restoration of early-phase insulin secretion and beta-cell function. As such, 42 % of patients maintained optimal glycaemic control after 2 years on diet alone [136]. A subsequent study led by Weng and colleagues randomised 410 newly diagnosed type 2 diabetes patients to multiple daily injections (MDI), continuous subcutaneous insulin infusion (CSII) or oral agents, and treatment was stopped after normoglycaemia was reached for 2 weeks [137]. The study demonstrated superior remission rates at 1 year in insulin-treated patients regardless of route (CSII 51 %, MDI 45 %) as compared with those treated with oral agents (27 %). Similar levels of A1c reduction were achieved in all three groups, suggesting the restoration of beta-cell function is not merely linked to amelioration of hyperglycaemia. These studies argue for a possible use of intensive insulin therapy to reverse acute glucotoxicity for preserving beta-cell function in Asian patients especially in those with early diabetes and without complications.

Given the phenotypic heterogeneity, subtle differences in disease mechanisms and lifestyle factors, the goal of a personalised regimen is to match the right drug to the right patient at the right time for the right outcome. In particular the risk-benefit of each therapeutic agent should be considered for in the individual in order to achieve the best outcomes [138].

Coordination and Delivery of Diabetes Care Services

In a meta-analysis, quality improvement initiatives targeting at patients, systems and care providers have been shown to reduce blood pressure, blood glucose and blood lipids although amongst these strategies, patient education, task delegation, self-care and case management were found to have the largest effect sizes [99]. Hong Kong is one of the most cosmopolitan cities in China with a population of seven million. It has a public health-care system delivered through the Hospital Authority which funds and governs all public hospitals and clinics, modelled after the UK National Health Scheme.

In response to the growing epidemic of diabetes since the early 1990s and given limited resources, clinical researchers and care providers used knowledge transfer and changed care settings to cope with the patient volume. By setting up a hospital-based diabetes centre, located away from the busy clinics, coordinated by specialised nurses and health-care assistants and supported by endocrinologists, the diabetes team offers regular risk assessment and education services to diabetic patients referred by all specialties. A key feature of this model is the use of protocols, task delegation and data management to establish the Hong Kong Diabetes Registry for risk stratification and quality assurance [139]. These data were used to generate personalised report for improving communications amongst specialists, doctors and patients as well as triaging patients into primary or hospital-based care. The Diabetes Center also serves as a central point for coordinating various activities including peer support, group medical follow-up and behavioural programmes for difficult-to-treat patients who need additional informational, medical and social support (Fig. 5.7) [140].

By combining service provision and epidemiological research, these cohorts, databases and biobanks have provided clinicians unique opportunities to track clinical progress, develop risk equations and identify treatment gaps such as the associations between hypoglycaemia, cancer and diabetic kidney disease [141] as well as interactions amongst genotypes, phenotypes, treatment and clinical outcomes [142, 143]. In 2009, the Hong Kong government fully adopted this integrated care model and introduced the risk assessment management programme and patient empowerment programme to the primary care clinics which were shown to improve control of all risk factors and reduce cardiovascular disease and all-cause death [144–146].

Using the JADE Registry to Promote Quality Assurance and Cooperative Learning

In 2007, this concept of using structured processes to personalise care [147], augmented by information technology and collaborative care [148], was digitalised through the establishment of the web-based Joint Asia Diabetes Evaluation (JADE) programme using private-public partnerships [139]. By joining the JADE programme, practitioners can establish their own clinic registry using built-in templates and protocols for quality assurance while contributing anonymous data to form the JADE Registry to identify treatment gaps and share best practices [139]. Using this regional registry, first of its kind, the researchers were able to confirm the high prevalence of young-onset diabetes (20%) in Asia and the treatment gaps [30] as well as the benefits of providing informational and social support on reducing clinical inertia, treatment non-adherence and hospitalisations [140, 149].

Future Directions

In 2009, the United Nations General Assembly identified diabetes, cardiovascular disease, cancer

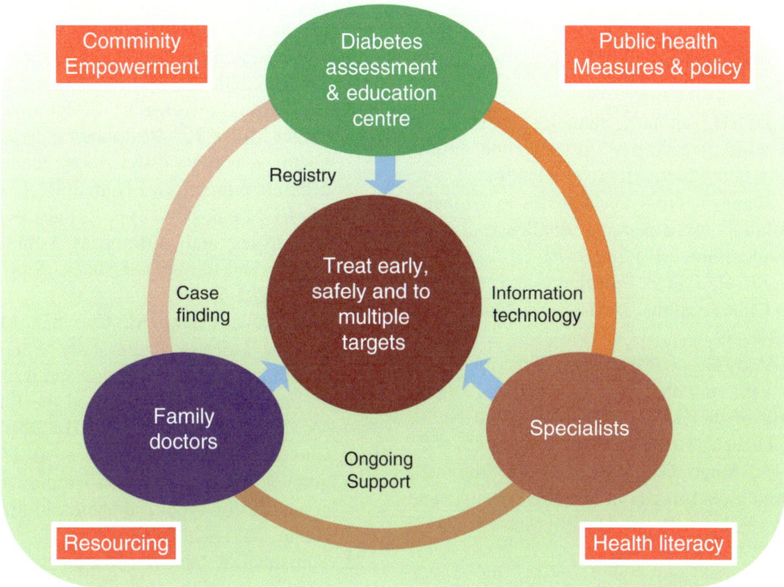

Fig. 5.7 A conceptual framework of using diabetes centres run by paramedical staff, supported by internists, to provide assessment, education, outreach and peer support programmes to complement medical care provided by specialists and family doctors. All parties concerned are linked by information technology and protocols to establish registry for quality assurance. Through community empowerment, capacity building and health-care policies, these centres can contribute towards early detection, prevention and control of diabetes and its comorbidities

and respiratory disease as the four NCDs as top priorities for prevention and control [150]. Recently, universal health coverage is ranked a top WHO agenda for ensuring people with NCD to have access to medications, technologies and basic medical care [151]. Given the diversity of the WP Region, different countries will have their unique transition patterns in terms of political, socio-economical, technological, cultural and health-care development which will interact to influence the diabetes landscapes in these countries. As such, each country/area will have to develop its own prevention and control strategies tailored to its special needs and circumstances to meet the mandates set by the WHO and UN Assembly.

Policies aside, from a more operational perspective, health-care providers who are equipped with knowledge about the nature of diabetes and stand between evidence and patients in need of evidence-based care, knowledge transfer and application become their armamentarium in the pursuit of health protection and disease prevention. In this regard, the IDF, as a global voice for people with diabetes, has established reference centres for education to develop, produce and disseminate diabetes education in order to enhance professional education for which two of the nine centres were located in the WP Region (Australia and Hong Kong) [152].

Conclusion

Although the definition of health by the WHO as a state of complete physical, mental and social well-being and not merely the absence of disease or infirmity [153] may not be easily attained, collective efforts through government mandates, clinical leaderships, intersectoral partnerships, community empowerment, ongoing research and advocacy and prevention and control of diabetes are aspiration that is feasible, achievable and indeed essential. To this end, with increasing globalisation, more countries/areas will undergo urbanisation and as such, the exposures to, and experiences gained with diabetes in the WP Region, will provide invaluable lessons in our common pursuit of prevention and control of diabetes and its comorbidities.

References

1. IDF Atlas 2015: International Diabetes Federation 2015.
2. Chan JC, Cho NH, Tajima N, Shaw J. Diabetes in the Western Pacific Region-past, present and future. Diabetes Res Clin Pract. 2014;103:244–55.
3. Chan JC, Zhang Y, Ning G. Diabetes in China: a societal solution for a personal challenge. Lancet Diabetes Endocrinol. 2014;2:969–79.
4. Xu Y, Wang L, He J, et al. Prevalence and control of diabetes in Chinese adults. JAMA J Am Med Assoc. 2013;310:948–59.
5. DeCODA Study Group. Prevalence of the metabolic syndrome in populations of Asian origin. Comparison of the IDF definition with the NCEP definition. Diabetes Res Clin Pract. 2007;76:57–67.
6. Stevens GA, Singh GM, Lu Y, et al. National, regional, and global trends in adult overweight and obesity prevalences. Popul Health Metrics. 2012; 10:22.
7. Khambalia A, Phongsavan P, Smith BJ, et al. Prevalence and risk factors of diabetes and impaired fasting glucose in Nauru. BMC Public Health. 2011; 11:719.
8. International Diabetes Federation, ed. International Diabetes Atlas 2013.
9. Hu FB. Globalization of diabetes: the role of diet, lifestyle, and genes. Diabetes Care. 2011;34: 1249–57.
10. Dancause KN, Dehuff C, Soloway LE, et al. Behavioral changes associated with economic development in the South Pacific: health transition in Vanuatu. Am J Hum Biol Off J Hum Biol Counc. 2011;23:366–76.
11. Ma RC, Lin X, Jia W. Causes of type 2 diabetes in China. Lancet Diabetes Endocrinol. 2014;2:980–91.
12. Kahn SE. The relative contributions of insulin resistance and beta-cell dysfunction to the pathophysiology of Type 2 diabetes. Diabetologia. 2004;46 :3–19.
13. Kodama K, Tojjar D, Yamada S, Toda K, Patel CJ, Butte AJ. Ethnic differences in the relationship between insulin sensitivity and insulin response: a systematic review and meta-analysis. Diabetes Care. 2013;36:1789–96.
14. Deurenberg-Yap M, Schmidt G, van Staveren WA, Deurenberg P. The paradox of low body mass index and high body fat percentage among Chinese, Malays and Indians in Singapore. Int J Obes. 2000;24:1011–7.
15. King GL, McNeely MJ, Thorpe LE, et al. Understanding and addressing unique needs of diabetes in Asian Americans, native Hawaiians, and Pacific Islanders. Diabetes Care. 2012;35:1181–8.
16. Suraamornkul S, Kwancharoen R, Ovartlarnporn M, Rawdaree P, Bajaj M. Insulin clamp-derived measurements of insulin sensitivity and insulin secretion in lean and obese Asian type 2 diabetic patients. Metab Syndr Relat Disord. 2010;8:113–8.
17. Yoon KH, Ko SH, Cho JH, et al. Selective beta-cell loss and alpha-cell expansion in patients with type 2 diabetes mellitus in Korea. J Clin Endocrinol Metab. 2003;88:2300–8.
18. Dickinson S, Colagiuri S, Faramus E, Petocz P, Brand-Miller JC. Postprandial hyperglycemia and insulin sensitivity differ among lean young adults of different ethnicities. J Nutr. 2002;132:2574–9.
19. Ma RC, Chan JCN. Type 2 diabetes in East Asians: similarities and differences with populations in Europe and the United States. Ann N Y Acad Sci. 2013;1281:64–91.
20. Hong KW, Chung M, Cho SB. Meta-analysis of genome-wide association study of homeostasis model assessment beta cell function and insulin resistance in an East Asian population and the European results. Mol Genet Genom MGG. 2014;289:1247–55.
21. Cho YS, Chen CH, Hu C, et al. Meta-analysis of genome-wide association studies identifies eight new loci for type 2 diabetes in East Asians. Nat Genet. 2011;44:67–72.
22. Yamauchi T, Hara K, Maeda S, et al. A genome-wide association study in the Japanese population identifies susceptibility loci for type 2 diabetes at UBE2E2 and C2CD4A-C2CD4B. Nat Genet. 2010; 42:864–8.
23. Ma RC, Lee HM, Lam VK, et al. Familial young-onset diabetes, pre-diabetes and cardiovascular disease are associated with genetic variants of DACH1 in Chinese. PLoS ONE. 2014;9, e84770.
24. Ma RC, Hu C, Tam CH, et al. Genome-wide association study in a Chinese population identifies a susceptibility locus for type 2 diabetes at 7q32 near PAX4. Diabetologia. 2013;56:1291–305.
25. Kong APS, Chan JCN. Other disorders with type 1 phenotype. In: Holt R, Goldstein B, Flyvbjerg A, Cockram CS, editors. Textbook of diabetes. 4th ed. Chichester: Wiley-Blackwell, Wiley; 2010. p. 152–9.
26. Kong AP, Xu G, Brown N, So WY, Ma RC, Chan JC. Diabetes and its comorbidities-where East meets West. Nat Rev Endocrinol. 2013;9:537–47.
27. Chambers JC, Loh M, Lehne B, et al. Epigenome-wide association of DNA methylation markers in peripheral blood from Indian Asians and Europeans with incident type 2 diabetes: a nested case-control study. Lancet Diabetes Endocrinol. 2015;3:526–34.
28. Lou S, Lee HM, Qin H, et al. Whole-genome bisulfite sequencing of multiple individuals reveals complementary roles of promoter and gene body methylation in transcriptional regulation. Genome Biol. 2014;15:408.
29. Ma RC, Tutino GE, Lillycrop KA, Hanson MA, Tam WH. Maternal diabetes, gestational diabetes and the role of epigenetics in their long term effects on offspring. Prog Biophys Mol Biol. 2015;118:55–68.
30. Yeung RO, Zhang Y, Luk A, et al. Metabolic profiles and treatment gaps in young-onset type 2 diabetes in Asia (the JADE programme): a cross-sectional study of a prospective cohort. Lancet Diabetes Endocrinol. 2014;2:935–43.

31. Chan JC, Yeung R, Luk A. The Asian diabetes phenotypes: challenges and opportunities. Diabetes Res Clin Pract. 2014;105:135–9.
32. Diamond JM. Diabetes running wild. Nature. 1992;357:362–3.
33. Li Y, Jaddoe VW, Qi L, et al. Exposure to the Chinese famine in early life and the risk of metabolic syndrome in adulthood. Diabetes Care. 2011;34:1014–8.
34. McCance DR, Pettitt DJ, Hanson RL, Jacobsson LTH, Knowler WC, Bennett PH. Birth weight and non-insulin dependent diabetes: thrifty genotype, thrifty phenotype, or surviving small baby genotype? Br Med J. 1994;308:942–5.
35. Neel JV. Diabetes mellitus: a "thrifty" genotype rendered detrimental by "progress"? Am J Hum Genet. 1962;14:353–62.
36. Boyko EJ, Fujimoto WY, Leonetti DL, Newell-Morris L. Visceral adiposity and risk of type 2 diabetes: a prospective study among Japanese Americans. Diabetes Care. 2000;23:465–71.
37. Wong MC, Leung MC, Tsang CS, Lo SV, Griffiths SM. The rising tide of diabetes mellitus in a Chinese population: a population-based household survey on 121,895 persons. Int J Public Health. 2013;58:269–76.
38. Demakakos P, Nazroo J, Breeze E, Marmot M. Socioeconomic status and health: the role of subjective social status. Soc Sci Med. 2008;67:330–40.
39. Ko GTC, Chan JCN, Cockram CS. A low socioeconomic class is associated with diabetes and metabolic syndrome in Hong Kong Chinese. Eur J Epidemiol. 2001;17:289–95.
40. Williams ED, Magliano DJ, Tapp RJ, Oldenburg BF, Shaw JE. Psychosocial stress predicts abnormal glucose metabolism: the Australian diabetes, obesity and lifestyle (AusDiab) study. Ann Behav Med Publ Soc Behav Med. 2013;46:62–72.
41. Harding JL, Backholer K, Williams ED, et al. Psychosocial stress is positively associated with body mass index gain over 5 years: evidence from the longitudinal AusDiab study. Obesity. 2014;22(1):277–86.
42. Ko GT, Chan JC, Chan AW, et al. Association between sleeping hours, working hours and obesity in Hong Kong Chinese: the 'better health for better Hong Kong' health promotion campaign. Int J Obes. 2007;31:254–60.
43. Cappuccio FP, D'Elia L, Strazzullo P, Miller MA. Quantity and quality of sleep and incidence of type 2 diabetes: a systematic review and meta-analysis. Diabetes Care. 2010;33:414–20.
44. Cho NH, Chan JC, Jang HC, Lim S, Kim HL, Choi SH. Cigarette smoking is an independent risk factor for type 2 diabetes: a four-year community-based prospective study. Clin Endocrinol. 2009;71:679–85.
45. Xu M, Zhou Y, Xu B, et al. Associations of smoking and alcohol consumption with impaired beta-cell function in Chinese men. J Diabetes. 2016;8(3):434–41.
46. Ko GT, So WY, Chow CC, et al. Risk associations of obesity with sugar-sweetened beverages and lifestyle factors in Chinese: the 'Better Health for Better Hong Kong' health promotion campaign. Eur J Clin Nutr. 2010;64:1386–92.
47. Qi Q, Chu AY, Kang JH, et al. Sugar-sweetened beverages and genetic risk of obesity. N Engl J Med. 2012;367:1387–96.
48. Pickup JC. Inflammation and activated innate immunity in the pathogenesis of type 2 diabetes. Diabetes Care. 2004;27:813–23.
49. Lao TT, Chan BC, Leung WC, Ho LF, Tse KY. Maternal hepatitis B infection and gestational diabetes mellitus. J Hepatol. 2007;47:46–50.
50. Cheng AY, Kong AP, Wong VW, et al. Chronic hepatitis B viral infection independently predicts renal outcome in type 2 diabetic patients. Diabetologia. 2006;49:1777–84.
51. Ueshima H, Sekikawa A, Miura K, et al. Cardiovascular disease and risk factors in Asia: a selected review. Circulation. 2008;118:2702–9.
52. Yu R, Woo J, Chan R, et al. Relationship between dietary intake and the development of type 2 diabetes in a Chinese population: the Hong Kong Dietary Survey. Public Health Nutr. 2011;14:1133–41.
53. Lim S, Cho YM, Park KS, Lee HK. Persistent organic pollutants, mitochondrial dysfunction, and metabolic syndrome. Ann N Y Acad Sci. 2010;1201:166–76.
54. Bi Y, Wang W, Xu M, et al. Diabetes genetic risk score modifies effect of bisphenol A exposure on deterioration in glucose metabolism. J Clin Endocrinol Metab. 2016;101:143–50.
55. Seshasai SR, Kaptoge S, Thompson A, et al. Diabetes mellitus, fasting glucose, and risk of cause-specific death. N Engl J Med. 2011;364:829–41.
56. Wu AY, Kong NC, de Leon FA, et al. An alarmingly high prevalence of diabetic nephropathy in Asian type 2 diabetic patients: the MicroAlbuminuria Prevalence (MAP) Study. Diabetologia. 2005;48:17–26.
57. Luk AO, So WY, Ma RC, et al. Metabolic syndrome predicts new onset of chronic kidney disease in 5,829 patients with Type 2 diabetes: a 5-year prospective analysis of the Hong Kong Diabetes Registry. Diabetes Care. 2008;31:2357–61.
58. Wen CP, Cheng TY, Tsai MK, et al. All-cause mortality attributable to chronic kidney disease: a prospective cohort study based on 462 293 adults in Taiwan. Lancet. 2008;371:2173–82.
59. Chan JC, So WY, Yeung CY, et al. Effects of structured versus usual care on renal endpoint in type 2 diabetes: the SURE study: a randomized multicenter translational study. Diabetes Care. 2009;32:977–82.
60. Win Tin ST, Gadabu E, Iro G, Tasserei J, Colagiuri R. Diabetes related amputations in Pacific Islands countries: a root cause analysis of precipitating events. Diabetes Res Clin Pract. 2013;100:230–4.
61. Morrish NJ, Wang S, Stevens LK, Fuller JH, Keen H. Mortality and causes of death in the WHO Multinational Survey of Vascular Diseases in Diabetes. Diabetologia. 2001;44:S14–21.

62. Yang X, Lee HM, Chan JC. Drug-subphenotype interactions for cancer in type 2 diabetes mellitus. Nat Rev Endocrinol. 2015;11:372–9.
63. Harding JL, Shaw JE, Peeters A, Cartensen B, Magliano DJ. Cancer risk among people with type 1 and type 2 diabetes: disentangling true associations, detection bias, and reverse causation. Diabetes Care. 2015;38:264–70. Diabetes care 2015;38:734–5.
64. Li HY, Jiang YD, Chang CH, Chung CH, Lin BJ, Chuang LM. Mortality trends in patients with diabetes in Taiwan: a nationwide survey in 2000–2009. J Formos Med Assoc Taiwan yi zhi. 2012;111: 645–50.
65. So WY, Yang X, Ma RC, et al. Risk factors in V-shaped risk associations with all-cause mortality in type 2 diabetes-The Hong Kong Diabetes Registry. Diabetes Metab Res Rev. 2008;24:238–46.
66. Chan JC, Malik V, Jia W, et al. Diabetes in Asia: epidemiology, risk factors, and pathophysiology. JAMA J Am Med Assoc. 2009;301:2129–40.
67. Chan JC, Lau ES, Luk AO, et al. Premature mortality and co-morbidities in young-onset diabetes – a 7 year prospective analysis. Am J Med. 2014;127: 616–24.
68. Luk AO, Lau ES, So WY, et al. Prospective study on the incidences of cardiovascular-renal complications in Chinese patients with young-onset type 1 and type 2 diabetes. Diabetes Care. 2014;37:149–57.
69. Diagnosis and classification of diabetes mellitus. Diabetes Care. 2010;33(Suppl 1):S62–9.
70. Federation WHOaID. Definition and diagnosis of diabetes mellitus and intermediate hyperglycemia: report of a WHO/IDF consultation. World Health Organization Geneva; 2006.
71. China Diabetes Society. China Guideline for Type 2 diabetes. 2010 edition (in Chinese) Beijing: Peking University Medical Press; 2011, p. 5.
72. Philippines United for Diabetes Philippine practice guidelines on diagnosis and management of diabetes mellitus. Compendium of Philippine Medicine, 16th edition 2014.
73. Seino Y, Nanjo K, Tajima N, et al. Report of the committee on the classification and diagnostic criteria of diabetes mellitus. J Diabetes Investig. 2010;1: 212–28.
74. Ko SH, Kim SR, Kim DJ, et al. 2011 clinical practice guidelines for type 2 diabetes in Korea. Diabetes Metab J. 2011;35:431–6.
75. International Expert Committee report on the role of the A1C assay in the diagnosis of diabetes. Diabetes Care. 2009;32:1327–34.
76. Buell C, Kermah D, Davidson MB. Utility of A1C for diabetes screening in the 1999 2004 NHANES population. Diabetes Care. 2007;30:2233–5.
77. Colagiuri S. Glycated haemoglobin (HbA1c) for the diagnosis of diabetes mellitus – practical implications. Diabetes Res Clin Pract. 2011;93:312–3.
78. Little RR, Rohlfing CL, Wiedmeyer HM, Myers GL, Sacks DB, Goldstein DE. The national glycohemoglobin standardization program: a five-year progress report. Clin Chem. 2001;47:1985–92.
79. Heianza Y, Hara S, Arase Y, et al. Impact of introducing HbA1c into the diagnostic criteria on prevalence and cardiovascular risk profiles of individuals with newly diagnosed diabetes in Japan: the Toranomon Hospital Health Management Center Study 2 (TOPICS 2). Diabetes Res Clin Pract. 2012;95: 283–90.
80. Venkataraman K, Kao SL, Thai AC, et al. Ethnicity modifies the relation between fasting plasma glucose and HbA1c in Indians, Malays and Chinese. Diabet Med. 2012;29:911–7.
81. Herman WH, Cohen RM. Racial and ethnic differences in the relationship between HbA1c and blood glucose: implications for the diagnosis of diabetes. J Clin Endocrinol Metab. 2012;97:1067–72.
82. Lee H, Oh JY, Sung YA, et al. Optimal hemoglobin A1C cutoff value for diagnosing type 2 diabetes mellitus in Korean adults. Diabetes Res Clin Pract. 2013;99:231–6.
83. Ko GT, Chan JC, Tsang LW, Cockram CS. Combined use of fasting plasma glucose and HbA1c predicts the progression to diabetes in Chinese subjects. Diabetes Care. 2000;23:1770–3.
84. Wu S, Yi F, Zhou C, et al. HbA1c and the diagnosis of diabetes and prediabetes in a middle-aged and elderly Han population from northwest China (HbA1c). J Diabetes. 2013;5:282–90.
85. Sabanayagam C, Khoo EY, Lye WK, et al. Diagnosis of diabetes mellitus using HbA1c in Asians: relationship between HbA1c and retinopathy in a multiethnic Asian population. J Clin Endocrinol Metab. 2015;100:689–96.
86. Qiao Q, Nakagami T, Tuomilehto J, et al. Comparison of the fasting and the 2-h glucose criteria for diabetes in different Asian cohorts. Diabetologia. 2000;43: 1470–5.
87. Ko GT, Chan JC, Yeung VT, et al. Combined use of a fasting plasma glucose concentration and HbA1c or fructosamine predicts the likelihood of having diabetes in high-risk subjects. Diabetes Care. 1998; 21:1221–5.
88. Ko G, Chan J, Cockram C. Use of a paired value of fasting plasma glucose and glycated hemoglobin in predicting the likelihood of diabetes in a community. Diabetes Care. 1999;22:1909.
89. Narayan KMV, Gregg EW, Engelgau MM, et al. Translation research for chronic diseases. The case for diabetes. Diabetes Care. 2000;23:1794–8.
90. Fisher EB, Chan JCN, Nan H, Sartorius N, Oldenburg B. Co-occurrence of diabetes and depression: conceptual considerations for an emerging global health challenge. J Affect Disord. 2012; 142(Suppl):S56–66.
91. Kong AP, Yang X, Ko GT, et al. Effects of treatment targets on subsequent cardiovascular events in Chinese patients with type 2 diabetes. Diabetes Care. 2007;30:953–9.

92. Leung WYS, So WY, Tong PCY, Chan NN, Chan JCN. Effects of structured care by a pharmacist-diabetes specialist team in patients with type 2 diabetic nephropathy. Am J Med. 2005;118:1414.e421–e427.
93. Chan JCN, Gagliardino JJ, Baik SH, et al. Multifaceted determinants for achieving glycaemic control: the International Diabetes Management Practice Study (IDMPS). Diabetes Care. 2009;32:227–33.
94. Chuang LM, Soegondo S, Soewondo P, et al. Comparisons of the outcomes on control, type of management and complications status in early onset and late onset type 2 diabetes in Asia. Diabetes Res Clin Pract. 2006;71:146–55.
95. David AM, Rubio JM, Luces PS, Zabala RV, Roberto JP. Getting the patients' perspective: a survey of diabetes services on Guam. Hawaii Med J. 2010;69:45–9.
96. Wagner EH, Groves T. Care for chronic diseases. Br Med J. 2002;325:913–4.
97. Marshall M, Pronovost P, Dixon-Woods M. Promotion of improvement as a science. Lancet. 2013;381:419–21.
98. Stock S, Pitcavage JM, Simic D, et al. Chronic care model strategies in the United States and Germany deliver patient-centered, high-quality diabetes care. Health Aff. 2014;33:1540–8.
99. Tricco AC, Ivers NM, Grimshaw JM, et al. Effectiveness of quality improvement strategies on the management of diabetes: a systematic review and meta-analysis. Lancet. 2012;379:2252–61.
100. Welin L, Wilhelmsen L, Bjornberg A, Oden A. Aspirin increases mortality in diabetic patients without cardiovascular disease: a Swedish record linkage study. Pharmacoepidemiol Drug Saf. 2009;18:1143–9.
101. Western Pacific Declaration on Diabetes (WPDD) Steering Committee, On behalf of International Diabetes Federation – Western Pacific Region, World Health Organization – Western Pacific Region, Secretariat of Pacific Community. Plan of Action (2006–2010) for the Western Pacific Declaration on Diabetes: from Evidence to Action: WHO-WPRO Publication Office. 2007.
102. Wang HH, Wang JJ, Wong SY, Wong MC, Mercer SW, Griffiths SM. The development of urban community health centres for strengthening primary care in China: a systematic literature review. Br Med Bull. 2015;116:139–54.
103. Chen Z. Launch of the health-care reform plan in China. Lancet. 2009;373:1322–4.
104. Willi C, Bodenmann P, Ghali WA, Faris PD, Cornuz J. Active smoking and the risk of type 2 diabetes: a systematic review and meta-analysis. JAMA J Am Med Assoc. 2007;298:2654–64.
105. Pan A, Wang Y, Talaei M, Hu FB. Relation of smoking with total mortality and cardiovascular events among patients with diabetes mellitus: a meta-analysis and systematic review. Circulation. 2015;132:1795–804.
106. Mackay J, Ritthiphakdee B, Reddy KS. Tobacco control in Asia. Lancet. 2013;381:1581–7.
107. Inzucchi SE, Sherwin RS. The prevention of type 2 diabetes mellitus. Endocrinol Metab Clin N Am. 2005;34:199–219, viii.
108. Brown N, Critchley J, Bogowicz P, Mayige M, Unwin N. Risk scores based on self-reported or available clinical data to detect undiagnosed Type 2 diabetes: a systematic review. Diabetes Res Clin Pract. 2012;98:369–85.
109. CDC Diabetes Cost-effectiveness Study Group. The cost-effectiveness of screening for Type 2 diabetes. J Am Med Assoc. 1998;280:1757–63.
110. Chan JC, So WY, Ma RCW, Tong P, Wong R, Yang XL. The complexity of both vascular and non-vascular complications of diabetes: the Hong Kong Diabetes Registry. Curr Cardiovasc Risk Rep. 2011;5:230–9.
111. Li JK, Ng MC, So WY, et al. Phenotypic and genetic clustering of diabetes and metabolic syndrome in Chinese families with type 2 diabetes mellitus. Diabetes Metab Res Rev. 2006;22:46–52.
112. Gong Q, Gregg EW, Wang J, et al. Long-term effects of a randomised trial of a 6-year lifestyle intervention in impaired glucose tolerance on diabetes-related microvascular complications: the China Da Qing Diabetes Prevention Outcome Study. Diabetologia. 2011;54:300–7.
113. Li G, Zhang P, Wang J, et al. Cardiovascular mortality, all-cause mortality, and diabetes incidence after lifestyle intervention for people with impaired glucose tolerance in the Da Qing Diabetes Prevention Study: a 23-year follow-up study. Lancet Diabetes Endocrinol. 2014;2:474–80.
114. Laatikainen T, Dunbar JA, Chapman A, et al. Prevention of type 2 diabetes by lifestyle intervention in an Australian primary health care setting: greater green triangle (GGT) diabetes prevention project. BMC Public Health. 2007;7:249.
115. Sukala WR, Page R, Cheema BS. Targeting the type 2 diabetes epidemic in Polynesia: historical perspective and rationale for exercise intervention trials. Ethn Dis. 2012;22:123–8.
116. World Health Organization. Updated revised draft global action plan for the prevention and control of noncommunicable diseases 2013–2020. 2013.
117. Tutino GE, Tam WH, Yang X, Chan JC, Lao TT, Ma RC. Diabetes and pregnancy: perspectives from Asia. Diabet Med J Br Diabet Assoc. 2014;31:302–18.
118. Urakami T, Suzuki J, Mugishima H, et al. Screening and treatment of childhood type 1 and type 2 diabetes mellitus in Japan. Pediatr Endocrinol Rev PER. 2012;10 Suppl 1:51–61.
119. Wei J, Sung F, Lin C, Lin R, Chiang C, Chuang L. National surveillance for type 2 diabetes mellitus in Taiwanese children. JAMA J Am Med Assoc. 2003;290:1345–50.
120. Toh C, Cutter J, Chew S. School based intervention has reduced obesity in Singapore. Br Med J. 2002; 324:427.

121. Chan JC, Deerochanawong C, Shera AS, et al. Role of metformin in the initiation of pharmacotherapy for type 2 diabetes: an Asian-Pacific perspective. Diabetes Res Clin Pract. 2007;75:255–66.
122. Nagi DK, Yudkin JS. Effects of metformin on insulin resistance, risk factors for cardiovascular disease, and plasminogen activator inhibitor in NIDDM subjects. A study of two ethnic groups. Diabetes Care. 1993;16:621–9.
123. Global guideline for type 2 diabetes. Diabetes Res Clin Pract. 2014;104:1–52.
124. Yang W, Weng J. Early therapy for type 2 diabetes in China. Lancet Diabetes Endocrinol. 2014;2:992–1002.
125. Chan JC, Chan KW, Ho LL, et al. An Asian multicenter clinical trial to assess the efficacy and tolerability of acarbose compared with placebo in type 2 diabetic patients previously treated with diet. Asian Acarbose Study Group. Diabetes Care. 1998;21:1058–61.
126. Yang W, Liu J, Shan Z, et al. Acarbose compared with metformin as initial therapy in patients with newly diagnosed type 2 diabetes: an open-label, non-inferiority randomised trial. Lancet Diabetes Endocrinol. 2014;2:46–55.
127. Chiasson JL, Josse RG, Gomis R, Hanefeld M, Karasik A, Laakso M. Acarbose for prevention of type 2 diabetes mellitus: the STOP-NIDDM randomised trial. Lancet. 2002;359:2072–7.
128. Kawamori R, Tajima N, Iwamoto Y, Kashiwagi A, Shimamoto K, Kaku K. Voglibose for prevention of type 2 diabetes mellitus: a randomised, double-blind trial in Japanese individuals with impaired glucose tolerance. Lancet. 2009;373:1607–14.
129. Chang CH, Chang YC, Lin JW, Chen ST, Chuang LM, Lai MS. Cardiovascular risk associated with acarbose versus metformin as the first-line treatment in patients with type 2 diabetes: a nationwide cohort study. J Clin Endocrinol Metab. 2015;100:1121–9.
130. Holman RR, Bethel MA, Chan JC, et al. Rationale for and design of the Acarbose Cardiovascular Evaluation (ACE) trial. Am Heart J. 2014;168:23–9.e2.
131. Cho YM. Incretin physiology and pathophysiology from an Asian perspective. J Diabetes Investig. 2015;6:495–507.
132. Kim YG, Hahn S, Oh TJ, Kwak SH, Park KS, Cho YM. Differences in the glucose-lowering efficacy of dipeptidyl peptidase-4 inhibitors between Asians and non-Asians: a systematic review and meta-analysis. Diabetologia. 2013;56:696–708.
133. Kim YG, Hahn S, Oh TJ, Park KS, Cho YM. Differences in the HbA1c-lowering efficacy of glucagon-like peptide-1 analogues between Asians and non-Asians: a systematic review and meta-analysis. Diabetes Obes Metab. 2014;16:900–9.
134. Scirica BM, Bhatt DL, Braunwald E, et al. Saxagliptin and cardiovascular outcomes in patients with type 2 diabetes mellitus. N Engl J Med. 2013;369:1317–26.
135. Green JB, Bethel MA, Armstrong PW, et al. Effect of sitagliptin on cardiovascular outcomes in type 2 diabetes. N Engl J Med. 2015;373:232–42.
136. Li Y, Xu W, Liao Z, et al. Induction of long-term glycemic control in newly diagnosed type 2 diabetic patients is associated with improvement of beta-cell function. Diabetes Care. 2004;27:2597–602.
137. Weng J, Li Y, Xu W, et al. Effect of intensive insulin therapy on beta-cell function and glycaemic control in patients with newly diagnosed type 2 diabetes: a multicentre randomised parallel-group trial. Lancet. 2008;371:1753–60.
138. Pozzilli P, Leslie RD, Chan J, et al. The A1C and ABCD of glycaemia management in type 2 diabetes: a physician's personalized approach. Diabetes Metab Res Rev. 2010;26:239–44.
139. Chan JC, Ozaki R, Luk A, et al. Delivery of integrated diabetes care using logistics and information technology – the Joint Asia Diabetes Evaluation (JADE) program. Diabetes Res Clin Pract. 2014;106 Suppl 2:S295–304.
140. Chan JC, Sui Y, Oldenburg B, et al. Effects of telephone-based peer support in patients with type 2 diabetes mellitus receiving integrated care: a randomized clinical trial. JAMA Intern Med. 2014;174:972–81.
141. Kong AP, Yang X, Luk A, et al. Severe hypoglycemia identifies vulnerable patients with type 2 diabetes at risk for premature death and all-site cancer: the Hong Kong diabetes registry. Diabetes Care. 2014;37:1024–31.
142. Ma RC, So WY, Tam CH, et al. Genetic variants for type 2 diabetes and new-onset cancer in Chinese with type 2 diabetes. Diabetes Res Clin Pract. 2014;103:328–37.
143. Kong AP, Yang X, So WY, et al. Additive effects of blood glucose lowering drugs, statins and renin-angiotensin system blockers on all-site cancer risk in patients with type 2 diabetes. BMC Med. 2014;12:76.
144. Jiao F, Fung CS, Wan YF, et al. Long-term effects of the multidisciplinary risk assessment and management program for patients with diabetes mellitus (RAMP-DM): a population-based cohort study. Cardiovasc Diabetol. 2015;14:105.
145. Fung CS, Wan EY, Jiao F, Lam CL. Five-year change of clinical and complications profile of diabetic patients under primary care: a population-based longitudinal study on 127,977 diabetic patients. Diabetol Metab Syndr. 2015;7:79.
146. Wong CK, Wong WC, Wan YF, et al. Patient Empowerment Programme in primary care reduced all-cause mortality and cardiovascular diseases in patients with type 2 diabetes mellitus: a population-based propensity-matched cohort study. Diabetes Obes Metabol. 2015;17:128–35.
147. Raz I, Riddle MC, Rosenstock J, et al. Personalized management of hyperglycemia in type 2 diabetes: reflections from a Diabetes Care Editors' Expert Forum. Diabetes Care. 2013;36:1779–88.

148. Institute of Medicine Crossing the quality chasm: a new health system for the 21st century. 2001. http://www.nap.edu/books/0309072808/html/.
149. Yin J, Wong R, Au S, et al. Effects of providing peer support on diabetes management in people with type 2 diabetes. Ann Fam Med. 2015;13 Suppl 1:S42–9.
150. United Nation General Assembly. Political declaration of the High-level Meeting of the General Assembly on the Prevention and Control of Non-communicable Diseases A/66/L.12011.
151. Holmes D. Margaret Chan: committed to universal health coverage. Lancet. 2012;380:879.
152. International Diabetes Federation Reference Centre of Education http://www.idf.org/centres-education. 2015. Accessed 9th Feb 2016, at http://www.idf.org/centres-education.
153. WHO. WHO definition of health. Preamble to the Constitution of the World Health Organization as adopted by the International Health Conference, New York, 19–22 June 1946, and entered into force on 7 April 1948. 1948.
154. Western Pacific Declaration on Diabetes Steering Committee. Plan of action (2006–2010) for the Western Pacific declaration on diabetes: from evidence to action. Manila: World Health Organization Western Pacific Regional Office; 2008. Available at www.wpdd.org.

Diabetes in India and Southeast Asia

6

Shashank R. Joshi and S.R. Aravind

Epidemiological Trends and Emerging Disease Burden

Diabetes is a multisystem disorder associated with complications, and the prevalence of which is increasing globally. Diabetes imposes immense public health burden with unacceptably high burdens on individuals, their families, and national economies. As the urban–rural divide narrows consistently, it adversely affects the lifestyle of populations. The rapid emerging economies of Southeast Asia (SEA) are a victim to the epidemiological transition which results in the shifting of the disease burden from the communicable to the non-communicable diseases. Moreover, Asians have a strong ethnic and genetic predisposition for diabetes and have lower thresholds for the environmental risk factors. There are 387 million people with diabetes in the world with 78.3 million people in the SEA region which is expected to rise to 131 million by the year 2040.

The last three decades have witnessed an epidemic rise in the number of people with diabetes, especially type 2 diabetes, and particularly in developing countries, where more than 80 % of the people with diabetes live. The recent landmark study for the pooled analysis across 751 studies with 4.4 million adults from 200 countries published in Lancet reflects that between 1980 and 2014 the number of adults with diabetes in the world increased fourfold from 108 million to 422 million. The increase has particularly been sharp in low- and middle-income countries. In 2014, 50 % of adults with diabetes lived in five

S.R. Joshi, MD,DM,FICP,FACP,FACE,FRCP (✉)
Joshi Clinic, Lilavati & Bhatia Hospital, Mumbai, India

Endocrine Society of India, New Delhi, India

Association of Physicians of India (API) (2014-15), Mumbai, India

Indian Academy of Diabetes, Mumbai, India

RSSDI (Research Society for the Study of Diabetes in India 2011), Mumbai, India

AIAARO (All India Association of Advancement for Research in Obesity), Mumbai, India
e-mail: shashank.sr@gmail.com

S.R. Aravind, MBBS,DNB,FRCP,FDRC,DHA,FRSSDI
Diacon Hospital, Bangalore, India

Columbia Asia Hospital, Yeshwanthpur, Bangalore, India

Post Graduate Studies in Diabetology (RGUHS & RSSDI), Bangalore, India

PESIMSR, Kuppam, India

RSSDI (Research Society for Study of Diabetes in India), Bangalore, India

DiabetesIndia, Hyderabad, India

KRSSDI, Bangalore, India

S. Dagogo-Jack (ed.), *Diabetes Mellitus in Developing Countries and Underserved Communities*,
DOI 10.1007/978-3-319-41559-8_6

countries: China, India, the USA, Brazil and Indonesia. The prevalence of diabetes in adults more than doubled for men in India and China (3.7–9.1 % in India, 3.5–9.9 % in China) but increased by 80 % amongst women in India (4.6–8.3 %) but only 50 % in women in China (5–7.6 %). The total number of adults with diabetes in India increased from 11.9 million in 1980 to 64.5 million in 2014. In China, the increase was from 20.4 million in 1980 to 102.9 million in 2014. While India contributed 15.3 % of the global share of adults with diabetes in 2014, it was 24.4 % for China. Across the region, approximately 72 million people have diabetes – close to one fifth of all adults with diabetes in the world. Overall, the rise of type 2 diabetes in South Asia is estimated to be more than 150 % between 2000 and 2035.

Economic and the Societal Impact of the Complications

Diabetes is increasingly affecting individuals in the region in their most productive years (refer to Fig. 6.1). This will pose a challenge to governments working to improve the economic situation in their countries. The scenario poses huge social and economic problems to most nations in the region and could impede national and, indeed, global development. More than half of the deaths due to diabetes occur in people under 60 years of age and one quarter in people under 50 years of age. India is the largest contributor to regional mortality, with 1.1 million deaths attributable to diabetes in 2015. Despite the huge number of people with diabetes in the Southeast Asia Region, health-care spending on diabetes was estimated to be only USD 6 billion, accounting for less than 1 % of the global total, with India estimated to have spent the largest proportion. The health-care spending appears to be low as government spending on healthcare is privatised less as predominant healthcare in India. There are an estimated 81,400 children under the age of 15 living with type 1 diabetes in the Southeast Asia Region. Approximately 13,100 children developed type 1 diabetes in the region during 2015. India is home to the second largest number of children with type 1 diabetes in the world (70,200), after the USA, and accounts for the majority of the children with type 1 diabetes in the region. More than half (53.2 %) of these deaths occurred in people under 60 years of age.

With an estimated 69.2 million people suffering from the condition, the largest in any country in the world, diabetes has become a major healthcare problem in India (refer to Figs. 6.2 and 6.3). Recent epidemiological studies from India point to the great burden due to diabetes and its micro- and macrovascular complications. This is primarily because the status of diabetes control in India is far from ideal. Based on the available data, the mean glycated haemoglobin levels are around 9 % which is at least 2 % higher than the goal currently suggested by international bodies. A balanced approach to improve awareness about diabetes and its control both amongst patients and the medical fraternity is an urgent need of the hour in India.

Factors Contributing to the Rapid Increase in Prevalence of Diabetes in Asia

Although ageing, urbanisation and associated lifestyle changes are the major determinants for the rapid increase, an adverse intrauterine environment and the resulting epigenetic changes could also contribute in many developing countries. More action is required to understand the drivers of the epidemic to provide a rationale for prevention strategies to address the rising global public health ‘tsunami’.

Urbanisation and Socioeconomic Transition

Diabetes burden in India is contributed by various factors. Genetic predisposition combined with lifestyle changes, associated with urbanisation and globalisation, contributes to this rapid rise of diabetes in India. The highest rates of

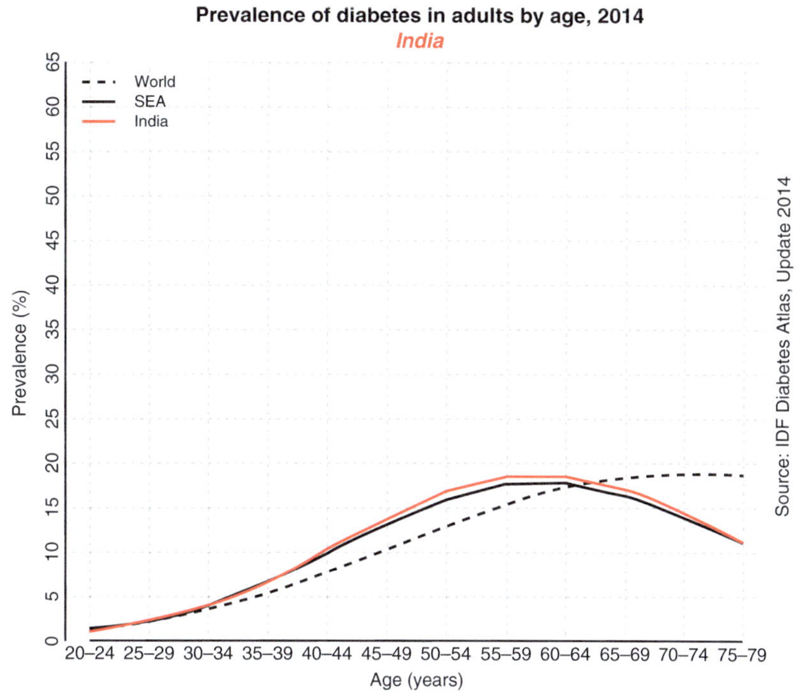

Fig. 6.1 Age-wise prevalence of diabetes

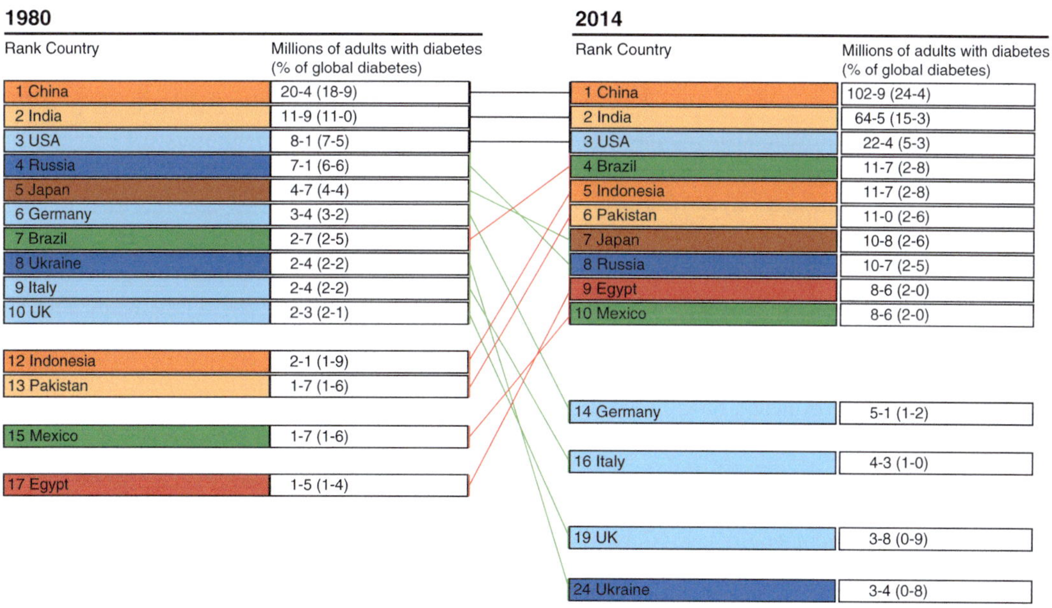

Fig. 6.2 Ten countries with the largest no. of diabetes in 1980 and 2014 [3]

urbanisation have been in Singapore, Korea, Malaysia, the Philippines and Indonesia (50 %). China, Pakistan, India and Thailand have intermediate rates (30 %) and Bangladesh and Sri Lanka have slow rates of urbanisation. The increase in urban population and ageing are the

2015

Rank	Country/territory	Number of people with diabetes
1	China	109.6 million [99.6–133.4]
2	India	69.2 million [56.2–84.8]
3	United States of America	29.3 million [27.6–30.9]
4	Brazil	14.3 million [12.9–15.8]
5	Russian Federation	12.1 million [6.2–17.0]
6	Mexico	11.5 million [6.2–13.7]
7	Indonesia	10.0 million [8.7–10.9]
8	Egypt	7.8 million [3.8–9.0]
9	Japen	7.2 million [6.1–9.6]
10	Bangladesh	7.1 million [5.3–12.0]

Fig. 6.3 Prevalence of diabetes in different countries (age 20–79 years) [1]

main determinants of the global rise in the prevalence of diabetes. Urbanisation and internal rural to urban migration result in several adverse impacts: physical activity decreases, diet habits shift towards high-energy foods and body mass index (BMI) and upper body adiposity increase considerably. The Indian Council of Medical Research (ICMR) study done in the 1970s reported a prevalence of 2.3 % in urban areas which has risen to 12–19 % in the 2000s. Correspondingly, in rural areas, prevalence rates have increased from around 1 to 4–10 % and even 13.2 % in one study. Thus it is clear that both in urban and rural India, prevalence rates of diabetes are rising rapidly with a rough urban–rural divide of 2:1 or 3:1 being maintained through the last two to three decades with the exception of Kerala where rural prevalence rates have caught up with or even overtaken urban prevalence rates. The postulates from the ICMR–INDIAB study predicted for the burden of diabetes which projected that in 2011, India would have 62.4 million people with diabetes and 77.2 million people with prediabetes.

Age

As compared to Western populations, Asian Indians develop diabetes at a younger age with more prevalence at the age of 60–69 years, whereas in the Chinese population, it peaks at 79–89 years. Indians also have a higher prevalence of impaired glucose tolerance at a younger age than the Chinese population. The findings from Pakistan and Sri Lanka also show similar results.

Anthropometry: Thin-Fat Phenotype

It is observed that amongst Asians, diabetes occurs at lower body mass index (BMI) levels than in Western populations, and small increments in weight trigger glucose intolerance in susceptible subjects. Especially Asian Indians have higher odds of developing diabetes, despite having a significantly lower BMI than the white population.

Several studies in Asian populations, particularly in Asian Indians, have highlighted the 'metabolically obese' phenotype amongst normal weight individuals. This phenotype, characterised by greater abdominal obesity despite a normal BMI, less muscle mass, higher percentage of body fat and increased propensity for insulin resistance compared with the Western population, renders higher susceptibility for diabetes in Asian populations.

The association of BMI and diabetes is well established and is usually modified by ethnicity. Ethnicity factors that contribute are genetic constitution, lifestyle, living environment and anthropometric characteristics. Body composition related to fat distribution is a stronger determinant of the metabolic milieu than BMI. The diabetes epidemiology, collaborative analysis of diabetes criteria in Europe/in Asia study group noted that the overall effect of age on the prevalence of diabetes differed considerably between the ethnic groups, even in the subjects with the same BMI. Asian populations are prone to have more intra-abdominal fat accumulation and low muscle mass. Asian Indians, in particular, have the above abnormalities which account for the high prevalence of insulin resistance and diabetes at low levels of BMI. The risk of diabetes increases progressively from a BMI of ≥ 23 kg/m^2 amongst

Indians. BMI in ≥ of 23 kg/m^2 is also considered overweight for most Asian populations. Asian Indians have small body size which has been named as 'thin-fat Indian'. Asian Indians have thinner limbs, which are suggestive of smaller muscle mass. However, despite their thinness, they are centrally obese, with higher waist–hip ratio (WHR) and higher subscapular–triceps skinfold ratio than their British counterparts. Many studies show that Asian Indians have more body fat for any given BMI compared with Caucasians and black Africans. Indians also have higher levels of central obesity (measured as waist circumference [WC], WHR, visceral fat and posterior subcutaneous abdominal fat). This is reflected in higher plasma nonesterified fatty acid (NEFA) and triglyceride concentrations, hyperinsulinaemia with fasting as well as post-glucose challenge states and higher insulin resistance. Thus, Asian Indians have an unusual thin-fat body composition associated with the insulin resistance syndrome, and this is the now popular 'thin-fat Indian' concept.

Smoking and Alcohol Use

Smoking increases the risk of central obesity and insulin resistance and the risk of diabetes is shown to be higher by 45 % in smokers than amongst nonsmokers. The increasing use of alcohol in Asian countries, especially amongst the middle class and rural population, also increases the risk for diabetes and other metabolic diseases and deleterious health effects.

Genetic Susceptibility

The genetic burden on Asian Indians makes the population more susceptible to diabetes. This risk is further increased due to interaction with environmental triggers. Exposure to a high fat diet and lower levels of physical activity trigger the gene–environmental interaction. Both the thrifty genotype and thrifty phenotype hypotheses appear to be the aetiology. The selective presence of 'thrifty genotypes' has been considered to be advantageous in certain populations during evolutionary selection by repeated famine and feast cycles. However, these genes have rendered them highly predisposed to obesity and diabetes during the modern era of continuous feasting. On the other hand, the 'thrift phenotype' hypothesis postulates that intrauterine malnutrition leads to metabolic and structural changes in the beta cells that are beneficial for early survival, but increases the risk of T2D and other chronic disorders in adulthood.

Screening

The prevalence of the micro- and macrovascular complications also influences the mortality rate due to diabetes. Unfortunately, more than 50 % of individuals with diabetes in India remain undiagnosed, and some may even present with macrovascular disease (coronary artery disease and cerebrovascular disease or stroke and peripheral vascular disease) and microvascular disease (retinopathy, nephropathy and neuropathy) at the time of diagnosis.

Data on various complications of diabetes have also been published by several authors. However, till recently, most of such data were hospital or clinic based and therefore subject to referral bias. The Chennai Urban Rural Epidemiology Study (CURES) and the Chennai Urban Population Study (CUPS) provide the first population-based data from India on virtually all complications of diabetes. CURES was a population-based study involving 26,001 participants aged 20 years or above based on a representative population of Chennai. The overall prevalence of diabetic retinopathy based on four-field stereo colour retinal photography was 17.6 %. The prevalence of overt nephropathy was 2.2 % while that of microalbuminuria was 26.9 %. Peripheral neuropathy based on biothesiometry was detected in 26.1 %.

In the CUPS study, coronary artery disease was evident in 21.4 % of diabetic subjects, 14.9 % of subjects with impaired glucose tolerance and in 9.1 % of people with normal glucose tolerance. In the same study, peripheral vascular disease was present in 6.3 % of diabetic subjects compared to 2.7 % amongst nondiabetic subjects. Diabetic subjects also had increased subclinical atherosclerosis as measured by intimal-medial thickness at every age point, compared to their nondiabetic counterparts. Assuming that 40 million people in India have diabetes, this translates to at least 7 million with retinopathy, 0.8 million with nephropathy, 10.4 million with neuropathy, 8.5 million with CAD and 2.5 million with PVD. Thus, the burden due to diabetic complications is very high in India due to the sheer number of people with diabetes. These figures are in fact very conservative, and it is possible that in rural areas, the prevalence of complications is much higher because of poorer control of diabetes and lack of access to healthcare.

Identifying accurate and low-cost screening methods is a necessary first step in assessing the cost-effectiveness of screening to detect undiagnosed diabetes. Indian Diabetes Risk Score (IDRS) is more effective and significantly less expensive for screening for undiagnosed T2DM compared to genotyping TCF7L2 SNPs, the strongest genetic marker for T2DM currently available. Using IDRS screening prior to OGTT reduces costs while still detecting a substantial portion of NDD individuals. A potential additional benefit of both the IDRS and genotyping is their ability to identify individuals who currently do not have diabetes but are at high risk of developing diabetes in the future. Thus an individual with an IDRS score of ≥60 at baseline was three times more likely to develop diabetes in the future than low-risk subjects (IDRS <30).

Awareness of Diabetes in India

The awareness of diabetes is a cornerstone of the prevention of this disease. CURES reported that nearly 25 % of the population was unaware of diabetes. Only around 40 % of the participants felt that the prevalence of diabetes was increasing, and only 22.2 % of the population and 41 % of known diabetic subjects felt that diabetes could be prevented. Though the awareness levels increased with education, only 42.6 % of postgraduates and professionals, which group included doctors and lawyers, knew that diabetes was preventable. The knowledge of risk factors of diabetes was even lower with only 11.9 % of the study subjects reporting obesity and physical inactivity as risk factors for diabetes. More alarming was the fact that even amongst known diabetic subjects, only 40.6 % were aware that diabetes could lead to some organ damage. There is another population-based study which was done to find out the levels and details regarding awareness on diabetes in urban adult Indian population aged ≥20 years. The knowledge regarding the causes of diabetes, its prevention and the methods to improve the health was significantly low amongst the general population. In the total study group, 41 % were unaware of the health being affected by diabetes, and only less than 30 % knew about the complications related to kidneys, eyes and nerves. Many persons with diabetes (46 %) felt it was a temporary phenomenon. Amongst the diabetic subjects, 92.3 % had sought the help of a general practitioner to take treatment. Only a small proportion went to a specialist.

Current Status of Diabetes Control in India

The next challenge in India is that the quality of diabetes care varies considerably depending upon the awareness levels, expertise available, attitudes and perceptions amongst diabetes care providers. An estimate based on sales of antidiabetic pharmaceutical agents shows that on an average only 10–12 % of people with diabetes receive modern pharmacological treatment in India. In 1998, the Diabcare–Asia study was carried out to investigate the relationship between diabetes control, management and late complications in a subset of urban Indian diabetes population treated at 26 tertiary diabetes care centres. A total of 2,269 patients participated in this study and it was observed that approximately half of the patients had poor control (HbA1c >2 % points above upper limit of normal), and the mean HbA1c was significantly higher (8.9 ± 2.1 %) than the levels recommended by the American Diabetes Association and the ICMR guidelines in India. Over 54 % of patients had diabetes-related complications. The mean HbA1c levels and frequency of complications were higher in patients with longer diabetes duration. This study also showed that 4 % of patients were on diet therapy, 53.9 % were receiving oral antidiabetic agents (OHAs), 22 % were receiving insulin and 19.8 % were receiving a combination of insulin and OHAs. This study concluded that with increasing duration of diabetes, glycaemic control deteriorates leading to late complications. It also confirmed that diabetes care in India leaves much to be desired and suggested the need for efforts to increase awareness amongst health professionals to improve diabetes care in India.

Non-pharmacologic Approach for the Management of Diabetes

Lifestyle modifications are the cornerstone of management of diabetes mellitus and include the prescription of a healthy diet, regular exercise, the management of stress and avoidance of tobacco. The aims of dietary management are to achieve and maintain ideal body weight, euglycaemia and desirable lipid profile, to prevent and postpone complications related to diabetes and to provide optimal nutrition during pregnancy, lactation, growth, old age and associated conditions, e.g. hypertension and catabolic illnesses. Recently the published STARCH study shows that Indians consume high carbohydrate in their diet compared to the Western population. The comparison of macronutrients (i.e. region-wise carbohydrate, fat and protein) revealed a similar pattern of dietary consumption, that is, high carbohydrate and a lower range of fat and protein. This study neutralises the myth that only the south Indian population consumes high carbohydrate in their diet (rice, idli, etc.). Dietary transition and a sedentary lifestyle have led to an increase in obesity and diet-related non-communicable diseases like T2DM, cardiovascular disease, etc. predominantly in urban, but also in rural areas. The dietary recommendations should be individualised according to the person's ethnicity, cultural and family background and personal preferences and associated comorbid conditions. It should be flexible in a variety and preparation of food choices and timing of meals according to the person's daily routine. Both the National Institute of Nutrition and expert group [2] have developed some broad Indian guidelines which recommend reduction intake of carbohydrate, higher intake of fibre, lower intake of saturated fat, optimal ratio of essential fatty acids, slightly higher protein intake, lower intake of salt and restricted intake of sugar.

The role of regular physical activity is well established in the management in persons with type 2 diabetes. A careful assessment of an individual should be made by the physician while incorporating an exercise programme in the management. Exercise programme should be individualised according to the individual capacity and disabilities. The person with diabetes must wear appropriate footwear.

'Clinical Inertia' in Diabetes: Failure to Achieve Tight Control

Failure of initiation of or intensification of therapy, when indicated, is termed 'clinical inertia'. Though we have well-defined management goals, effective therapies and practice guidelines, there is often a failure to take appropriate action despite recognition of the problem. This is a common problem in the management of patients with asymptomatic chronic illnesses. The use of 'soft' reasons to avoid intensification of therapy and lack of education, training and practice organisation aimed at achieving therapeutic goals are the common reasons for clinical inertia. Clinical inertia in achieving glycaemic targets in Indian diabetic subjects could be expected to be even more than in the West, where it has been reported that 65 % of the patients diagnosed with diabetes, only 73 % are prescribed pharmacologic therapy and only 33 % of those treated achieve a haemoglobin A1C value of less than 7 % by the ADA goal. This may be due to the low rates of awareness of diabetes and its complications in India resulting in poor glycaemic control seen in Indians with diabetes. Moreover, other factors like poverty, lack of accessibility to health services and inadequate follow-up are additional factors in developing countries like India.

Consequently, insulin is delayed until it is absolutely necessary. Most patients are initiated on insulin after a course of multiple oral antidiabetic drugs. Insulin therapy is initiated only when the HbA1c levels had deteriorated further to around 9 %. Physicians often delay insulin therapy worrying that the daily injections, modification of lifestyle due to insulin and dependence on insulin for life and that patients may feel that insulin therapy indicates the last stage of diabetes. However, patients who had moved on to insulin seemed to have a more positive approach towards his/her treatment due to the improvement in quality of life and better control despite the issues outlined above.

Pharmacologic Therapy in Diabetes: Is It Different?

A proactive approach to treating type 2 diabetes is recommended: therapy should be individualised with early consideration of combination therapy and ongoing reinforcement of lifestyle modification messages. Indeed, the conservative stepwise approach to type 2 diabetes management involves lifestyle modification, followed by treatment with a single oral antidiabetic agent, often up-titrated to maximal recommended doses before combination therapy is introduced. Very often there is a delay between stepping up from monotherapy (e.g. metformin alone) to combination therapy (e.g. metformin plus other OADs, often sulphonylurea), and this can result in unacceptable delays in achieving and maintaining glycaemic goals with the potential for long periods of hyperglycaemia. Periods of hyperglycaemia long or even short can increase the risk of micro- and macrovascular complications. The current understanding of the complex pathophysiology of the disease and the progressive deterioration in glycaemic control over time supports the philosophy of earlier intervention with a more comprehensive initial therapy. The major classes of antidiabetic agents that may be combined with metformin include sulphonylurea (SU), thiazolidinedione (TZD), dipeptidyl peptidase-4 inhibitor (DPP4-i), insulin and glucagon-like peptide-1 (GLP-1) receptor agonist. Few studies have investigated the effect of metformin-based early combination therapy. There are several different types of insulin available, but as a minimum, regular quick-acting human insulin and longer-acting NPH insulin should be available to everyone in all parts of the world.

In India, which is a resource-limited country, all therapies are available and it is a predominantly non-reimbursed market. Usually sulphonylureas, metformin, alpha glucosidase inhibitors and glitazone form the cornerstone of therapy with insulin. However, recently gliptins including the low-cost one as well as SGLT2 inhibitors are also available. Biosimilar insulin is also available but not popular and premixed insulin is still used widely. Cost and dose play a role in resource-limited environment. Indian usually requires lower doses and is more insulin resistant.

Translating Primary Prevention of Diabetes

The Indian Diabetes Prevention Programme (IDPP) has been a unique prospective study which has provided several pathways and strategies for the prevention of diabetes in India including the importance of the lifestyle modification and metformin which independently could reduce the incidence of diabetes in Asian Indians with impaired glucose tolerance. Also, these have been proposed as the cost-effective benchmarks amongst high-risk individuals with high degree of insulin resistance and may be useful in other developing countries as well. It is important to control the persistent IGT as it is demonstrated to add to the higher incidence of diabetes with other risk factors for diabetes, such as high BMI, waist circumference and body fat percentage. In a recent collaborative work across South Asia, Latin America and South Africa to compare the prevalence, awareness, treatment and control of diabetes and assess the relationship between diabetes and prediabetes with known cardiovascular and metabolic risk factors, it has been demonstrated that propensity for South Asians to develop diabetes and prediabetes at a younger age and lower body mass index compared with individuals from other low- and middle-income countries. Therefore, it is important that the long-term impact and the complications are prevented, and the health systems and policy makers must make concerted efforts to improve diabetes prevention and detection in the targeted population. Ramachandran A et al. have suggested that it is important to develop precise predictors for incident diabetes amongst Asian men. The analysis of the data from the combined cohorts of the Indian Diabetes Prevention Programmes 1 and 2 demonstrates that the baseline HbA (1c) was highly predictive of future diabetes in Asian Indian subjects with impaired glucose tolerance and nearly 60 % of the incidence occurred with values ≥6.0. Diagnostic sensitivity of ≥6.5 % for new diabetes was only 51 % using the oral glucose tolerance test as the standard for comparison. The combination of gamma-glutamyltransferase (GGT) and fasting plasma glucose (FPG) offers a simple and sensitive tool to identify subjects at high risk of developing diabetes. Similarly, several other markers including adiponectin, IL-6, retinol-binding protein 4, and hypertriglyceridaemic waist phenotype have been proposed to independently associate with incident diabetes. Prospective, intervention studies have demonstrated that increased compliance to lifestyle goals especially with the modification of the diet habits, independent of the physical activity, could result in the decrease in the incident of prediabetes. The mechanistic insights now ascribe these benefits through improvement in insulin sensitivity and beta-cell preservation. Prospective, parallel-group, randomised controlled trial across close to 9,000 subjects have demonstrated that mobile phone messaging is an effective and acceptable method to deliver advice and support towards lifestyle modification to prevent type 2 diabetes in men at high risk. Evidence from the DPP, and other prevention trials conducted in patients with prediabetes, shows that appropriate lifestyle modification including physical activity could lead to risk reduction in the incidence of T2DM by almost 58 %. Studies have shown that resistance and aerobic exercise is effective in improving metabolic profile of adults with T2DM. Previous research has reported improved insulin sensitivity/resistance and reductions in hyperglycaemia-related medications as a result of exercise training. In particular, supervised resistance training (max. ten repetitions for >3 days per week) has been shown to lead to significant improvement in insulin sensitivity and values of glycosylated haemoglobin, lipid profile and truncal and peripheral subcutaneous adipose tissue in Asian Indians with T2DM. It has been reported that children and adolescents with type 1 diabetes should complete a minimum of 30–60 min of moderate-intensity physical activity daily. Additional physical activity beyond 60 min/day would be helpful in maintaining glycaemic profile for T2DM patients. The practice of yoga is a traditional Indian practice that helps therapeutically and promotes physical and mental health. Yoga-based lifestyle modification programme helps in the reduction of blood glucose, HbA1c, triglycerides, total cholesterol and VLDL. Mindfulness eating and yoga exercise had health benefits on glycaemic control in pregnant women with GDM in some studies. Yogic exercises have enhanced the antioxidant defence mechanism in diabetics by reducing oxidative stress. Unless drastic steps are taken through national prevention programmes to curb the escalating trends in all of the countries, the social, economic and health-care challenges are likely to be insurmountable.

Organising and Conducting Diabetes Research in the Region

RSSDI (Research Society for the Study of Diabetes in India) is the largest organisation of diabetes health-care professionals and researchers in Asia, which was formed in 1972. Currently, there are more than 5,500 life members from across the country representing 29 Indian states and Union territories. Every year, RSSDI organises the national annual meeting, which not only provides a platform for its members to listen to the leaders in the field of diabetes from within the country as well as from abroad but also to interact amongst themselves and exchange knowledge and ideas. Annual meetings of RSSDI have been a regular feature for more than four decades and are very well attended. RSSDI has a nationwide presence through its 14 state chapters. All state chapters carry on the work of RSSDI at the state and local level. In addition, these chapters carry out independent activities including CMEs for member physicians, local research grants and awareness programmes for public as well as diabetes patients. RSSDI regularly publishes a newsletter, both in print and electronic format, which serves as an important link between the national body and its membership to keep the members informed of various activities, research grants and educational initiatives. The *International Journal of Diabetes in Developing Countries* (IJDDC) is the prestigious indexed publication of RSSDI and is an important resource of research work done in the field of diabetes in India. RSSDI funds research proposals from Indian scientists interested in conducting research in the field of diabetes mellitus. For providing research grants, RSSDI invites proposals from Indian scientists interested in conducting original research in the field of diabetes mellitus. Furthermore, limited grants are also available for the students of medical colleges for smaller projects. Recently, RSSDI has developed a simple user-friendly novel approach to decide the appropriate antidiabetic agent to be used in type 2 diabetes through the 'therapeutic wheel'. The best choices can be determined from the outer rings of the wheel (orange and red), and the choices can be further streamlined by an 'individualised approach' (Fig. 6.4).

Future Directions: Unmet Needs, Unanswered Questions and Unquestioned Answers

There have been rapid epidemiological transitions translating into a huge disease burden in diabetes in the SEA region. Prevention of diabetes through consistent awareness about the disease in population would be a critical step forward which would have tremendous implications that halt the progress of disease. One of the global targets for non-communicable disease is to halt by 2025 the rise in the prevalence of diabetes to its 2010 levels. A better understanding for the basis for the gene–environment interaction, in which beta-cell dysfunction, typically on the background of insulin resistance, is critical for the increase in glucose levels observed in impaired glucose metabolism and for the development of the hyperglycaemia of type 2 diabetes, would be explored to target effective therapies. Prevention is of utmost importance, but for the more than 420 million people currently living with diabetes, managing their disease must remain the priority. The recent WHO's report recommends a multidisciplinary approach with patient education, medication and consistent follow-up. For primary prevention, the challenge lies in raising awareness, promoting health literacy and identifying individuals at high risk of diabetes for early intervention. For secondary prevention, poor access to care, clinical inertia and treatment non-adherence are major barriers in evidence-based practice. Given the phenotypic heterogeneity of diabetes, and thus the pluralistic needs of those affected, clinical acumen to identify problems and sufficient contact time to empower the person to change behaviour and adhere to treatment are key to successful management.

Screening in young-onset diabetes in India for CV risk factors and complications would be vital to curb the impact of the microvascular and macrovascular complications. This has been clearly demonstrated in the landmark CINDI and CINDI 2 trials published recently for the clinic-based

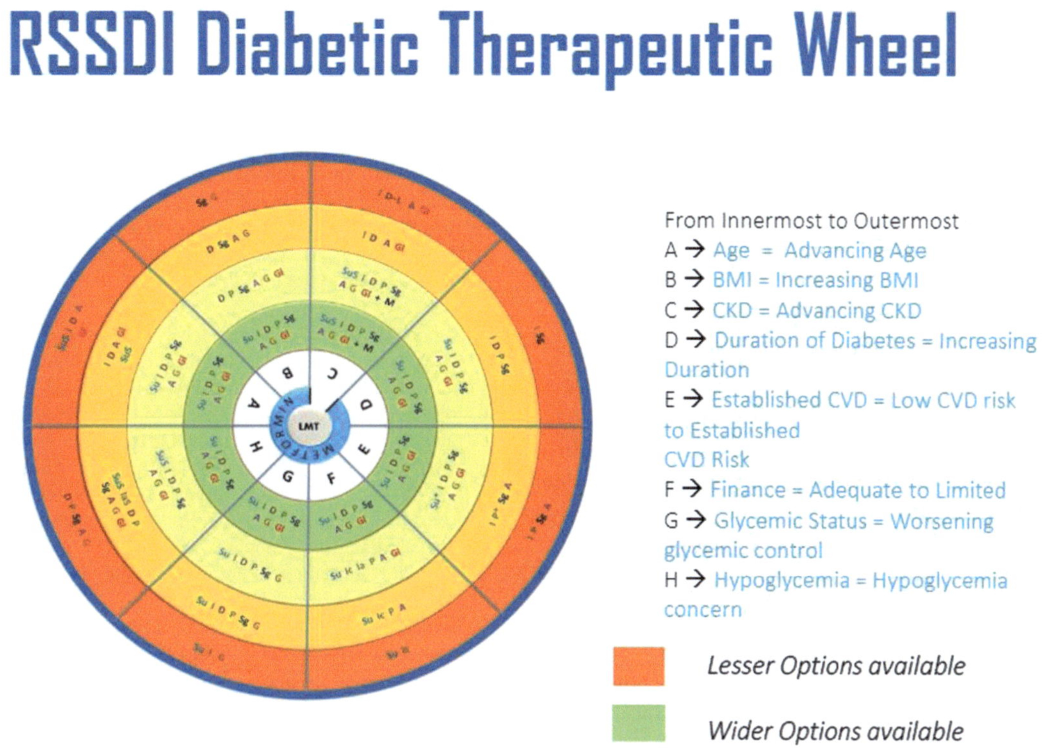

Fig. 6.4 The RSSDI therapeutic wheel

survey amongst 4,600 patients for diabetes-related complications and a retrospective cross-sectional study of 1,500 patients with newly detected young-onset diabetes, respectively.

Conclusions

Considering the enormous burden due to diabetes in India, it is important to realise the cost-effective measures of diabetes care like early screening, tight metabolic control, monitoring of risk factors and assessing of the organ damage. The study done for economic analysis in diabetes care in India has also shown that the cost of providing routine care is only a fraction of the overall cost and is perhaps still manageable. However, when this is not available or its quality is poor, the overall direct and indirect costs escalate with disastrous health and economic consequences to the individual, his family and society particularly due to the onset of the micro- and macrovascular complications of diabetes. Published data from several epidemiological, experimental human and animal studies as well as the data from several mega-trials have convincingly proved the importance of tight metabolic control in arresting and preventing the progression of target organ damage. In the last two decades, there is a better understanding of the pathophysiology of type 2 diabetes and availability of newer oral drugs for diabetes; newer insulin and improved delivery systems should translate to improve diabetes control. However, the survey described above indicates the gaps between the guidelines and real-life practice. In view of this, appreciation and understanding of both patient and physician barriers regarding proper monitoring and judicious use of therapeutic options including insulin therapy for optimising diabetes management should be encouraged in order to improve control of diabetes in India. Result-oriented organised programmes involving patient education, updating medical fraternity on various developments in the management of diabetes and providing them the opportunity to use and analyse these newer treatment options in the form of observational studies are required to combat the diabetes epidemic currently threatening to affect the lives of millions of people in India. Coordination, patient education and ongoing support are important components of quality diabetes care, but most health-care systems are created to provide acute and episodic care rather than chronic care. The effectiveness of team-based chronic care management is well established but not widely implemented. Thus, the challenge lies in designing alternative care models that identify people with undetected diabetes, define individual needs, provide interdisciplinary care and measure effectiveness to make diabetes prevention and control programmes accessible, affordable and sustainable. It is time to evaluate existing policies to address diabetes and devise a strategy and accountability framework for short-, medium- and long-term solutions to address the growing unmet needs in diabetes prevention and control. Immediate action is needed to avert this escalating health disaster.

References

1. International Diabetes Federation. Diabetes Atlas. 7th ed. 2015 Update. http://www.diabetesatlas.org/resources/2015-atlas.html. Last accessed on 21 Apr 2016.
2. Misra A, Sharma R, Gulati S. Consensus dietary guidelines for healthy living and prevention of obesity, the metabolic syndrome, diabetes, and related disorders in Asian Indians. Dia Tec Ther. 2011;13(6):683–94.
3. NCD Risk Factor Collaboration (NCD-RisC). Worldwide trends in diabetes since 1980: a pooled analysis of 751 population-based studies with 4·4 million participants. Lancet. 2016;387:1513–30.

Further Reading

4. Sicree R, Shaw J, Zimmet P. Diabetes and impaired glucose tolerance in India. In: Gan D, editor. Diabetes atlas. Belgium: International Diabetes Federation; 2006. p. 15–103.
5. Mohan V, Sandeep S, Deepa R, et al. Epidemiology of type 2 diabetes: Indian scenario. Indian J Med Res. 2007;125:217–30.
6. Mohan V, Alberti KGMM. Diabetes in the tropics. In: Alberti KGMM, Zimmet P, Defronzo RA, et al., editors. International text book of diabetes mellitus. 2nd ed. Chichester: Wiley; 1997. p. 171–87.
7. Nakagami T, Qiao Q, Carstensen B, The DECODE -DECODA Study Group, et al. Age, body mass index and type 2 diabetes-associations modified by ethnicity. Diabetologia. 2003;46:1063–70.
8. Banerji MA, Faridi N, Atluri R, et al. Body composition, visceral fat, leptin, and insulin resistance in Asian Indian men. J Clin Endocrinol Metab. 1999;84:137–44.
9. Zargar AH, Wani AI, Masoodi SR, et al. Mortality in diabetes mellitus—data from a developing region of the world. Diabetes Res Clin Pract. 1999;43:67–74.
10. Mohan V, Shanthirani CS, Deepa M, et al. Mortality rates due to diabetes in a selected urban south Indian population – the Chennai Urban Population Study (CUPS-16). J Assoc Phys India. 2006;54:113–7.
11. Rema M, Deepa R, Mohan V. Prevalence of retinopathy at diagnosis among type 2 diabetic patients attending a diabetic centre in South India. Br J Ophthalmol. 2000;84:1058–60.
12. Ramachandran A, Snehalatha C, Satyavani K, et al. Prevalence of vascular complications and their risk factors in type 2 diabetes. J Assoc Physicians India. 1999;47:1152–6.
13. Tripathy BB, Panda NC, Tej SC, et al. Survey for detection of glycosuria, hyperglycaemia and diabetes mellitus in urban and rural areas of Cuttack district. J Assoc Physicians India. 1971;19:681.
14. Ahuja MMS, Sivaji L, Garg VK, et al. Prevalence of diabetes in northern India (Delhi area). Horn Metab Res. 1974;4:321.
15. Gupta OP, Joshi MH, Dave SK. Prevalence of diabetes in India. Adv Metab Disord. 1978;9:147–65.
16. Murthy PD, Pullaiah B, Rao KV. Survey for detection of hyperglycaemia and diabetes mellitus in Tenali. In: Bajaj JS, editor. Diabetes mellitus in developing countries. New Delhi: Interprint; 1984. p. 55.
17. Patel JC. Prevalence of hypertension and diabetes mellitus in a rural village. J Diabet Assoc India. 1986;26:68.
18. Ramachandran A, Jali MV, Mohan V, et al. High prevalence of diabetes in an urban population in South India. Br Med J. 1988;297:587–90.
19. Deurenberg P, Deurenberg-Yap M, Guricci S. Asians are different from Caucasians and from each other in their body mass index/body fat per cent relationship. Obes Rev. 2002;3:141–6.
20. Rao PV, Ushabala P, Seshiah. The Eluru survey: prevalence of known diabetes in a rural Indian population. Diabetes Res Clin Pract. 1989;7:29–31.
21. McKeigue PM, Shah B, Marmot MG. Relation of central obesity and insulin resistance with high diabetes prevalence and cardiovascular risk in South Asians. Lancet. 1991;337:382–6.
22. Wander GS, Khurana SB, Gulati R, et al. Epidemiology of coronary heart disease and risk factors in a rural Punjab population: prevalence and

correlation with various risk factors. Ind Heart J. 1994;46:319–23.
23. Ramachandran A, Snehalatha C, Dharmaraj D, et al. Prevalence of glucose intolerance in Asian Indians. Urban–rural difference and significance of upper body adiposity. Diabetes Care. 1992;15:1348.
24. Ramankutty V, Joseph A, Soman CR. High prevalence of type 2 diabetes in an urban settlement in Kerala, India. Ethn Health Med. 1999;4:231–9.
25. Zargar AH, Khan AK, Masoodi SR, et al. Prevalence of type 2 diabetes mellitus and impaired glucose tolerance in the Kashmir Valley of the Indian subcontinent. Diabetes Res Clin Pract. 2000;47:135.
26. Ramachandran A, Snehalatha C, Kapur A, Diabetes Epidemiology Study Group in India (DESI), et al. High prevalence of diabetes and impaired glucose tolerance in India: National Urban Diabetes Survey. Diabetologia. 2001;44:1094.
27. Misra A, Pandey RM, Devi JR, et al. High prevalence of diabetes, obesity and dyslipidaemia in urban slum population in northern India. Int J Obes. 2001;25:1722–9.
28. Mohan V, Shanthirani CS, Deepa R. Glucose intolerance (Diabetes and IGT) in a selected South Indian population with special reference to family history, obesity and lifestyle factors- the Chennai Urban Population Study (CUPS 14). J Assoc Physicians India. 2003;51:771.
29. Sadikot SM, Nigam A, Das S, et al. The burden of diabetes and impaired glucose tolerance in India using the WHO 1999 criteria: prevalence of diabetes in India study (PODIS). Diabetes Res Clin Pract. 2004;66:301–7.
30. Gupta A, Gupta R, Sarna M, et al. Prevalence of diabetes, impaired fasting glucose and insulin resistance syndrome in an urban Indian population. Diabetes Res Clin Pract. 2003;61:69.
31. Agrawal RP, Singh G, Nayak KC, et al. Prevalence of diabetes in camel milk consuming 'RAICA' Rural Community of North West Rajasthan. Int J Diabetes Dev Countries. 2004;24:109–14.
32. Ramachandran A, Snehalatha C, Baskar AD, et al. Temporal changes in prevalence of diabetes and impaired glucose tolerance associated with lifestyle transition occurring in the rural population in India. Diabetologia. 2004;47:860–5.
33. Mohan V, Deepa M, Deepa R, et al. Secular trends in the prevalence of diabetes and glucose tolerance in urban South India-the Chennai Urban Rural Epidemiology Study (CURES- 17). Diabetologia. 2006;49:1175.
34. Basavanagowdappa H, Prabhakar AK, Prasannaraj P, Gurudev KC, Virupaksha S. Study of prevalence of diabetes mellitus and impaired fasting glucose in a rural population. Int J Diabetes Dev Countries. 2005;25:98–101.
35. Prabhakaran D, Shah P, Chaturvedi V, et al. Cardiovascular risk factor prevalence among men in a large industry of northern India. Natl Med J India. 2005;18:59–65.
36. Reddy KS, Prabhakaran D, Chaturvedi V, on behalf of the Sentinel Surveillance System for Indian Industrial Populations Study Group, et al. Methods for establishing a surveillance system for cardiovascular diseases in Indian industrial populations. Bull WHO. 2006;84:461–9.
37. Deo SS, Zantye A, Mokal R, et al. To identify the risk factors for high prevalence of diabetes and impaired glucose tolerance in Indian rural population. Int J Diabetes Dev Countries. 2006;26: 19–23.
38. Menon VU, Kumar KV, Gilchrist A, et al. Prevalence of known and undetected diabetes and associated risk factors in central Kerala – ADEPS. Diabetes Res Clin Pract. 2006;74:289.
39. Chow CK, Raju PK, Raju R, et al. The prevalence and management of diabetes in rural India. Diabetes Care. 2006;29:1717–8.
40. Raghupathy P, Antonisamy B, Fall CH, et al. High prevalence of glucose intolerance even among young adults in south India. Diabetes Res Clin Pract. 2007;77:269–79.
41. Mohan V, Mathur P, Deepa R, et al. Urban rural differences in prevalence of self reported diabetes in India-The WHO-ICMR Indian NCD risk factor surveillance. Diabetes Res Clin Pract. 2008;80:159–68.
42. Ramachandran A, Mary S, Yamuna A, et al. High prevalence of diabetes and cardiovascular risk factors associated with urbanization in India. Diabetes Care. 2008;31:893–8.
43. Rema M, Ponnaiya M, Mohan V. Prevalence of retinopathy in non insulin dependent diabetes mellitus in southern India. Diabetes Res Clin Pract. 1996;24: 29–36.
44. Dandona L, Dandona R, Naduvilath TJ, et al. Population based assessment of diabetic retinopathy in an urban population in southern India. Br J Ophthalmol. 1999;83:937–40.
45. Narendran V, John RK, Raghuram A, et al. Diabetic retinopathy among self reported diabetics in southern India: a population based assessment. Br J Ophthalmol. 2002;86:1014–8.
46. Rema M, Premkumar S, Anitha B, et al. Prevalence of diabetic retinopathy in Urban India: the Chennai Urban Rural Epidemiology Study (CURES) Eye Study-1. Invest Ophthalmol Vis Sci. 2005;46:2328–33.
47. John L, Sundar Rao PSS, Kanagasabhapathy AS. Prevalence of diabetic nephropathy in non insulin dependant diabetes mellitus. Indian J Med Res. 1991;94:24–9.
48. Gupta DK, Verma LK, Khosla PK, et al. The prevalence of microalbuminuria in diabetes: a study from north India. Diabetes Res Clin Pract. 1991;12:125–8.
49. Yajnik CS, Naik SS, Raut KN, et al. Urinary albumin excretion rate (AER) in newly-diagnosed type 2 Indian diabetic patients is associated with central obesity and hyperglycaemia. Diabetes Res Clin Pract. 1992;17:55–60.

50. Vijay V, Snehalatha C, Ramachandran A, et al. Prevalence of proteinuria in non-insulin dependent diabetes. J Assoc Physicians India. 1994;42: 792–4.
51. Mohan V, Meera R, Premalatha G, et al. Frequency of proteinuria in type 2 diabetes mellitus seen at a diabetes centre in Southern India. Postgrad Med J. 2000;76:569–73.
52. Varghese A, Deepa R, Rema M, et al. Prevalence of microalbuminuria in type 2 diabetes mellitus at a diabetes centre in Southern India. Postgrad Med J. 2001;77:399–402.
53. Ranjit Unnikrishnan I, Rema M, Pradeepa R, et al. Prevalence and risk factors of diabetic nephropathy in an Urban South Indian population. The Chennai Urban Rural Epidemiology Study (CURES-45). Diabetes Care. 2007;30(8):2019–24.
54. Mohan V, Premalatha G, Sastry NG. Ischaemic heart disease in south Indian NIDDM patients – a clinic based study on 6597 NIDDM patients. Int J Diabetes Dev Countries. 1995;15:64–7.
55. Ramachandran A, Snehalatha C, Latha E, et al. Clustering of cardiovascular risk factors in urban Asian Indians. Diabetes Care. 1998;21:967–71.
56. Mohan V, Deepa R, Shanthirani CS, et al. Prevalence of coronary artery disease and its relationship to lipids in a selected population in South India. J Am Coll Cardiol. 2001;38:682–7.
57. Premalatha G, Shanthirani CS, Deepa R, et al. Prevalence and risk factors of peripheral vascular disease in a selected south Indian population – the Chennai Urban Population Study (CUPS). Diabetes Care. 2000;23:1295–300.
58. Ashok S, Ramu M, Deepa R, et al. Prevalence of neuropathy in type 2 diabetic patients attending a diabetes centre in south India. J Assoc Physicians India. 2002;50:546–50.
59. Pradeepa R, Rema M, Vignesh J, et al. Prevalence and risk factors for diabetic neuropathy in an urban south Indian population: the Chennai Urban Rural Epidemiology Study (CURES-55). Diabet Med. 2008;25:407–12.
60. Mohan V, Ravikumar R, Shanthirani S, et al. Intimal medial thickness of the carotid artery in south Indian diabetic and non diabetic subjects: the Chennai Urban Population Study (CUPS). Diabetologia. 2000;43:494–9.
61. Deepa M, Deepa R, Shanthirani CS, et al. Awareness and knowledge of diabetes in Chennai— the Chennai Urban Rural Epidemiology Study [CURES-9]. J Assoc Physicians India. 2005;53:283–7.
62. Murugesan N, Snehalatha C, Shobhana R, et al. Awareness, about diabetes and its complications in the general and diabetic population in a city in southern India. Diabetes Res Clin Pract. 2007;77: 433–7.
63. Kapur A, Shishoo S, Ahuja MMS, et al. Diabetes care in India: patient's perceptions attitudes and practices (DIPPAP-1 study). Int J Diabetes Dev Countries. 1997;17:2–12.
64. Raheja BS, Kapur A, Bhoraskar A, et al. DiabCare Asia—India Study: diabetes care in India—current status. J Assoc Physicians India. 2001;49:717–22.
65. American Diabetes Association (ADA) Recommendations Regarding Glycated Hemoglobin Standardization. American diabetes association position statement. Tests of glycemia in diabetes. Diabetes Care. 2004;27:S91–3.
66. Dilley J, Ganesan A, Deepa R, et al. Association of A1C with cardiovascular disease and metabolic syndrome in Asian Indians with normal glucose tolerance. Diabetes Care. 2007;30:1527–32.
67. Phillips LS, Branch WT, Cook CB, et al. Clin Inertia Ann Intern Med. 2001;135:825–34.
68. Couzin J. Clinical research: deaths in diabetes trial challenge a long-held theory. Science. 2008; 884–885:15.
69. Kapur A. Economic analysis of diabetes care. Indian J Med Res. 2007;125:473–82.
70. Nagpal J, Bhartia A. Quality of diabetes care in the middle and high-income group populace: the Delhi Diabetes Community (DEDICOM) survey. Diabetes Care. 2006;29:2341–8.
71. Kapur A, Shishoo S, Ahuja MMS, et al. Diabetes care in India: physicians perceptions, attitudes and practices. Int J Diabetes Dev Countries. 1998;18: 124–30. 72.
72. Chuang LM, Tsai ST, Huang BY, Tai TY. The status of diabetes control in Asia—a cross-sectional survey of 24 317 patients with diabetes mellitus in 1998. Diabet Med. 2002;19:978–85.
73. Mohan V, Goldhaber-Fiebert JD, Radha V, et al. Screening with OGTT alone or in combination with the Indian diabetes risk score or genotyping of TCF7L2 to detect undiagnosed type 2 diabetes in Asian Indians. Indian J Med Res. 2011;133:294–9.
74. Engelgau MM, Narayan KMV, Herman WH. Screening for type 2 diabetes. Diabetes Care. 2000;23(10):1563–80.
75. Joshi SR, Das AK, Vijay VJ, Mohan V. Challenges in diabetes care in India: sheer numbers, lack of awareness and inadequate control. J Assoc Physicians India. 2008;56:443–50.
76. Misra A, Nigam P, Hills AP, et al. Consensus physical activity guidelines for Asian Indians. Diabetes Technol Ther. 2012;14(1):83–98.
77. Cuff DJ, Meneilly GS, Martin A, et al. Effective exercise modality to reduce insulin resistance in women with type 2 diabetes. Diabetes Care. 2003; 26(11):2977–82.
78. Ishii T, Yamakita T, Sato T, et al. Resistance training improves insulin sensitivity in NIDDM subjects without altering maximal oxygen uptake. Diabetes Care. 1998;21(8):1353–5.
79. Silverstein J, Klingensmith G, Copeland K, et al. Care of children and adolescents with type 1 diabetes:

a statement of the American Diabetes Association. Diabetes Care. 2005;28(1):186–212.
80. Joshi SR, Bhansali A, Bajaj S, et al. Results from a dietary survey in an Indian T2DM population: a STARCH study. BMJ Open. 2014;4(10):e005138.
81. Sadikot SM, Nigam A, Das S, et al. Diabetes India. The burden of diabetes and impaired fasting glucose in India using the ADA1997 criteria: prevalence of diabetes in India study (PODIS). Diabetes Res Clin Pract. 2004;66:293–30.
82. Research India Diabetes(ICMR-INDAB) study (phase I): Indian Council of Medical Research India Diabetes 4. Indian J Endocrinol Metab. 2014;18:379–85.
83. The Diabetes Prevention Program Research Group. The diabetes prevention program. Diabetes Care. 2002;25:2165–71.
84. Lindstorm J, Louheranta A, Mannelin M, et al. The Finnish diabetes prevention study. Diabetes Care. 2003;26:3230–6.
85. Misra A, Alappan NK, Vikram N. Effect of supervised progressive resistance-exercise training protocol on insulin sensitivity, glycemia, lipids, and body composition in Asian Indians with type 2 diabetes. Diabetes Care. 2008;31(7):1282–7.
86. Thangasami SR, Chandani AL, Thangasami S. Emphasis of yoga in the management of diabetes. J Diabetes Metab. 2015;6:10.
87. Youngwanichsetha S, Phumdoung S, Inqkathawornwong T. The effects of mindfulness eating and yoga exercise on blood sugar levels of pregnant women with gestational diabetes mellitus. Appl Nurs Res. 2014;27(4):227–30.
88. The DCCT Research Group. The effect of intensive treatment of diabetes on the development and progression of long-term complications in insulin dependent diabetes mellitus. N Engl J Med. 1993; 329:977–86.
89. Okhubo Y, Hideki K, Araki E, et al. Intensive insulin therapy prevents the progression of diabetic microvascular complications in Japanese patients with non-insulin dependent diabetes mellitus. A randomized prospective six year study. Diabetes Res Clin Pract. 1995;28:103–17.
90. UKPDS Study Group. Intensive blood glucose control with SU and insulin compared with conventional treatment and risk of complications in patients with type 2 diabetes. (UKPDS 33). Lancet. 1998;352:837–53.
91. Pung OJ, Sobieraj DM, Engel SS. Early combination therapy for the treatment of type 2 diabetes mellitus: systematic review and meta-analysis. Diabetes Obes Metab. 2014;16(5):410–7.
92. Screening for Diabetes. American diabetes association. Diabetes Care. 2002;25(1):s21–4.
93. Sosale B, Sosale AR, Mohan AR. (CINDI 2). Cardiovascular risk factors, micro and macrovascular complications at diagnosis in patients with young onset type 2 diabetes in India: CINDI 2. Indian J Endocrinol Metab. 2016;20(1):114–8.
94. Sosale A, Prasanna Kumar KM, Sadikot SM. (CINDI). Chronic complications in newly diagnosed patients with Type 2 diabetes mellitus in India. Indian J Endocrinol Metab. 2014;18(3):355–60.
95. Krug EG. Trends in diabetes: sounding the alarm. Lancet. 2016;387:1485–6.
96. Madhu SV, et al. Guideline development group. Int J Diabetes Dev Countries. 2015;35 Suppl 1:S1–71.
97. Nanditha A, et al. Diabetes in Asia and the Pacific: implications for the global epidemic. Diabetes Care. 2016;39(3):472–85.
98. Shen J, Prabhakaran D, Tandon N, et al. A multiethnic study of pre-diabetes and diabetes in LMIC. Glob Heart. 2016;11(1):61–70.
99. Ramachandran A, et al. Combining fasting plasma glucose with gamma-glutamyl transferase improves the sensitivity to predict incident diabetes in Asian Indian men with impaired glucose tolerance. J Assoc Physicians India. 2014;62(11):18–22.
100. Vinitha R, Johnston DG, Ramachandran A, et al. Adiponectin, leptin, interleukin-6 and HbA1c in the prediction of incident type 2 diabetes: a nested case-control study in Asian Indian men with impaired glucose tolerance. Diabetes Res Clin Pract. 2015;109(2): 340–6.
101. Ram J, Snehalatha C, Ramachandran A, et al. Retinol binding protein-4 predicts incident diabetes in Asian Indian men with prediabetes. Biofactors. 2015;41(3):160–5.
102. Ramachandran A, et al. Improvement in diet habits, independent of physical activity helps to reduce incident diabetes among prediabetic Asian Indian men. Diabetes Res Clin Pract. 2014;106(3):491–5.
103. Ramachandran A, et al. Hypertriglyceridaemic waist phenotype as a simple predictive marker of incident diabetes in Asian-Indian men with prediabetes. Diabet Med. 2014;31(12):1542–9.
104. Ramachandran A, et al. Effectiveness of mobile phone messaging in prevention of type 2 diabetes by lifestyle modification in men in India: a prospective, parallel-group, randomised controlled trial. Lancet Diabetes Endocrinol. 2013;1(3):191–8.
105. Ramachandran A, et al. Predictive value of HbA1c for incident diabetes among subjects with impaired glucose tolerance – analysis of the Indian Diabetes Prevention Programmes. Diabet Med. 2012;29(1): 94–8.
106. Anjana RM, ICMR–INDIAB Collaborative Study Group, et al. Prevalence of diabetes and prediabetes (impaired fasting glucose and/or impaired glucose tolerance) in urban and rural India: phase I results of the Indian Council of Medical Research-INdia DIABetes (ICMR-INDIAB) study. Diabetologia. 2011;54(12):3022–7.
107. Ramachandran A, Indian Diabetes Prevention Programme (IDPP), et al. The Indian Diabetes

Prevention Programme shows that lifestyle modification and metformin prevent type 2 diabetes in Asian Indian subjects with impaired glucose tolerance (IDPP-1). Diabetologia. 2006;49(2):289–97.

108. Ramachandran A, et al. Persistent impaired glucose tolerance has similar rate of risk factors as for diabetes – results of Indian diabetes prevention programme (IDPP). Diabetes Res Clin Pract. 2006;73(1):100–3.

109. Ramachandran A, et al. Cost-effectiveness of the interventions in the primary prevention of diabetes among Asian Indians: within-trial results of the Indian Diabetes Prevention Programme (IDPP). Diabetes Care. 2007;30(10):2548–52.

110. Snehalatha C, et al. Beneficial effects of strategies for primary prevention of diabetes on cardiovascular risk factors: results of the Indian Diabetes Prevention Programme. Diabetes Vasc Dis Res. 2008;5(1):25–9.

111. Unnikrishnan R, Anjana RM, Mohan V. Diabetes mellitus and its complications in India. Nat Rev Endocrinol. 2016. doi:10.1038/nrendo.2016.53. [Epub ahead of print]. Online ahead of print.

Diabetes in Latin America

7

Omar Y. Bello-Chavolla
and Carlos A. Aguilar-Salinas

Classification and Unique Aspects of the Pathophysiology of Type 1 and Type 2 Diabetes in the Region

The Latin America (LA) region is comprised of 21 countries, including Mexico, six countries in Central America, ten countries in South America, and three countries in the Caribbean islands spanning a total population of almost 600 million people. The region is composed of low- and middle-income countries with populations mainly composed of young adults. Ethnic diversity and the preservation of the Amerindian heritage are unique features of the Latin American populations. Meanwhile, the Amerindian component is the dominant genetic background in Peru and Guatemala; its contribution is minimal in areas of Argentina or Uruguay. In urban areas of Colombia and Mexico, the average proportion of Native American and European admixture are 50–60 % and 30–45 %, respectively. In addition, an ongoing demographic transition has modified the age structure of Latin American populations with important increases in the adult (15–59 years) population and especially for populations of older populations (aged 60 years and over) [1].

The rapid growth of the number of inhabitants in the Latin American population observed in the first half of the preceding century was reverted in the past few decades (2.8 % growth per year in 1950, 1.3 % in the early 2000s). This trend resulted from birth control campaigns, migratory movements, and economic phenomena. On the other hand, a trend for decreasing all-cause mortality started to occur within Latin America 50 years ago. Life expectancy in the region has increased by 21.6 years on average reaching 73.4 years for the 2005–2010 period. The variation of life expectancy is wide within the region, ranging from 65.5 in Bolivia to >78 years in Chile and Costa Rica. As a result, the percentage of elder population has increased in the last 50 years. It is expected that, by the year 2050, the percentage of elders move from 8.8 to 23.6 %. The demographic modifications pose a remarkable challenge for the local healthcare systems. The increase of life expectancy will lead to increased number of susceptible cases for having

O.Y. Bello-Chavolla, MD, PhD (PECEM)
Department of Endocrinology and Metabolism, Instituto Nacional de Ciencias Médicas y Nutrición Salvador Zubirán, Mexico City, Mexico

Facultad de Medicina, Universidad Nacional Autónoma de México, Mexico City, Mexico

C.A. Aguilar-Salinas (✉)
Departamento de Endocrinologia y Metabolismo, Instituto Nacional de Ciencias Médicas y Nutricion, Vasco de Quiroga 15, Mexico City 14000, Mexico
e-mail: caguilarsalinas@yahoo.com

S. Dagogo-Jack (ed.), *Diabetes Mellitus in Developing Countries and Underserved Communities*,
DOI 10.1007/978-3-319-41559-8_7

non-transmissible chronic diseases (i.e., type 2 diabetes mellitus), which already are the major health burden within Latin American countries.

Type 2 Diabetes

Close to 80 % of 415 million T2DM cases live in middle- and low-income countries. A significant proportion of them (41.1 millions) reside in LA. This number is expected to increase to 69.4 in 2040. The International Diabetes Federation (IDF) estimated that the age-adjusted prevalence for the region was 9.2 % for adults (aged 20–79 years) in 2014. Only North America (10.5 %) and southern Asia (10.9 %) had a greater prevalence of diabetes than LA. Two of the ten leading countries for the number of cases are located in the region (Brazil (14.3 million) and Mexico (11.5 million)) (Table 7.1). In addition, the increment in the number of cases is expected to be greater in this region compared to other areas.

According to the Global Burden of Disease group, the mean fasting plasma glucose of the adults living in LA has increased 3.06 mg/dl every decade since 1980 [2]. The end result has been a rapidly increasing prevalence of diabetes. The epidemic growth is expected to continue since the prevalence of several preceding conditions of T2D (i.e., obesity and glucose intolerance) is higher in LA than in other regions. According to the latest report by the Food and Agriculture Organization of the United Nations (FAO) [3] and the World Health Organization (WHO), the worldwide prevalence of obesity in 2013 was 11.7, whereas the prevalence of obesity for the Latin American was reported to be 23.4 %, distributed in 30.4 % for Central America and 21.6 % for South America (Table 7.2). The countries with the highest obesity prevalence in the LA region are Mexico, followed by Venezuela, Argentina, and Chile. The reported prevalence for obesity in Mexican women proves to be higher than the same figure reported for the USA in 2008 (31.8 %). A high percentage of patients with excess body weight have central fat accumulation, arterial hypertension as well as abnormal concentrations of total cholesterol, HDL and triglycerides, and abnormal fasting glucose. When three or more of these abnormalities are present, individuals are diagnosed as having the metabolic syndrome. This condition is associated with a fivefold increase for having T2D. Several metabolic syndrome definitions have been proposed. Using the ATP-III criteria, the age-adjusted prevalence for the region is 28.3 %. Population-based data are available for Brazil (29 %), Peru (18.1 %), Colombia (34.8 %), Venezuela (35.3 %), and Mexico (36.8 %). Higher percentages are found if the IDF definition is applied (for Mexican adults, the prevalence changes from 36.8 to 49.8 %). The prevalence of the metabolic syndrome traits is different in LA compared to that reported in Caucasian populations; low HDL cholesterol, abdominal obesity, and hypertriglyceridemia are significantly more common in LA subjects.

The clinical expression of T2D has several peculiarities that have been consistently reported in LA populations. Especially among mestizo individuals, the disease is expressed at an earlier age and with a lower body mass index (BMI) compared to that reported in Caucasians. The premature age of onset increases the social and economic burden because of the higher prevalence of chronic complications and premature disability during productive years. In Mexico, 22.7 % of people with T2D are under the age 40. Individuals with early-onset T2D comprise a heterogeneous population [4]. Two thirds of them have BMI >25 kg/m^2; these cases had an increased prevalence of several metabolic syndrome traits (e.g., hypertension and hypoalphalipoproteinemia) and can be controlled using oral glucose-lowering agents. In contrast, a large proportion of the lean cases require insulin as part of their treatment. Compared to the overall population with T2D, the young T2D population had a higher prevalence of underdiagnosis, more school years but a lower socioeconomic level, and higher alcohol and tobacco consumption. Few young patients undertake preventive measures, with very few receiving statins, acetylsalicylic acid, or follow-up with an ophthalmologist. This group has specific barriers to adhere treatment programs (e.g., depression,

Table 7.1 Prevalence of diabetes in Latin America

Country	Number of cases (20–79 years)	Prevalence	Annual death rate due to diabetes (20–79 years)	Annual treatment cost per subject (US dollars)	Estimated number of undiagnosed cases	Annual increment of the number of cases
Argentina	1,570,200	5.57	15,416	966.44	722,290	29,000
Bolivia	325,220	6.89	4,732	124.63	149,600	–
Brazil	14,300,000	10.52	129,226	1,031.44	6,164,590	377,000
Chile	1,442,610	12.78	10,459	992.13	755,600	28,000
Colombia	2,067,870	7.26	14,602	482.72	951,220	95,000
Costa Rica	259,350	8.81	1,659	937.20	119,300	–
Cuba	872,950	8.58	7,560	823.71	401,560	19,000
Ecuador	563,840	6.89	5,492	335.41	259,360	19,000
El Salvador	312,430	9.88	3,233	333.58	143.72	–
French Guiana	12,610	9.60	–	–	5,800	–
Guatemala	589,140	9.93	7,202	311.52	271,010	27,000
Honduras	239,590	7.16	2,338	209.40	110,210	–
Mexico	11,500,000	14.4[a]	80,000[a]	815.53	3,452,410	323,000
Nicaragua	309,320	11.58	3,001	172.21	142,290	–
Panama	184,580	8.59	1,399	732.45	84,910	–
Paraguay	222,220	6.81	2,174	283.14	102,220	–
Peru	1,108,610	6.81	8,150	307.31	509,960	–
Puerto Rico	391,870	12.98	–	–	108,590	–
Dominican Republic	405,580	7.36	5,183	419.28	186,570	–
Uruguay	157,330	6.02	1,122	922.68	72,370	–
Venezuela	1,764,900	10.39	13,380	914.01	811,850	61,000

Modified from: Whiting et al. [23]. International Diabetes Federation Atlas 2012
[a]Villalpando et al. [93]

work-related stress, and alcoholism) that should be intentionally sought.

On the other hand, the mean BMI of recently diagnosed populations is lower in LA patients (e.g., for Mexico, 27.9 kg/m^2 in males and 28.9 kg/m^2 in females) compared to that reported in the USA (usually above 30 kg/m^2). Mestizo populations are less tolerant to excess body weight because fat is accumulated in ectopic organs and in the intra-abdominal cavity instead of the subcutaneous adipose tissue [5].

T2D coexists frequently with other comorbidities. Taking as an example the Mexican population, a high percentage of patients with T2D had at least one cardiovascular risk factor (86.7 %) (e.g., hypercholesterolemia, family history of cardiovascular mortality, arterial hypertension, and smoking). Nearly half the patients had hypertension, but almost half of them are unaware of the presence of arterial hypertension. Smoking persists as a common risk factor in the patients with diabetes. Dyslipidemia is one of the most common comorbidities in T2D, with higher levels of triglycerides and non-HDL cholesterol compared with values of the general population. LDL cholesterol (LDL-C) levels >100 mg/dL are observed in 74.8 % (95 % CI 72.5–76.9 %) of previously diagnosed patients [6]. Similar percentages have been reported by the Qualidiab network using data from several South American countries [7].

A high percentage of women with T2D had at least one pregnancy during their lifetimes (94.7 %); this proportion was similar to the one found in patients without T2D. However, the number of women who had suffered at least one abortion was significantly higher in the group with diabetes (OR 1.62, 95 % CI 1.53–1.83) with

Table 7.2 Average body mass index (BMI) standardized for age by age and country for the years 1980 and 2008

	Men (kg/m^2)		Women (kg/m^2)		Prevalence of obesity in adults (%)
	1980	2008	1980	2008	2008
Argentina	25.4	27.5	23.8	27.5	29.4
Bolivia	23.0	24.4	23.6	26.9	18.9
Brazil	22.6	25.8	24.1	26.0	19.5
Chile	24.5	27.0	24.0	27.9	29.1
Colombia	22.1	24.9	23.4	26.2	18.1
Costa Rica	23.7	26.5	23.4	27.0	24.6
Cuba	22.7	25.1	23.8	26.6	20.5
Ecuador	23.8	25.6	24.7	27.1	22.0
El Salvador	23.8	26.4	23.7	27.8	26.9
Guatemala	23.2	25.3	22.9	26.8	20.7
Honduras	23.1	25.1	23.0	26.7	19.8
Mexico	24.5	27.4	24.6	28.7	32.8
Nicaragua	24.0	25.8	24.4	27.6	24.2
Panama	23.5	26.3	23.9	27.7	25.8
Paraguay	23.4	25.5	23.5	25.9	19.2
Peru	23.0	24.8	25.1	26.0	16.5
Dominican Republic	22.9	25.2	22.6	26.9	21.9
Uruguay	24.2	26.4	23.3	26.6	23.6
Venezuela	24.6	27.4	24.7	28.1	30.8

Adapted from: Finucane MM, Stevens GA, Cowan MJ, et al., and the Food and Agriculture Organization of the United Nations. The State of Food and Agriculture 2013

a similar trend found in the risk of stillbirth (OR 1.99, 95 % CI 1.75–2.3); these differences were held significant when adjusted by age. A high percentage of women with T2D during their reproductive years did not use contraceptive methods (42.5 %); this rate was not significantly different in women without T2D (38.8 %). A quarter of patients with T2D had a current or previous history of a urinary tract infection during the previous year. Additionally, the risk of suffering an accident is higher for T2D patients (OR 1.42, 95 % CI 1.25–1.60) with half of the accidents occurring within the patient's house. The risk of accidental falls in patients with T2D is not held significant when stratified by age group [8].

The elder patient with T2D is a growing group in the region. Two major profiles are found among them. The first is composed of T2D patients with a long exposure to the disease and chronic complications, third-party dependence, and requiring a more complex management. The second group is composed of T2D patients diagnosed after the age 70; these patients have a low prevalence of microvascular complications and their glucose levels can be kept stable with one or two oral hypoglycemic agents. Both groups are represented in similar proportions. Cardiovascular risk factors were common in this age group; 60 % had hypertension, 88.7 % was taking one or more antihypertensive agents, and microalbuminuria was detected in 48.4 % of cases. These patients have a higher prevalence of geriatric syndromes (falls, motor limitations, cognitive dysfunction, and polypharmacy) [9].

T2DM patients in Latin America are exposed to endemic and highly prevalent infectious diseases (such as tuberculosis, influenza, HIV, and hepatitis C), which represent a serious comorbidity within this group. T2D increases the risk for having tuberculosis, and it is associated with a decreased rate of eradication. The epidemiologic transition from infectious to noncommunicable chronic diseases has created a unique environment in Latin American countries where the interaction of both disease trends increases morbidity and mortality associated with noncommunicable diseases [10].

Gestational Diabetes

Gestational diabetes is a common obstetric complication in the LA region. Prevalence depends on the sampling approach and the diagnostic criteria applied. It varies between 4.3 and 30.1 %; the majority of reports inform percentages close to 10 %. The use of the recently introduced IADPSG criteria results in remarkably higher percentages [11]. According to the 2015 IDF Atlas, the age-adjusted prevalence of hyperglycemia during pregnancy is 11.5 % (crude 13.2 %) in the LA region; it means that close to 0.9 million live births are affected by this condition.

Macrosomia is frequently associated with gestational diabetes. In a multinational survey, the prevalence of macrosomia was between 2.8 and 9.3 % in the LA region. This percentage was greater than that reported in Asia and Africa. Macrosomia is a strong risk factor for having cesarean section and various adverse perinatal outcomes (e.g., fetal distress and cephalopelvic disproportion).

Type 1 Diabetes Mellitus (T1D)

The IDF reported that 542,000 children (<15 years) worldwide are affected by this disease; 86,000 new cases are diagnosed every year. Prevalence of T1DM has been increasing in recent years worldwide. An annual increase in incidence of 3 % has been recorded.

The estimated number of cases in LA is 45,100; 7,300 new cases are diagnosed every year. Two of the top ten countries with the highest number of cases are located in the region (Brazil (30,900) and Mexico (13,500)). However, none of the countries with the highest number of new cases per year are located in LA. Readers should be aware that it is likely that these numbers are underestimated due to the lack of national registries in the majority of the countries of the region. The information about the epidemiology of T1DM in this region is scant [12].

In most high-income countries, the majority of diabetes in children and adolescents is caused by T1DM. This statement does not apply for the LA region. The growth in the number of children with diabetes is mainly caused by T2D. In Mexico, half of the children with diabetes are obese, do not have positive titers of GAD antibodies, and are controlled with oral glucose-lowering agents.

The WHO coordinated a Multinational Project for Childhood Diabetes (DIAMOND) from 1990 to 1999 in order to monitor the patterns of worldwide incidence of T1DM in children up to the year 2000 [13]. The Diabetes and Genetic Epidemiology Unit of the National Public Health Institute in Helsinki, Finland served as the coordinator unit, and 100 centers from 50 countries around the world headed by a principal investigator were recruited. To be eligible, the center must have an accurate, well-defined, population-based registry. The inclusion criteria considered children 0–14 years with residency in the study area. Fifty countries participated in this program. Seventy-five million children fitted the inclusion criteria and 19,164 were diagnosed with T1DM from 1990 to 1994, according to WHO classification and diagnostic criteria. Ten Latin American countries (Argentina, Brazil, Chile, Colombia, Paraguay, Peru, Uruguay, Venezuela, Cuba, and Mexico) participated with 13 centers. The overall age-adjusted incidence of T1D varied from 0.1/100,000 per year in Zunyi, China, and Venezuela to 36.8/100,000 in Sardinia and 36.5/100,000 in Finland (350-fold variation among 100 populations around the world). The incidence among populations in South America ranged from intermediate to very low. The highest incidence rates were among European and North American populations [14, 15]. The incidence rates for T1DM in Latin American countries are lower than those described in Spain (12.4/100,000 (11.7–13.1)) or Portugal (14.6/100,000 (10.6–19.6)), suggesting that the Amerindian genetic background might be protective against T1DM development. Native unmixed minority groups remain in rural areas of Mexico,

Table 7.3 Incidence of type 1 diabetes in Latin America per 100,000 persons aged 14 years or younger

Country	Study period	Incidence (%) (95 % CI)	Annual change of incidence	Estimate of ascertainment (%)
Puerto Rico	1990–1999	16.8 (16.0–17.6)	−1.0 (−2.7; 0.7)	90–97
Uruguay (Montevideo)	1992	8.3 (5.4–11.7)	[a]	97
Brazil (Sao Paulo)	1990–1992	8.0 (5.53–11.14)	−16 (−48.6; 37.2)	70–95
Argentina (Avellaneda)	1990–1996	6.3 (5.7–11.1)	0.4 (−8.8; 10.5)	88–100
Argentina (Tierra del Fuego)	1993–1996	10.3 (5.5–18.5)	[a]	100
Colombia (Bogota)	1990	3.8 (2.9–4.9)	[a]	97
Colombia (Cali)	1995–1999	0.5 (0.3–0.7)	[a]	–
Chile (Santiago)	1990–1999	3.7 (3.4–4.0)	7.5 (4.3; 10.9)	100
Cuba	1990–1999	2.3 (2.2–2.5)	−10.8 (−13.4; −8.2)	25–100
Mexico (Veracruz)	1990–1993	1.5 (0.7–2.9)	–	100
Paraguay	1990–1999	0.9 (0.8–1.0)	−0.5 (−5.7; 4.9)	[a]
Peru (Lima)	1990–1994	0.5 (0.4–0.64)	12.1 (−7.5; 35.8)	[a]
Dominican Republic	1995–1999	0.5 (0.4–0.7)	12.6 (−11.4; 43.0)	[a]
Venezuela (Caracas)	1990–1994	0.1 (0.1–0.2)	−6.8 (−24.6; 15.3)	[a]
Hispanics in the USA	1990–1999	11.4 (10.1–12.9)	–	51–100

Adapted from *The DIAMOND Project Group* and Gómez-Díaz et al.
[a]Missing data

Bolivia, Peru, and Guatemala; very low incidence of T1DM has been reported in these groups. Furthermore, T1DM prevalence seems to be related to the proportion of Caucasoid populations in a certain country (Table 7.3).

Genomic Landscape of Diabetes in the Region

Type 2 Diabetes

Amerindian populations have an increased risk for having T2D. Populations with Amerindian ancestry comprise 27.6–63 % of the genetic background of the LA countries. The Slim Initiative in Genomic Medicine for the Americas (SIGMA) Type 2 Diabetes Consortium was set out to characterize the genetic factors that explain the higher T2DM prevalence registered within this population. The SIGMA consortium genotyped 8,214 Mexicans and Latin Americans, which included 3,848 T2DM patients (cases) and 4,366 controls and have Native American and European ancestry [16]. The higher susceptibility of the admixed Latin American population can be explained both by the high prevalence of Caucasian- and ethnic-specific risk alleles. Fifty-six of the 68 known genetic associations identified in Caucasians were replicated. The *TCF7L2* and *KCNQ1* risk alleles are highly prevalent in mestizos. In addition, two ethnic-specific associations were found. The strongest novel association was found at chromosome 17p13.1, specifically an *SLC16A11* haplotype (OR 1.29 (95 % CI 1.20–1.38)). Individuals with the risk haplotype develop T2DM 2.1 years earlier ($p = 3.1 \times 10^{-4}$) and had 0.9 kg/m^2 lower BMI than noncarriers. This frequency of this variant is very small in Europeans and Africans, moderate in Asians (~10 %), and high in the Americas' native population (50 %). This newly discovered risk allele is thought to be derived from Neanderthal introgression. Approximately 20 % of the difference in prevalence of T2DM among people with Amerindian and European ancestry can be explained by the presence of the risk allele. The second risk allele associated with T2DM in the Latin American population is the p. E508K variant of the hepatocyte nuclear factor 1-α (HNF-1α). It is present in 2.1 % of T2DM patients [17]. The p.E508K variant partially reduces transactivation activity. Although the affected gene is the cause of MODY (maturity-onset diabetes of the young)-3, the clinical profile of the patient with the p.E508K variant is undistinguishable from T2D.

Several polymorphisms have been studied among other populations; in Brazilians the *TCF7L2* rs7903166 (C/T) was associated with T2DM risk among the southern-Brazilian population. The frequency of the minor allele was 38 % in the type 2 diabetes group and 31 % in nondiabetic subjects, and this allele was significantly associated with type 2 diabetes risk (OR = 1.42, 95 % CI 1.15–1.76 for the dominant model of inheritance).

Gestational Diabetes

Few genetic studies have been focused in women with gestational diabetes in LA. Recently, Chagoya and coworkers found an association between gestational diabetes and two of the most frequently replicated T2D loci: a TCF7L2 haplotype (rs7901695, rs4506565, rs7903146, rs12243326; $P = 2.16 \times 10\text{-}06$; OR = 2.95) and a KCNQ1 haplotype (rs2237892, rs163184, rs2237897; $P = 1.98 \times 10\text{-}05$; OR = 0.55). This finding is in accordance with the strong relation that exists between T2D and gestational diabetes.

Type 1 Diabetes

As recognized by the Diabetes Epidemiology Research International Group, the ethnic diversity of the Latin American populations yields an opportunity to identify the existence of protective genotypes or the absence of susceptibility variants in the Amerindians. T1DM is a multifactorial and polygenic disease that exerts a high genetic susceptibility trait with a concordance rate in twins of about 30–50 %. Genetic variants of the human leukocyte antigen (HLA) on chromosome 6p21.3, particularly combinations of DR3/DR4, produce the highest risk, which explains nearly 50 % of the genetic contribution. Other non-HLA T1DM susceptibility genes have been identified also.

Cruz-Tapias et al. published a meta-analysis designed to estimate the risk associated with variations in HLA class II in some autoimmune diseases, including T1DM in Latin American countries. Major risk alleles related to T1DM incidence showed to be DQA1*301/*501, DQB1*201/*302/*301, and DQB1*401/*402/*405, while the protective ones were DQB1*501, DQB1*602/*603, and DQB1*11/*13/*14/*15. Meanwhile, Gorodezky et al. identified HLA haplotypes with a strong association with T1DM in Mexicans which included DRB1*0301-DQA1*0501-DQB1*0201 (OR = 21.4), DRB1*0405-DQA1*0301-DQB1*0302 (OR = 44.5), and the same DQA1/DQB1 with the HLA haplotype DRB1*0404/*0401 conferring lower risk, increasing the risk of an earlier age at onset (OR = 61.3). Finally, a meta-analysis limited to LA patients with T1D (21 studies, 1,138 cases, and 1,920 controls) found that DRB1*0301 (OR: 9.65; 95 % CI: 5.69–16.36; $p < 0.0001$), DRB1*1201 (OR: 4.84; 95 % CI: 1.97–11.91; $p = 0.001$), DQB1*0302 (OR: 4.58; 95 % CI: 3.36–6.26; $p < 0.0001$), DQA1*0301(OR: 3.02; 95 % CI: 1.37–6.65; $p = 0.0059$) and DQB1*0602 (OR: 0.19; 95 % CI: 0.11–0.33; $p < 0.0001$), DRB1*14 (OR: 0.18; 95 % CI: 0.06–0.55; $p = 0.0024$), and DQB1*0501 (OR: 0.47; 95 % CI: 0.26–0.83; $p = 0.0097$) were the most significant alleles associated with T1D. Despite of the above, Latin American populations and the Amerindian individuals have been underrepresented in the T1DM genetic studies. Future GWAS study may consider the inclusion of ethnic diverse populations composed by both high (i.e., Caucasian) and low (i.e., Amerindians) incidence groups [18–20].

Diagnosis of Diabetes and Prediabetes in the Region

T2D

Prevalence data are available for the majority of the countries of the region [21–25]. However, the design of the surveys is heterogeneous leading to contrasting conclusions even in the same country [26]. Table 7.1 shows the prevalence reported by IDF which is derived mainly from population-based surveys. Twelve Latin American countries have prevalence higher than the world average (8.3 %). More than 10 % of the adult population is affected in Chile, Puerto Rico, Nicaragua, Venezuela, Mexico, and Brazil. Prevalence is higher in urban settings, native Amerindian communities (>25 % in Canada and the USA), low-income/low-education groups, and populations that have undergone migratory movements (e.g., 25.7 % in the US/Mexico border). In Mexico, the mean age of onset is 48 years, being lower in women. The highest prevalence is found in the 55–60-year-old group. The time since diagnosis is 9.3 years in males and 8.4 years in females [27].

There is a lack of data about the prevalence of prediabetes in LA [28]. This term encloses three conditions (i.e., impaired fasting glucose (100–125.9 mg/dl), impaired glucose tolerance (2 h post-challenge plasma glucose between 140 and 199 mg/dl), and abnormal HbA1c (5.7 to 6.4 %) associated with an increased risk for having T2D in the next 10 years. The prevalence of prediabetes in Hispanics living in the USA was 36.8 % (95 % CI 32.1–41.7 %) in 2011–2012 NHANES. Regrettably, no comparable information is available in the region because only fasting glycemia has been registered in the majority of the LA population-based surveys. In the Mexican 2006 National Health and Nutrition Survey (ENSANUT, in Spanish), the prevalence of impaired fasting glucose was 19.1 % in adults aged 20–69 years old. The corresponding rate in Peru is 22.4 % [29]. This information is in clear contrast with the remarkably lower prevalence of impaired glucose tolerance (7.9 %, 42.2 million) reported for the region by the IDF.

A high percentage of T2DM patients remain undiagnosed. For example, in Mexico, half of the patients with diabetes were unaware of their condition. The undiagnosed proportion of cases in the region is not different from the rest of the developing countries but remarkably higher compared to some European countries (nearly 6 %). This percentage is even higher in young adults (70 %) or low-income groups. Several countries have implemented screening programs. The strategies are diverse. For example, Brazil had a massive screening program in 2001, based in capillary glucose tests ($n = 22{,}069{,}905$). It covered 73 % of the target population [30]. In Mexico, the adult population who attended for T2D screening in the previous year increased from 10.5 % in 2000 to 22.7 % in 2006. However, a major limitation of the screening programs is the lack of a systematic inclusion of the detected cases into treatment programs.

Incidence data are scant in the region. In the Mexico City study, Gonzalez Villalpando and coworkers found an incidence rate of 1.4 cases per 100,000 persons per year in low-income subjects [31]. Meza and coworkers using a Markov model estimated that incidence rates may vary between five and 25 cases per 100,000 persons per year among adults aged 30–90 years living in Mexico during 2010 [32]. Clearly, an unmet need in the LA area is the existence of representative cohorts of patients with and without diabetes with a long-term follow-up. Incidence data are critical to design and validate public policies.

T2DM in Mexico

Mexico has four population-based, nationwide surveys in which the prevalence of T2D has been measured (National Chronic Disease Survey [ENEC] in 1993, National Health Survey [ENSA] in 2000, and the National Health and Nutrition Surveys (ENSANUT) performed in 2006 and 2012) [33–35]. The surveys (Fig. 7.1) have

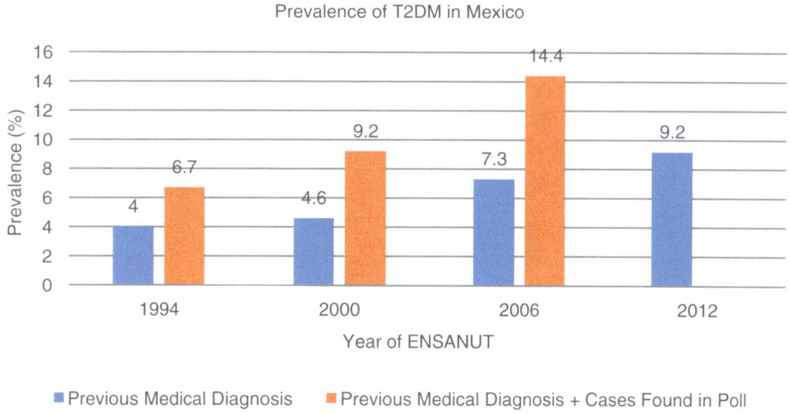

Fig. 7.1 Comparison of T2DM prevalence reported for the National Health and Nutrition Polls in Mexico for the years 1994, 2000, 2006, and 2012, comparing the cases with previous medical diagnosis and the cases with both previous medical diagnosis and the cases found by the polls (Adapted from: Hernández-Ávila et al.)

proved an increase in prevalence from 6.7 % in 1993 (previously diagnosed (PD) 4.6 % and undiagnosed (UD) 2.1 %) to 7.5 % in 2000 (PD 5.8 % and UD 1.7 %) to 14.4 % in 2006 (PMD 7.3 % and 7.1 % FP). The increases were similar for both sexes and for rural and urban areas. The growing trend in T2DM prevalence is multifactorial; aging of the population, the large proportion of Amerindian ethnic background, and an increase in the prevalence of obesity attributable to changes in the lifestyle are the most obvious explanations. Results from ENSANUT 2012 show that the prevalence of T2DM by PD is 9.2 % in adults over 20 years of age; this implies that 6.4 million Mexican adults have the diagnosis of T2DM which shows an overall doubling up from the prevalence recorded in the year 2000. A recent IDF report estimates that 11.5 million (95 % CI 6.2–13.7 million) Mexican adults are affected.

Several complimentary sources of information should be highlighted. The diabetes study of Mexico City is a population-based cohort study of subjects from six low-income colonies located within the periphery of the ABC hospital in Mexico City [36]. The recruitment of adults without T2DM diagnosis started in 1990 reaching 1,754 subjects with an average follow-up period of 11 years; after the follow-up period, an incidence of 1.42 per 100 person-years for men and 1.21 per 100 person-years for women was obtained. The resulting incidence was inferior to those obtained by a similar study undertaken in San Antonio, TX, in which an incidence of 2.7 and 2.86 per 100 person-years was obtained for men and women, respectively, despite taking into consideration different diabetes-associated risk factors. In addition, Mexico City was among the cities included in the CARMELA study, a multinational survey designed to assess the prevalence of diabetes, dyslipidemias, and other cardiovascular risk factors. Mexico City had the highest prevalence of T2D in the region.

T2DM in Brazil

According to data from the IDF, Brazil ranks fourth among countries with the largest number of people with T2DM, comprising nearly 14.3 million cases; the T2DM prevalence in Brazil has been estimated by the IDF to be 10.52 % in 2012. There is significant variability between regions ranging from 5.2 % (Brasilia) to 13.5 % (São Carlos). The Surveillance of Risk and Protective Factors for Chronic Diseases Telephone Survey (VIGITEL, in Portuguese) is a telephone surveillance system to identify risk and protective factors for noncommunicable chronic diseases in subjects aged 18 years or older; through this system, a trend of increasing prevalence rates for all NCCDs has been identified. In 2013, VIGITEL reported a prevalence of self-reported T2DM of 6.9 %. The trend of increasing prevalence has also been demonstrated for different age groups as shown in Fig. 7.2, where the prevalence ranges from 8.5 % in the 45–54-year group to 17.1 % in the 55–64-year group and 22.1 % in the groups with 65 years or older. The rates of self-reported diabetes through VIGITEL have also shown a

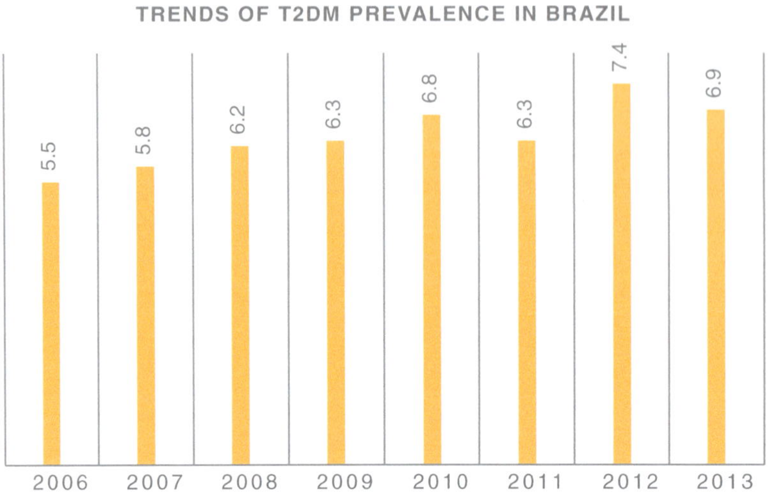

Fig. 7.2 Comparison of self-reported T2DM prevalence trends from 2006 to 2013 in the Brazilian population as reported by the VIGITEL strategy (Adapted from Almeida-Pititto et al.)

difference in its distribution: northern Brazil, characterized by lower incomes, reports T2DM rates of 3.6–5.5 %, whereas southern Brazil, with higher incomes, reports rates ranging from 6.7 to 8.2 %. The rates of T2DM have been reported to be higher specifically in Japanese Brazilians and in Native American groups (28 % of Xavantes has T2D).

Obesity rates in Brazil have similarly been escalating across all age groups; serial data from the Household Budget Survey showed that BMI >25 kg/m^2 have increased from 16 to 50 % in men and from 28 to 48 % in women. Likewise, the prevalence of BMI >30 kg/m^2 has increased from 8.9 to 12.5 % in men and from 13.1 to 16.9 % in women. Other risk factors include physical inactivity and sedentary lifestyle; in Brazil nearly 41 % of the adult population is not sufficiently active to achieve health benefits. VIGITEL has reported the prevalence of T2DM risk factors as follows: high frequency of soft drink consumption (23.3 %), alcohol abuse (16.4 %), cigarette smoking (11.3 %), and physical inactivity (33.8 %). The health system provides the full range of services for diabetes care and prevention but not universally. The federal government covers 50–80 % of costs, including basic medicines under prescription and testing strips for people with T1DM. Similar to what has been happening in other Latin American countries, the epidemiologic transition motivated by populations concentrating in urban areas, along with nutritional changes and population aging, has contributed to an accumulation of cardiovascular risk factors that have led to a general increase in the prevalence of T2DM [37–39].

T2DM in Central America

The epidemiologic transition from infectious diseases to noncommunicable chronic diseases has also changed the epidemiologic landscape within Central America. The top three countries with the highest prevalence are Nicaragua, Guatemala, and El Salvador [40]. The Central American Diabetes Initiative (CAMDI) 2010 is a study by the Pan American Health Organization with the objective to determine the prevalence of T2DM and hypertension in people 20 years or older (n = 10,822) in a sample taken from six Central American populations (urban areas of San José, Costa Rica; Santa Tecla, San Salvador, El Salvador; Villanueva, Guatemala City, Guatemala; Tegucigalpa, Honduras; Managua, Nicaragua; and the national population of Belize) [41]. Prevalence of previously diagnosed T2DM was similar among males and females (4.9 vs 5.3 %); the overall prevalence of diagnosed hypertension was higher among women (19.0 %. 95 %-CI = 16.9–21.4) than among men (10.9 %, 95 %-CI = 9.6–12.5). Overall 5.1 % of participants reported diagnosed diabetes while 3.4 % were found to have newly

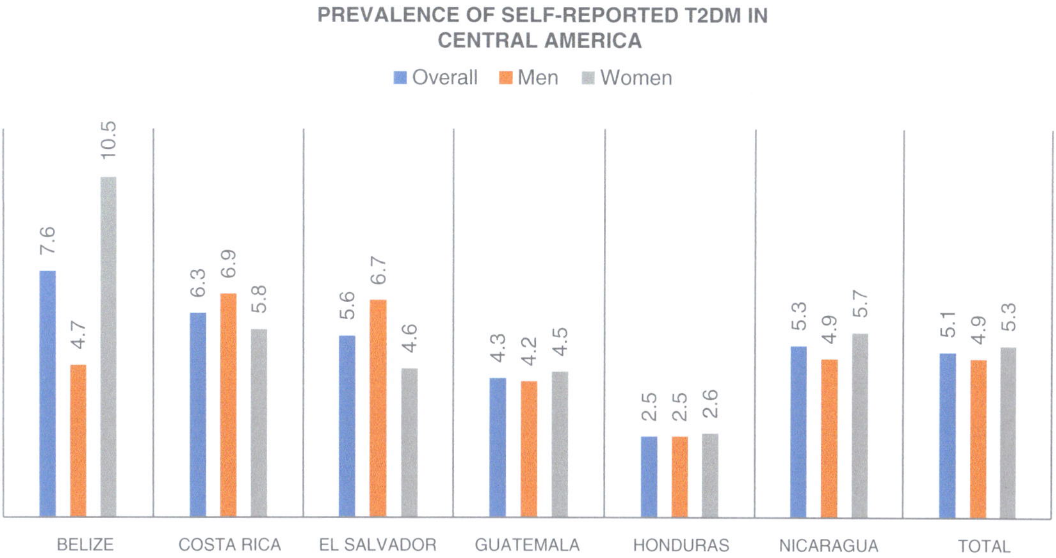

Fig. 7.3 Comparative prevalence of the sites studied by CAMDI, comparing the overall prevalence with prevalence among men, women, and overall (Adapted from: The Central America Diabetes Initiative (CAMDI): Survey of Diabetes, Hypertension and Chronic Disease Risk Factors. Belize, San José, San Salvador, Guatemala City, Managua, Tegucigalpa, and Washington, D.C.: PAHO, © 2011)

diagnosed diabetes for a total prevalence of 8.5 %. An additional 18.6 % was reported to have prediabetes (IFG and/or IGT). The prevalence of previously or newly diagnosed diabetes and prediabetes was comparable in men and women. As shown for all participant sites in Fig. 7.3, the prevalence of known and newly diagnosed T2DM was the lowest in Tegucigalpa (2.5 % and 2.9 %, respectively); the lowest prevalence of prediabetes was found in Managua (12.4 %).

In the case of Guatemala for the year 2014, the IDF reports that the prevalence in adults aged 20–79 years was 8.9 % with a total number of T2DM cases of 680,000 where nearly 107,500 cases are undiagnosed. The number of deaths attributable to T2DM in Guatemala during 2014 was 7,965 implying a cost (both direct and indirect) of 385.4 USD. For Nicaragua in the year 2014, the IDF reports a prevalence of T2DM in adults aged 20–79 years of 10.3 % with a total number of T2DM cases of 356,100, where 98,900 are undiagnosed; the number of deaths attributable to T2DM during 2014 in Nicaragua was 54.7 with a cost per person with diabetes of 221.3 USD.

T2DM in South America

After Brazil, the countries with the highest prevalence are Colombia, Chile, Argentina, and Venezuela. The CARMELA study, conducted in seven cities of South America and Mexico, found no difference in the prevalence between Barquisimeto (Venezuela), Bogotá (Colombia), Quito (Ecuador), Buenos Aires (Argentina), and Santiago (Chile) with a significantly lower prevalence only for Lima (Peru) [42].

A population-based, nationwide survey done in Peru in 2012 found a T2D prevalence of 7 % (95 % CI 5.3–8.7 %). It was estimated that 763,600 Peruvians may live with diabetes. The prevalence of previously diagnosed cases was 4.2 and 22.4 % for impaired fasting glucose. The capital city (Lima) has a higher prevalence compared to the rest of Peru (8.4 vs 6 %). Peru showed a twofold difference in the prevalence of T2DM in the urban population (8.2 %) with respect to suburban areas in the mountain and in the jungle.

In Colombia, several cross-sectional surveys have measured the prevalence of T2D in urban or rural populations. The highest prevalence (8.93 %) was reported in Cartagena in 2006. A

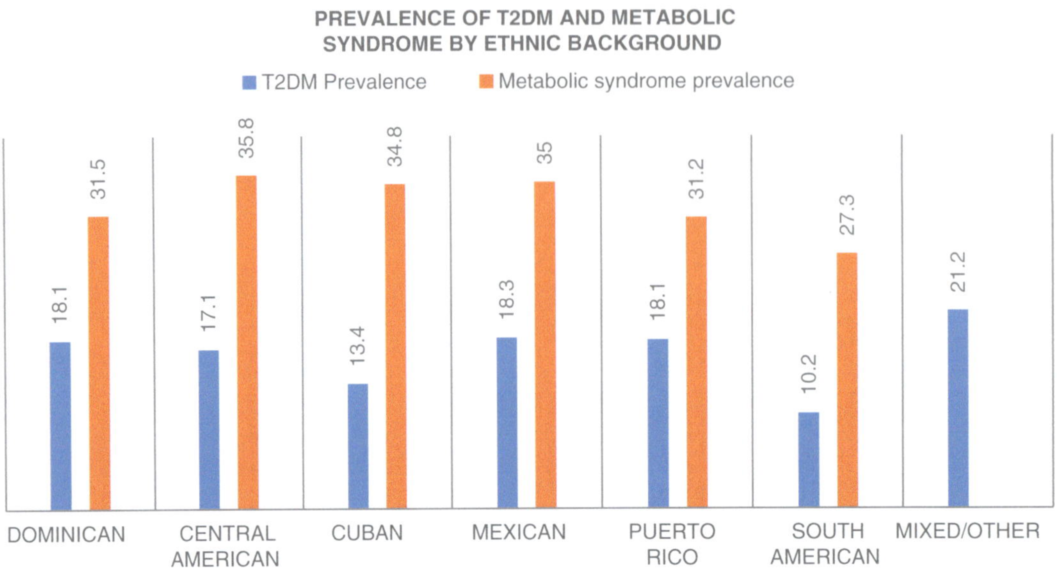

Fig. 7.4 Comparative prevalence of T2DM and metabolic syndrome by Hispanic/Latino background, comparing the overall prevalence among different ethnic backgrounds (Adapted from: Schneiderman et al. [44])

growing trend in the prevalence of the disease was observed in the time period 2009–2012 based on the number reported by institutions of the federal government. The magnitude of the increment varies from 26 % (in the Amazonas) to 153 % in Bogota [43]. Still a low prevalence has been found in rural communities.

In Argentina, the prevalence of T2D changed from 8.4 to 9.6 % between 2005 and 2009. These numbers are based on patient self-report and a nationwide survey. Argentina, Venezuela, and Uruguay have more than 90 % of their population living within urban areas.

T2DM in Hispanics/Latinos Living in the USA

The Hispanic/Latino population comprises nearly 16 % of the total US population. They are the ethnic group with the highest prevalence of T2D (22.6 % (95CI % 18.4–27.5 % in 2012 NHANES)) despite that they are not the group with the biggest mean body mass index (29.7 kg/m^2, 95 % CI 29.2–30.1) [44, 45]. Also, they are the group in which the proportion of undiagnosed cases is greater (49 %, 95 % CI 40.8–57.2 %) and the achievement of treatment goals is the lowest. Isolation, language barriers, and lack of access to medical care are among the particular challenges that should be overcome in this group [46]. The prevalence is not homogeneous between Hispanics in the USA (Fig. 7.4). Additional problems are faced when they return to their countries; it is well recognized that glycemic control deteriorates, but, there is scant data on this topic. More studies are required to understand the interaction between genetic and environmental risk factors that contribute to the increased prevalence within these minority groups and between the ethnic groups living within their country and those living in the USA.

Gestational Diabetes

The gestational diabetes screening programs applied in the region are under debate. Universal screening is the recommended approach in nearly 80 % of the reviewed guidelines. Although settings with weak health systems might struggle to implement a universal screening approach, selective screening would risk missing up a large proportion of cases. Selection would be complicated given the nature of some of the most common risk factors used to determine the need for screening. For example, history of previous GDM is likely to be missed. Likewise, ethnicity as a risk factor would qualify all patients in African, Asian, and Latin American settings as high risk.

Type 1 Diabetes

There is a lack of national registries and large cohort studies in the region. Evidence is derived mainly from single-center studies. Diagnoses and treatment of T1D are limited to reference centers. Ketoacidosis remains as a common initial T1D manifestation. A Brazilian registry (2008–2010) informed that T1D diagnosis was made based on the presence of ketoacidosis in 42.3 %; this percentage is greater than that reported in the USA (29 %) or in some countries of Europe (<20 %). Positive titers of anti-GAD antibodies were found in 64 % of recently diagnosed Brazilian T1D patients. There is no information regarding the number of at-risk individuals (based on the presence of positive titers of antibodies and/or an abnormal insulin secretion).

A growing challenge is the differential diagnosis of new-onset hyperglycemia in pediatric populations. Nearly half of children with diabetes are obese and resistant to ketoacidosis and could be treated with oral glucose-lowering agents.

T1DM in Chile

Between 1980 and 1993, a study conducted in a native aboriginal Mapuche population from Chile showed a very low incidence (0.43/100,000 per year CI 95 % 0–0.95) of T1DM in children under the age of 14 [47]. These data were significantly different from that reported for the Caucasian Chilean population in the same study (1.58/100,000 CI 95% 1.11–2.04; $p<0.0016$). Even though Caucasian heritage came mainly from Spain, incidence of T1DM in this Chilean subgroup was seven times lower than that reported for Madrid or Catalonia. A significant increase in incidence was observed in the period 2001–2004 (5.4 vs 8.33/100,000 inhabitants per year, $p<0.04$). Higher rates were observed in higher-income strata, urbanized counties, and those with low Amerindian admixture. Temporal patterns and interaction with environmental factors were postulated as potential explanations for the changes in incidence rates [48, 49].

T1DM in Uruguay

The Uruguayan population is, demographically, a mixture of Caucasian (Spain, Italy, France, Portugal, and Lebanon), Negroid (Congo and Angola), and Amerindian (mainly Charrúas, Minuanes, and Guaranies) groups; during the seventeenth and eighteenth centuries, their groups were admixed, making it impossible nowadays to find native unmixed ethnic groups as opposed to most Latin American countries. Interestingly, 92 % of the population in Montevideo is of Caucasian origin, representing one of the cities with the highest T1DM incidence according to the DIAMOND study in Latin America: 8.3 % (CI95 % 5.4–11.7) [50].

T1DM in Mexico

Limited information regarding T1DM in Mexico has been published. Data collected in the years 1978–1992 revealed a low incidence that was consistent with the figures issued by the DIAMOND project group. The study was conducted under standardized methodology proposed by the WHO in an urban area at Boca del Rio, a port located on the Gulf of Mexico in between 1990 and 1993 [51]. The average incidence rate was 1.15/100,000 per year (CI95 % 0.75–1.9). These results have positioned Mexico as the country with the lowest rates of T1D incidence. Nevertheless, Gómez-Díaz et al. [52] recently reported remarkably greater incidence rates using as source of documentation the registries of the Mexican Institute for Social Security (IMSS, in Spanish), the largest social healthcare provider within the country. Incidence among children younger than 19 years of age was calculated for a 10-year period (2000–2010); the number of new T1DM cases increased from 3.4 to 6.2 per 100,000 insured cases during the study. The highest incidence rate was observed in 2006, with 1,029 new cases within a population of 11,739,112 (8.8 new cases/100,000 insured pediatric subjects). The age groups with the biggest increment in number of cases were between the ages of 10–14 years (2.1-fold increase between 2003 and 2010) and 15–19 years (1.9-fold increase between 2003 and 2010). This study revealed a substantial increasing trend in T1DM incidence in Mexican children less than 19 years. Even though causative factors such as perinatal infections, weight gain in the first months of life, and increased maternal age might be related to the outcome, it must be considered that inclusion criteria were different for both studies.

T1DM in Argentina

Four Argentinean centers were included in the DIAMOND project. Avellaneda was the most representative city of Caucasian population; data were obtained from a retrospective study conducted from 1985 to 1988 (obtained from the national census). In addition a prospective survey was conducted from 1988 to 1994; the primary sources were preprimary and primary schools with secondary sources considering pediatric hospitals, private diabetologists, and pediatricians in Avellaneda, its surroundings, and Buenos Aires City. An annual incidence rate ranging from 6.89/100,000 per year (CI95 % 4.38–9.4) in 1985 to 7.59/100,000 per year (CI95 % 6.41–8.77) in 1990 was observed [53].

Hispanics Living in the USA

Data regarding T1DM prevalence in Hispanics living within the USA is scarce. Orchard et al. analyzed the NHANES 1999–2010 sample ($n=59{,}130$). The population-based design of the survey and the small number of cases limited the ability of the authors to provide precise estimates of the prevalence. The Hispanic population had half the prevalence of that reported in Caucasians and African Americans. The same conclusion was reached when the Mexican American subjects were analyzed as a separate group [54].

The T1DM incidence has been compared in US samples between groups with different ethnic backgrounds. One of the first studies reporting incidence was published in 1985 and was conducted in southern California between 1978 and 1981; the observed incidence rates showed an excess of cases in the Caucasian population and a lower-than-expected number of cases among Mexicans, Blacks, and Oriental populations. Other comparative ethnic studies include the SEARCH study, the Philadelphia Registry, and the Allegheny and Colorado IDDM studies [55].

Complications of Diabetes in the Region

Information regarding diabetes-related chronic complications is scant in LA. Screening procedures for retinopathy, nephropathy, and foot problems are performed without proper systematization. In the 2012 ENSANUT survey, screening for albuminuria, retinopathy, and foot abnormalities were performed in 34.2 %, 38.6 %, and 59.3 % of the T2D cases, respectively, during the previous year. In the same population-based survey, 14.6 % referred having some degree of visual problems, 13.4 % had lost sensitivity in at least one part of their bodies, 9.4 % reported having had ulcers in legs or feet, 4.9 % were blind, 3 % had some amputation, 2.3 % had been diagnosed with a diabetic foot, and 1.2 % were on dialysis [56].

T2D is the main cause of premature disability, blindness, end-stage renal disease (ESRD), and nontraumatic amputations as well as one of the ten most frequent cases of hospitalization in adults.

ESRD is a major cause of premature disability and premature mortality in the region. Registries are available in many LA countries, but in few instances the contributions of diabetes and hypertension (main causes of ESRD in all countries) are estimated separately [57]. The Latin American Dialysis and Renal Transplant Registry, founded in 1991, collected the available evidence in 2010. The ESRD prevalence has increased in the region from 119 patients per million in 1991 to 660 patients per million in 2010. The highest prevalence was reported in Puerto Rico (1,355 patients per million) followed by Mexico, Argentina, Uruguay, and Chile (between 777 and 1,136 patients per million). The higher incidence rates were reported for Mexico (458 patients per million year), Puerto Rico, Argentina, Brazil, and

Chile. The most common alternative to replace kidney function is hemodialysis (75 % of treated ESRD cases), but large differences exist between countries and health systems. The kidney transplant rate increased from 3.7 to 6.9 patients per million in the 1991–2010 period. Among countries in which the ESRD cause is registered, the contribution of diabetes is the highest in Puerto Rico (66.8 %) and Mexico (61.8 %). The smallest contributions were found for Cuba (26.2 %) and Uruguay (23.2 %).

The ESRD incidence reported for Mexico is the highest worldwide. This observation is in accordance with the increased susceptibility for having microvascular complications found in Hispanics in the USA. This population has a threefold increased risk compared to Caucasians. Furthermore, the disease burden of ESRD in the population with diabetes is remarkably bigger in Mexico compared against reported in the USA. The disability-adjusted life years (DALYs) rate due to diabetic kidney disease is several times greater in Mexico (103.1 vs 880.5 per 100,000 inhabitants). The same is true for the annual change of DALYs rate (2.5 vs 6.5 % in the 1990–2013 period) and the years of life lost (YLL) (836.2 vs 42.9 per 100,000 individuals). In contrast, the years lost due to disability (YLD) are greater in the USA (44.3 vs 60.2 per 100,000 subjects). Thus, the distribution of the disease burden is different between Mexico and the USA. While in Mexico the burden is caused mainly by premature mortality, premature disability is the main contributor in the USA.

There is a lack of information about the incidence of diabetic nephropathy and the prevalence of the various stages of the disease using as source of evidence population-based surveys.

The prevalence of diabetic retinopathy was estimated at the LA region in 1999. Sixteen countries and 7,715 patients participated. Any kind of diabetic retinopathy was found in 42 % of the cases; 17 % required immediate treatment. A large percentage had no previous eye exam [58]. Other efforts in the region have use as outcome the functional loss of vision. Using information from 15 countries and 55,643 patients (2010–2013), Limburg and coworkers found that 0.9–2.2 % of the adults older than age 50 were functionally blind. Diabetic retinopathy was responsible of 19 % of the cases in which the cause was recorded. Other common causes were age-related macular degeneration (26 %) and glaucoma (26 %). The contribution of diabetic retinopathy varied between countries, being the highest (>30 %) in Argentina, Paraguay, and Colombia. Furtado and coworkers collected the evidence published until 2012 regarding the prevalence of diabetic retinopathy in the LA region. He found 63 studies from 11 countries. However, a large proportion of the reports are based in relatively small, biased populations (studied in reference centers).

Prevalence of diabetic retinopathy is higher in Mexican Americans than in Caucasians, but this difference was not statistically significant in the 2005–2008 NHANES survey. Despite that, Mexican Americans have a significantly higher risk for having blindness as a result of diabetic retinopathy (odds ratio 3.6 (95 % CI 1.05–12.56)). There is scant information about the incidence of diabetic retinopathy. The Mexico City Diabetes Study found a 3-year incidence of 23 % in 164 cases [59].

Lower-limb amputations remain as a major cause of premature disability in the region. Diabetes is the cause of 70 % of nontraumatic lower extremity amputations. Despite that, population-based information is scant. In the Mexican ENSANUT 2012 report, 2 % of the T2D participants had an amputation and 7.2 % had at least one ulcer in the lower limbs in the past. In Costa Rica, the incidence of lower-limb amputations was 6.02 per 1,000 patients per year among the population treated by a social security system (2001–2007). This rate is unacceptably high; it is similar to that informed in other developing countries (13.7 per 1,000 cases per year) and several times higher than that reported in Great Britain (2.8 per 1,000 cases per year) and the USA (0.8 per 1,000 cases per year). Similar rates have informed in Brazil (4.3 %) and for Mexicans living in the US/Mexico border. In clinic-based cohorts, the percentage of amputee subjects is remarkably greater (13 % in a cohort from

Chile). In Mexico, 12 % of the hospital admissions among T2D patients were due to lower-limb ulcers.

Cardiovascular events are the major cause of mortality in the T2D population. The contribution of T2D among cases with an acute myocardial infarction is greater than that found in Caucasians. In the RENASICA II registry (the largest registry of acute coronary syndrome in LA, $n = 4{,}555$), 42 % of cases had T2D [60]. This percentage is greater than that found in the ACCESS (33 %) and the INTERHEART (7.2 %) studies. The same conclusion was proposed by the authors of the REACH study [61] (1,816 stable outpatients with established vascular disease). In this report, the prevalence of T2D among cases with coronary artery disease, cerebrovascular disease, and peripheral artery disease was 37.2, 37.5, and 56.8 %, respectively.

Based on T2D patients' data from the Mexican ENSANUT 2006, Reynoso-Noverón and coworkers estimated that 112 cases per 1,000 persons with T2D will suffer at least one ischemic coronary event within the next 20 years. In the same period, there will be 889,433 new cases of heart failure, 2,048,996 events of myocardial infarction, 798,188 stroke events, and 491,236 nontraumatic amputations attributable to T2D. The expected mortality rate is 539 per 1,000 persons with T2D with an average life expectancy of 10.9 years [62].

In less than 30 years (1970–2000), T2DM moved from the fifteenth to the first position among the main causes of death. This remarkable change is multifactorial. The coding system of the death certificates was adjusted to fully represent the contribution of chronic diseases (instead of the attribution of death to the final event). Recent data indicated that the mortality rate for T2DM has progressively increased. In 2013, 89,420 of the 717,357 reported deaths (12.46 %) occurred in T2D patients. The diabetes mortality rate was 73.95 per 100,000 inhabitants. Mortality rates have had a larger increase for men; the average age at death was 66.7 years [63].

The impact of diabetes in health systems should be assessed following the "Global Burden of Disease group (GBD)" approach. It considers not only the contribution of the disease to total mortality but also YLL (years of life lost) and YLD (years of life with disability). Individual profiles of each one of the countries of the region are available at the Web page of the GBD group (www.healthmetricsandevaluation.org). For Mexico, diabetes is the third cause of YLL due to premature death; this parameter grew 32 % in the time period 1990–2013. Also it is the leading cause of DALY (with an increment of 50 % from 1990 to 2013) and the fourth cause of YLDs (with a growth of 102 % in the same time period).

Brazil T2DM accounts for 5.1 % of disability-adjusted life years, according to the Global Burden of Disease project; when compared to other countries, Brazil showed a higher proportion of life years with disability among total disability-adjusted life years for T2DM. Registry data suggests that mortality standardized for age and gender in people with diabetes was 57 % higher than that of the general population. The Brazilian Study on Diabetes Costs (ESCUDI) estimated the costs of diabetes care in the public healthcare system by interviewing 1,000 patients and a retrospective analysis of their medical records; data suggests that 70.4 % of patients had at least one microvascular complication, 17 % had at least one macrovascular complication, and 16 % had at least one of both. ESCUDI estimated that the direct and indirect costs of T2DM were 1,144 USD per patient at the primary care level, reaching 2,810 USD at the tertiary level. T2DM is the fifth cause of death in Brazil. The control of hypertension, tobacco use, and dyslipidemia in recent years has decreased cardiovascular mortality in T2DM patients from an 11 % increase in the 1996–2000 period to an 8 % reduction from 2000 to 2007.

In Argentina, the crude diabetes mortality increased from 19.6 to 21.3 per 100,000 inhabitants. It is the seventh cause of death (7,701 deaths per year). The main cause of mortality is cardiovascular death. Chronic complications are common. Among patients with more than 20 years of exposure, 2.6 % had ESRD, 15.7 % had an amputation, and 6.9 % were blind. Diabetes caused in 2005 1,328,802 DALYs; it is the ninth and 11th cause of YLL for women and men, respectively.

Coordination and Delivery of Diabetes Care Services

Healthcare systems in Latin America have evolved in synchrony with the socioeconomic and political system [64]. At the end of the 1980s, several countries in Latin America thrived for a reduction in poverty and income inequalities. Despite that, big disparities persist in the region and within countries. The gross domestic product (GDP) per capita varies from close to 4,000 USD (Honduras) to 21,000 USD (Chile). In the process of those reforms, also, the organization and philosophy of their individual healthcare systems changed. Several Latin American healthcare systems have implemented or are in the process to implement healthcare reforms. Brazil, Cuba, and Costa Rica currently have unified healthcare systems with parallel subsystem organizations; other countries introduced a government-financed insurance scheme and healthcare provision to attempt a reduction at care inequalities. Despite that, four main barriers should be addressed: (1) the structural fragmentation of healthcare systems, which reduces efforts of mitigating inequalities in standards of care throughout the region; (2) the centralized decision-making processes; (3) the lack of regulation within the healthcare system, especially in terms of the quality of health-related services and quality of drugs in health systems; and (4) high costs and low efficiency. The percentage of the GDP allocated to cover health expenditures is below 10 % in the region (being Brazil the highest (9.7 %) and Venezuela the lowest (3.6 %)). A detailed analysis of the health systems of the region is beyond the scope of this manuscript. Interested readers may consult reference [65] for additional information.

In a great proportion of the LA countries, three independent sectors (public, social security, and private) provide health services. The public sector covers the population not attended by the two other providers. In many instances, the public sector offers a basic package of services that covers the ambulatory care of the main chronic disease in primary care units at a low cost or free of charge. The packages usually include generic forms of metformin, sulphonylureas, statins, acetyl salicylic acid, and regular NPH insulin. In some countries, materials required for self-glucose monitoring are provided. Limited or no access to specialists, certified laboratories, and reference centers and the lack of coverage for ESRD or other major complications are common deficiencies in this sector. The social security sector is financed by a fixed contribution by the employee, employers, and the government. A large proportion of patients with chronic diseases are treated at primary care units. Although patients may have access to specialized services, a major challenge is to avoid delays in giving access to services. Finally, the private sector offers prepaid medical plans or independent medical services.

The Pan American Health Organization has published several documents to help governments and organizations to improve the quality of diabetes care and to provide services to underserved communities [66]. Recommendations are based in the chronic care model using a patient-centered approach. With their support, several pilot studies have been implemented in Mexico [67], Chile, and Bolivia with good results. However, their impact has not been enough to change local practices.

Several health systems have launched initiatives to provide specialized care at a low cost. In Mexico, the health ministry started the UNEMES program, which is a network of primary care units operated by a multidisciplinary team (dietitian, psychologist, internist) that applies a standardized intervention against T2D and other chronic diseases [68]. Some countries (e.g., Brazil and Mexico) have developed Internet-based monitoring systems of the interventions (SysHiperDia) and policies focused in T2D [69]. In addition, reforms in the health insurance coverage have been implemented to stimulate the adoption of a healthy lifestyle among T2D patients (e.g., in Colombia) or to improve the performance of health providers (e.g., in Chile) [70]. Some conditional cash transfer programs have been linked to preventive health programs.

The direct and indirect costs of T2D treatment are remarkable [71, 72]. In the region, the annual cost of diabetes healthcare is between 34.6 and 59.9 billion US dollars; it represents close to 12 % of the total healthcare budget. This proportion is the same than mean percentage worldwide. The average annual cost per person is between 1,169 and 2,027 US dollars, which is lower to that reported in the USA and Europe (5,374–9,641 USD). There are large differences in the amount of money spent in diabetes healthcare costs between countries. In 2010, the biggest budgets were estimated for Mexico (4,836 million USD) and Brazil (4,296 million USD).

In 2010, researchers from the National Institute of Public Health in Mexico calculated that the greater direct costs correspond to medications (133,143,734 USD), followed by complication costs (110,410,928 USD), consult/diagnosis-related costs (59,734.448 USD), and hospitalization costs (39,937,331 USD). Indirect costs are mainly due to permanent disability (409,205,846 USD), followed by costs due to premature mortality (19,623,029 USD) and costs due to temporal disability (6,372,059 USD). Thus, more than half of the cost is due to indirect costs; as a result, conclusions are heavily dependent on the methodology applied to estimate the indirect costs. Out-of-pocket payments are a major challenge in the region. The average annual cost per person was 3,193 USD; the cost is bigger for cases with chronic complications (2,749 vs 3550 USD). These numbers may be underestimated. The cost of covering diabetes-related ESRD is not properly included in these estimations because a large percentage of cases do not receive a substitutive therapy of renal function. Similar numbers have been informed several reports from Argentina (reviewed in detail in Gonzalez et al. [73]).

Non-pharmacological Management

More than 80 % of T2D cases are treated by primary care physicians in the public and social security sectors. In many cases, there are significant delays in getting an appointment, and the time spent in each consultation is too short to provide proper care. A major problem of the region is lack of access to structured and efficacious treatment programs. Providers are not properly trained and do not have stimulus to improve the quality of their services and their knowledge regarding T2D. Clinical inertia is a major challenge in the region. Many health systems have dietitians involved in the treatment of T2D cases in primary care units, but, only a few have multidisciplinary teams. Access to electronic medical records is limited to some social security systems. Referral to an endocrinologist is usually late and limited to cases with chronic complications. There are not enough endocrinologists in the region. For example, Mexico has close to 800 endocrinologists that are insufficient to treat the 11.5 million cases. Despite of the above, the services provided by specialists are underutilized due to lack of awareness of the public, their primary care physicians, and the health systems. In many countries, diabetes educators are not included in the structure of health services. Certified HbA1c measurements are not available for a large proportion of the primary care clinics. Screening for chronic complications and other preventive actions (e.g., retinopathy screening) are performed at lower than expected rates. Table 7.4 shows the percentage of cases in Mexico (nationwide) and Argentina (Qualidiab network) in which preventive actions are implemented. Although the representativeness of

Table 7.4 Implementation of preventive actions against diabetes-related chronic complications in Mexico and Argentina

Preventive action (percentage, 95 % CI)	Mexico 2006	Mexico 2012 (Ref. [56])	Argentina Qualidiab 2006 (Ref. [73])
Four or more medical evaluations per year	58.8 (58.5–59.2)	65.4 (64.9–66.0)	–
HbA1c testing (at least two times per year)	3.7 (3.6–3.8)	7.7 (7.3–8.2)	40
Blood pressure measurements	50.5 (50.2–50.8)	67.9 (67.4–68.3)	99
Plasma lipid measurements	27.3 (27.0–27.6)	79.2 (78.7–79.7)	61
Microalbuminuria detection	6.6 (6.5–6.7)	12.6 (11.9–13.3)	8
Retinopathy detection	12.3 (12.1–12.4)	8.6 (8.1–9.0)	45
Diabetic foot detection	9.4 (9.2–9.5)	14.7 (14.1–15.2)	55
Follow a dietary and exercise plan	3.7 3.6–3.7)	6.8 (6.5–7.4)	2.3

these reports is different, some deficiencies are shared. Retinopathy screening and foot exams are not scheduled as needed despite that patients have frequent contacts with the medical units. A very small proportion of patients have received and implemented a dietary/exercise plan. These deficiencies could be reverted in a short period of time by quality assurance programs and training of the health providers.

Some countries have organized support networks coordinated by patients and health professionals. In addition, educational Web pages and 24-h phone lines are available. However, some of these efforts are mainly focused in providing information rather than modifying behaviors. Their impact at community level has not been measured in a systematic manner. Telemedicine is available in some countries to provide services to communities with limited access. It includes medical consultation and screening for some chronic complications (e.g., diabetic retinopathy, diabetic foot). In some countries (i.e., Argentina) legislation has been modified to give the right to patients to have continuous access to insulin and glucose strips.

Inequality is a major challenge of the region. Diabetes care is not an exemption. Despite of the above, there are highly qualified reference centers that provide state-of-the-art care of their patients in the majority of the countries of the LA region. However, the percentage of the population that has access to them is small due to limited infrastructure or economic reasons.

Rational Selection of Anti-diabetes Medications

Multiple diabetes guidelines are available in the region. Every country has legal documents that regulate local practices. In addition, most national diabetes societies have position documents, which contain the opinions of the local experts. Furthermore, the Latin American Diabetes Association (ALAD) published a set of evidence-based guidelines that take in consideration the existing information and local resources. Also, the most frequently cited international guidelines are widely disseminated among primary care physicians. Despite of the above, a large proportion of them do not have an in-depth knowledge of any of these documents.

More than 80 % of patients receive pharmacologic treatment for hyperglycemia control. It is based mainly in oral glucose-lowering drugs (generally metformin with or without sulphonylureas). The most recently introduced drugs (DPP-IV inhibitors, SGLT2 inhibitors, GLP1 agonists) are available in the Latin American markets, but, not in the majority of the public or social security systems. The proportion of insulin-treated patients (6–20 %) [74, 75] is below the international standards (30–50 %). Insulin is usually administered as a single bedtime dose in combination with oral agents. Insulin analogs are available in some social security systems. There is no information regarding the pattern of use of insulin based on nationwide surveys or registries. In addition, close to 10 % of cases are treated with herbal medicine.

As a result, the achievement of the treatment goals is lower to that reported in other regions. For example, in the 2012 Mexican ENSANUT survey, only 25 % of the patients had an HbA1c below 7 % despite that the vast majority of them have more than two medical visits per year and were treated with oral agents. Still, 50 % of patients had an A1c above 9 %. According to the Qualidiab network, 57 % of T2D cases have fasting plasma glucose above 140 mg/dl in South America [76]. In Brazil, a nationwide cross-sectional study evaluating 5,750 T2DM patients in between 2006 and 2011 found mean HbA_{1c} levels of 8.6 ± 2.2 %, with a median of 8.1 % where only 48.5 % of patients had HbA_{1c} levels <8 %.

Treatment of comorbidities share the same problems than that mentioned for the management of hyperglycemia. Statins or antiplatelet agents are prescribed in a lower than expected percentage of cases. In Mexico, according to the ATP-III guidelines, 71 % of T2D patients qualify for statin therapy; in contrast, less than 10 % of the cases were treated and controlled at the moment of the survey. In addition, nearly 50 % of T2D cases had high blood pressure; less than 10 % are treated and controlled. Similar rates have been found in Colombia. A large proportion of the hypertensive or dyslipidemic cases receive drug therapy, but only a few achieve treatment targets. The achievement of treatment goals is below to that reported in the USA [77, 78].

The Qualidiab network analyzed the efficacy of T1D treatment in patients living in several cities of Argentina and South America. A quarter of them had a blood glucose level of <80 mg/dl, and 41 % had a glucose value >140 mg/dl. Only one-quarter of the patients could play an active, effective role in DM control and treatment. Half of them were treated with a mixed dose of insulin (NPH + regular insulin), administered in two daily injections; only 9 % received three daily insulin injections.

The lack of effectiveness of the diabetes management programs is a multifactorial phenomenon. Explanations are classified as related to the healthcare provider, the service organization, and the patient. Clinical inertia, the lack of decision-making tools, and the absence of competence-based training programs are the most common barriers for the healthcare provider. With respect to the healthcare system, obstacles include attention processes designed to treat acute conditions, insufficient access to multidisciplinary teams, and other basic services and overcrowded facilities. Depression, alcoholism, physical limitations, economic problems, and lack of awareness and knowledge of the disease are the most common barriers among patients.

Translating Primary Prevention of Type 2 Diabetes

The region has undergone rapid socioeconomic changes moving from a predominantly rural society to a westernized lifestyle in less than half a century. Migratory movements to urban centers and to the more developed countries exist in a large proportion of the LA countries [79]. As a result, dramatic shifts in food availability, food preferences, and physical activity have happened. LA countries, especially Mexico, are among the biggest consumers of soft drinks and caloric-dense processed food. The proportion of the Mexican adult population who does not meet the minimum WHO-advised physical activity has increased by 6 % between 2006 and 2012. Only 28.8 % of Mexican adults had more than 150 min per week of moderate-intensity physical activity. As a result, the adoption of a healthy lifestyle for at-risk subjects and T2D cases is a challenging process. A growing trend in the region is to reduce the duration of the lactation period due to lack of adequate facilities at the work places. As a result, women do not return to the preconception weight leading to an increased risk for having T2D. In addition, there is a lack of

T2D-preventive programs applicable for women with gestational diabetes. Finally, air pollution and exposure to several environmental contaminants (e.g., arsenic, lead) are highly prevalent in some areas of the region. These are known risk factors for having T2D. Each one of these risk factors is a target for intervention to prevent chronic diseases.

Several countries have enforced action plans to mitigate the impact of diabetes. The Pan American Health Organization proposed a set of potential actions for the region in accordance with the recommendations by the World Health Organization. Taxes for sugary beverages and caloric-dense industrialized products [80], mass media campaigns, school-based interventions [81], various forms of food labeling [82], worksite interventions, food advertising regulation, changes in urban settings, and public transportation [83] are some examples. In some countries (e.g., Mexico, Brazil, Argentina, Guatemala, and others), these proposals have become public policies, and they have been integrated in a national plan against chronic diseases [84]. Still, no sufficient evidence has been published to assess the impact of these interventions. A PAHO group published the estimated impact based on a simulation model (the chronic disease prevention model) for Brazil, Mexico, and Canada. At the individual level, intervention should increase the consumption of fruits and vegetables, decrease the fat intake, raise the time devoted to physical activity, and decrease the mean body mass index, cholesterol, and systolic blood pressure of the population. According to them, fiscal measures are the public policy with the biggest impact (nearly 80,000 life years gained per year). Mass media campaigns and school-based interventions resulted in half of the effect estimated for taxation. In Mexico, primary care counseling was the most effective intervention to modify the number of disability-adjusted life years (DALYs) in the middle term. Some of these policies may take two decades or more to have a significant impact on DALYs. The intervention that requires more time to become cost-effective is the school-based lifestyle modification. The authors assume that the implementation cost will be recovered in a 10-year period. For Brazil, the estimated cost of the integrated package of preventive actions is 0.4 USD per year per capita per DALY. However, the individual cost of each public policy is remarkably different and varies between countries. A "health in all policies" approach and a coordinating body at the highest social and governmental level are critical to assure the success of the prevention plans.

National and regional (Asociación Latinoaméricana de Diabetes) nongovernmental associations are active stakeholders in the region [85]. Several academic bodies have published pro-action documents; some include critical analyses of the current approaches and alternative proposals [86].

Organizing and Conducting Diabetes Research in the Region

The remarkable impact of diabetes in the region has raised the attention of several international and regional agencies. For example, The European-Latin American and the Caribbean Health (EU-LAC Health) consortia, funded by the European Union, have sponsored calls for projects to develop low-threshold interventions to tackle diabetes and other chronic diseases [87]. The Global Alliance for Chronic Diseases, a network funded by several countries, facilitates the interaction between LA researchers and groups from developed countries to design and validate high-impact interventions in developing countries [88]. Some national funding agencies (i.e., CONACYT) have funded problem-specific calls to tackle diabetes-related issues. Although these efforts are remarkable, an integrated approach is needed to have a significant impact in the short term.

Several regional initiatives should be highlighted. The CARMEN network addresses health determinants and health equity [89]. Their products include implementation and evaluation of public policies, social mobilization, community-based interventions, epidemiological surveillance of risk conditions, and preventive healthcare services. The Slim Initiative in Genomic

Medicine for the Americas (SIGMA) Type 2 Diabetes Consortium, a collaboration between the Broad Institute, the University of Southern California, and several Mexican institutions funded by a private source, has identified ethnic-specific risk variants that explain a large proportion of the genetic susceptibility for having T2D of the Amerindian communities [16]. Finally, FunPrecal is a collaborative network between several countries of the region with Finnish and US centers to validate preventive and therapeutic interventions [90].

Innovation is a common requirement in the call for proposals published in the region. As a result, a growing number of groups are working on nanotechnology, new multidisciplinary patient-centered treatment schemes [91], telemedicine, cell-phone-based interventions or new diagnostic devices, or population-specific prognostic tests.

Future Directions: Unmet Needs, Unanswered Questions, and Unquestioned Answers

In summary, three major challenges exist in the region to mitigate the impact of T2D. First, a large proportion of the population has preceding conditions that increase their risk in the midterm. Second, half of the patients are undiagnosed, precluding the implementation of preventive actions against chronic complications. Third, the effectiveness of the treatment programs is below the international standards, resulting in high expenditures without changing the rates of premature disability and mortality. The number of preventable hospital admissions and deaths could be greatly diminished by the implementation of nationwide quality assurance programs. Budget allocation should be based on economic models and cost-effective interventions. Incentive programs may be helpful to increase productivity and quality of services; those programs should be adapted to the local culture and needs in order to create win-win relationships. A detailed analysis of the potential solutions is beyond the scope of this manuscript; interested readers should consult references [70, 86, 92].

Research is a critical component to plan and implement policies against diabetes. Still, there are several LA countries in which population-based, nationwide epidemiological information is not available. In addition, there is scant or no information in the region regarding the prevalence of T2D in pediatric or unserved populations (e.g., Native Americans or migrants). Additional studies are needed about the epidemiology of gestational diabetes, prediabetes, monogenic diabetes, and the majority of chronic complications. No incidence data exists in the majority of countries for many of the diabetes-related outcomes. National registries and translational research are at an early stage in the region. Few papers had informed the use of services or the development of diabetes-related economic models.

Despite of the above, there are unique research opportunities for the study of diabetes in Latin America. The region has peculiarities that may be used to generate new local and global knowledge to the field. For example, the ethnic composition of many countries of the region contains a large proportion of Amerindian heritage, a group that has not been sufficiently represented in the genetic consortia. In addition, the study of the interaction between infectious diseases with diabetes may offer new insights about the effects of diabetes-related abnormalities on the immune response. Environmental phenomena linked to T2D (e.g., migration, exposure to pollutants or caloric dense foods and beverages) are rapidly evolving in the region. Public policies against T2D could be tested in a shorter period of time than in other areas due to the large number of diabetes-related outcomes occurring in LA.

Actions to control the T2D outbreak in LA should come from the whole society. Although it is critical to have the support of the authorities at the highest level, it is unlikely that governmental plans could be sufficient to mitigate the health and economic consequences of the disease. Academic institutions, NGOs, and social leaders are crucial for keeping T2D among the top health priorities. Also, they introduce the innovation and the scientific background of the action plans. Everybody could contribute. At the end, prevention and treatment of T2D heavily depend on personal choices that determine people's lifestyle.

References

1. Saad PM. Demographic trends in Latin America and the Caribbean. In: CEPAL 2010. http://www.cepal.org/celade/noticias/documentosdetrabajo/6/48786/Demographic_Trends_in_LAC_PAULO_SAAD_ED_12_7_09.pdf. Accessed 26 Sept 2015.
2. Danaei G, Finucane MM, Lu Y, Singh GM, Cowan MJ, Paciorek CJ, Lin JK, Farzadfar F, Khang YH, Stevens GA, Rao M, Ali MK, Riley LM, Robinson CA, Ezzati M, Global Burden of Metabolic Risk Factors of Chronic Diseases Collaborating Group (Blood Glucose). National, regional, and global trends in fasting plasma glucose and diabetes prevalence since 1980: systematic analysis of health examination surveys and epidemiological studies with 370 country-years and 2·7 million participants. Lancet. 2011;378:31–40.
3. Food and Agriculture Organization of the United Nations. The state of food and agriculture 2013. In: FAO 2013. http://www.fao.org/docrep/018/i3300e/i3300e.pdf. Accessed 25 Sept 2015.
4. Aguilar-Salinas CA, Rojas R, Gómez-Pérez FJ, García E, Valles V, Ríos-Torres JM, et al. Early onset type 2 diabetes in a Mexican, population-based, nation-wide survey. Am J Med. 2002;113:569–74.
5. Del Brutto OH, Mera RM, Atahualpa Project Investigators. Indices of abdominal obesity may be better than the BMI to discriminate Latin American natives/mestizos with a poor cardiovascular status. Diabetes Metab Syndr. 2014;8(2):115–8.
6. Rojas R, Aguilar-Salinas CA, Jimenez A, Shamah T, Rauda J, Avila-Burgos L, Villalpando S, Lazcano Ponce E. Metabolic syndrome in mexican adults. Results from the national health and nutrition survey 2006. Salud Publica Mex. 2010;52(supl1):S11–8.
7. Gagliardino JJ, de la Hera M, Siri F. Evaluation of the quality of care for diabetic patients in Latin America. Rev Panam Salud Publica. 2001;10(5):309–17.
8. Aguilar-Salinas CA, Velazquez Monroy O, Gómez-Pérez FJ, Gonzalez Chávez A, Lara Esqueda A, Molina Cuevas V, Rull-Rodrigo J, Tapia Conyer R, ENSA 2000 Group. Characteristics of the patients with type 2 diabetes in México: results from a large population-based, nation-wide survey. Diabetes Care. 2003;26:2021–6.
9. Mehta R, Del Moral ME, Aguilar Salinas CA. Epidemiologia de la diabetes en el anciano. Rev Invest Clin. 2010;62:305–11.
10. Delgado-Sánchez G, García-García L, Castellanos-Joya M, Cruz-Hervert P, Ferreyra-Reyes L, Ferreira-Guerrero E, Hernández A, Ortega-Baeza VM, Montero-Campos R, Sulca JA, Martínez-Olivares ML, Mongua-Rodríguez N, Baez-Saldaña R, González-Roldán JF, López-Gatell H, Ponce-de-León A, Sifuentes-Osornio J, Jiménez-Corona ME. Association of pulmonary tuberculosis and diabetes in Mexico: analysis of the national tuberculosis registry 2000–2012. PLoS One. 2015;10(6):e0129312.
11. Chan JCN, Gagliardino JJ, Baik SH, Chantelot J-M, Ferreira SRG, Hancu N, et al. Multifaceted determinants for achieving glycemic control: the International Diabetes Management Practice Study (IDMPS). Diabetes Care. 2009;32:227–33.
12. Collado-Mesa F, Barceló A, Arheart KL, Messiah SE. An ecological analysis of childhood-onset type 1 diabetes incidence and prevalence in Latin America. Rev Panam Salud Publica. 2004;15(6):388–94.
13. Karvonen M, Viik-Kajander M, Moltchanova E, Libman I, LaPorte R, Tuomilehto J, Diabetes Mondiale (DIAMOND) Project Group. Incidence of childhood type 1 diabetes worldwide. Diabetes Care. 2000;23(10):1516–26.
14. Stanescu DE, Lord K, Lipman T. The epidemiology of type 1 diabetes in children. Endocrinol Metab Clin N Am. 2012;41(4):679–94.
15. The DIAMOND Project Group. Incidence and trends of childhood type 1 diabetes worldwide 1990–1999. Diabet Med. 2006;23(8):857–66.
16. The SIGMA Type 2 Diabetes Consortium. Sequence variants in SLC16A11 are a common risk factor for type 2 diabetes in Mexico. Nature. 2014;506:97–101.
17. The SIGMA Type 2 Diabetes Consortium. Association of a low-frequency variant in HNF1A with type 2 diabetes in a Latino population. JAMA. 2014;311(22):2305–14.
18. Lorenzi M, Cagliero E, Schmidt NJ. Racial differences in incidence of juvenile-onset type 1 diabetes: epidemiologic studies in Southern California. Diabetologia. 1985;28(10):734–8.
19. Vehik K, Hamman R, Lezotte D, Norris JM, Klingensmith G, Bloch C, Rewers M, Dabelea D. Increasing incidence of type 1 diabetes in 0–17 year-old Colorado youth. Diabetes Care. 2007;30(3):503–9.
20. Pettitt DJ, Talton J, Dabelea D, Divers J, Imperatore G, Lawrence JM, Liese AD, Linder B, Mayer-Davis EJ, Pihoker C, Saydah SH, Standiford DA, Hamman RF, SEARCH for Diabetes in Youth Study Group. Prevalence of diabetes mellitus in U.S. youth in 2009: the SEARCH for diabetes in youth study. Diabetes Care. 2014;37:402–8.
21. Aschner P. Diabetes trends in Latin America. Diabetes Metab Res Rev. 2002;18 Suppl 3:S27–31.
22. Atun R, Odorico-Monteiro de Andrade L, Almeida G, Cotlear D, Dmytraczenko T, Frenz P, Garcia P, Gómez-Dantés O, Knaul F, Muntaner C, Braga de Paula J, Rígoli F, Castell-Florit P, Wagstaf A. Health-system reform and universal health coverage in Latin America. Lancet. 2015;385:1230–47.
23. Whiting D, Guariguata L, Weil C. IDF diabetes atlas: global estimates of the prevalence of diabetes for 2011 and 2030. Diabetes Res Clin Pract. 2011;94:311–21.
24. Wild S, Roglic G, Green A, Sicree R, King H. Global prevalence of diabetes: estimates for the year 2000 and projections for 2030. Diabetes Care. 2004;27:1047–53.
25. International Diabetes Federation. South and Central America Region. In: IDF Atlas. 2015. http://www.idf.

org/regions/south-central-america. Accessed 12 Dec 2015.
26. Barcelo A, Rajpathak S. Incidence and prevalence of diabetes mellitus in the Americas. Pan Am J Publ Health. 2001;10(5):300–8.
27. ALAD Guidelines 2013. In: ALAD Latinoamerica. 2013. http://www.alad-latinoamerica.org. Accessed 26 Sept 2015.
28. Serrano R, García-Soidán FJ, Díaz-Redondo A, Artola S, Franch J, Díez J, et al. Estudio de cohortes en atención primaria sobre la evolución de sujetos con prediabetes (PREDAPS). Fundamentos y metodología. Rev Esp Salud Publica. 2013;87:121–35.
29. Seclen SN, Rosas ME, Arias AJ, et al. Prevalence of diabetes and impaired fasting glucose in Peru: report from PERUDIAB, a national urban population based longitudinal study. BMJ Open Diabetes Res Care. 2015;3:e000110. doi:10.1136/bmjdrc-2015-000110.
30. Nucci LB, Toscano CM, Maia ALM, Fonseca CD, Britto MMB, Duncan BB, Schmidt MI, Brazilian National Campaign for Diabetes Mellitus Detection Working Group. A nationwide population screening program for diabetes in Brazil. Rev Panam Salud Publica. 2004;16(5):320–7.
31. González-Villalpando C, Dávila-Cervantes CA, Zamora-Macorra M, Trejo-Valdivia B, González-Villalpando ME. Risk factors associated to diabetes in Mexican population and phenotype of the individuals who will convert to diabetes. Salud Publica Mex. 2014;56:317–22.
32. Meza R, Barrientos-Gutierrez T, Rojas-Martinez R, Reynoso-Noverón N, Palacio-Mejia LS, Lazcano-Ponce E, Hernández-Ávila M. Burden of type 2 diabetes in Mexico: past, current and future prevalence and incidence rates. Prev Med. 2015;81:445–50.
33. Olaiz-Fernández G, Rojas R, Aguilar-Salinas C, Rauda J, Villalpando S. Diabetes mellitus in Mexican adults: results from the 2000 National Health Survey. Salud Publica Mex. 2007;49:331–7.
34. Villalpando S, Rojas R, Shamah-Levy T, Avila MA, Gaona B, De la Cruz V, et al. Prevalence and distribution of type 2 diabetes mellitus in Mexican adult population. A probabilistic survey. Salud Publica Mex. 2010;52 Suppl 1:S19–26.
35. Gutierrez JP, Dommarco J, Shamah T, Villalpando S, Franco A, Cuevas L, Romero M, Hernández M. Encuesta Nacional de Salud y Nutrición 2012. Resultados Nacionales. In: Instituto Nacional de Salud Pública. 2012. http://ensanut.insp.mx/informes/ENSANUT2012ResultadosNacionales.pdf. Accessed 11 Oct 2015.
36. Burke JP, Williams K, Haffner SM, Villalpando CG, Stern MP. Elevated incidence of type 2 diabetes in San Antonio, Texas, compared with that of Mexico City. Mex Diabetes Care. 2001;24(9):1573–8.
37. Almeida-Pititto, Lourenço Dias M, Franco de Moraes A, Ferreira A, Reis-Franco D, Goldberg-Eliaschewitz F. Type 2 diabetes in Brazil: epidemiology and management. Diabetes Metab Syndr Obes Targets Ther. 2015;8:17–28.
38. Mendes ABV, Fittipaldi JAS, Neves RCS, et al. Prevalence and correlates of inadequate glycemic control: results from nationwide survey in 6,671 adults with diabetes in Brazil. Acta Diabetol. 2010;47:137–45.
39. Viana LV, Leitão CB, Kramer CK, et al. Poor glycaemic control in Brazilian patients with type 2 diabetes attending the public healthcare system: a cross-sectional study. BMJ Open. 2013;3:e003336.
40. Aschner P, Aguilar-Salinas CA, Aguirre L, Franco L, Gagliardino JJ, Seclen S, Vinocour M, on behalf of the IDF Diabetes Atlas. Diabetes in South and Central America: an update. Diabetes Res Clin Pract. 2014;103:238–43.
41. The Central America Diabetes Initiative (CAMDI): survey of diabetes, hypertension and chronic disease risk factors. Belize, San José, San Salvador, Guatemala City, Managua and Tegucigalpa PAHO. 2011. http://www.paho.org/hq/index.php?gid=16710&option=com_docman&task=doc_view. Accessed 12 Oct 2015.
42. Schargrodsky H, Hernández-Hernández R, Champagne BM, Silva H, Vinueza R, Silva Ayçaguer LC, Touboul PJ, Boissonnet CP, Escobedo J, Pellegrini F, Macchia A, Wilson E, CARMELA Study Investigators. CARMELA: assessment of cardiovascular risk in seven Latin American cities. Am J Med. 2008;121(1):58–65.
43. Aschner P. Eídemiologia de la diabetes en Colombia. Av Diabetol. 2010;26:95–100.
44. Schneiderman N, Llabre M, Cowie CC, Barnhart J, Carnethon M, Gallo LC, Giachello AL, Heiss G, Kaplan RC, LaVange LM, Teng Y, Villa-Caballero L, Avilés-Santa ML. Prevalence of diabetes among Hispanics/Latinos from diverse backgrounds: the Hispanic Community Health Study/Study of Latinos (HCHS/SOL). Diabetes Care. 2014;37(8):2233–9.
45. Heiss G, Snyder ML, Teng Y, Schneiderman N, Llabre MM, Cowie C, Carnethon M, Kaplan R, Giachello A, Gallo L, Loehr L, Avilés-Santa L. Prevalence of metabolic syndrome among Hispanics/Latinos of diverse background: the Hispanic Community Health Study/Study of Latinos. Diabetes Care. 2014;37(8):2391–9.
46. Cusi K, Ocampo GL. Unmet needs in Hispanic/Latino patients with type 2 diabetes mellitus. Am J Med. 2011;124 Suppl 10:S2–9.
47. Carrasco E, Pérez-Bravo F, Dorman J, Mondragón A, Santos JL. Increasing incidence of type 1 diabetes in a population from Santiago of Chile: trends in a period of 18 years (1986–2003). Diabetes Metab Res Rev. 2006;22(1):34–7.
48. Carrasco E, Ángel B, Codner E, García D, Ugarte F, Bruzzone ME, Pérez F. Type 1 diabetes mellitus incidence in Santiago, Chile. Analysis by counties in the period 2000–2004. Rev Med Chile. 2006;134(10):1258–64.
49. González RN, Torres-Avilés F, Carrasco E, Salas F, Pérez F. Association of the incidence of type 1 diabetes mellitus with environmental factors in Chile

during the period 2000–2007. Rev Med Chile. 2013;141(5):595–601.
50. Mimbacas A, Pérez-Bravo F, Hidalgo PC, Javiel G, Pisciottano C, Grignola R, Jorge AM, Gallino JP, Gasagoite J, Cardoso H. Association between diabetes type 1 and DQB1 alleles in a case control study conducted in Montevideo. Uruguay Genet Mol Res. 2003;2(1):29–35.
51. Aude Rueda O, Libman IM, Altamirano N, Robles C, LaPorte RE. Low incidence of IDDM in children of Veracruz-Boca del Rio, Veracruz. Diabetes Care. 1998;21(8):1372–3.
52. Gómez-Díaz RA, Pérez-Pérez G, Hernández-Cuesta IT, Rodríguez-García Jdel C, Guerrero-López R, Aguilar-Salinas CA, Wacher NH. Incidence of type 1 diabetes in Mexico: data from an institutional register 2000–2010. Diabetes Care. 2012;35(11):e77.
53. Sereday M, Martí M, Damiano M, Moser M. Establishment of a registry and incidence of IDDM in Avellaneda, Argentina. Diabetes Care. 1994;17(9):1022–5.
54. Menke A, Orchard TJ, Imperatore G, Bullard KM, Mayer-Davis E, Cowie CC. The prevalence of type 1 diabetes in the United States. Epidemiology. 2013;24(5):773–4.
55. Orchard TJ, Secrest AM, Miller GR, Costacou T. In the absence of renal disease, 20 year mortality risk in type 1 diabetes is comparable to that of the general population: a report from the Pittsburgh epidemiology of diabetes complications study. Diabetologia. 2012;53(11):2312–9.
56. Flores-Hernández S, Saturno-Hernández PJ, Reyes-Morales H, Barrientos-Gutiérrez T, Villalpando S, Hernández-Ávila M. Quality of diabetes care: the challenges of an increasing epidemic in Mexico. Results from two national health surveys (2006 and 2012). PLoS One. 2015;10(7):e0133958.
57. Machado-Alba JE, Moncada-Escobar JC, Gaviria H. Quality and effectiveness of diabetes care for a group of patients in Colombia. Rev Panam Salud Publica. 2009;26(6):529–35.
58. Villena JE, Yoshiyama CA, Sánchez JE, Hilario NL, Merin LM. Prevalence of diabetic retinopathy in Peruvian patients with type 2 diabetes: results of a hospital-based retinal telescreening program. Rev Panam Salud Publica. 2011;30(5):408–14.
59. González-Villalpando C, González-Villalpando ME, Rivera Martínez D, Stern MP. Incidence and progression of diabetic retinopathy in low income population of Mexico City. Rev Invest Clin. 1999;51(3):141–50.
60. Juárez-Herrera Ú, Jerjes-Sánchez C. Risk factors, therapeutic approaches, and in-hospital outcomes in Mexicans with ST-elevation acute myocardial infarction: the RENASICA II multicenter registry. Clin Cardiol. 2013;36(5):241–8.
61. Cantú-Brito C, Chiquete E, Ruiz-Sandoval JL, Gaxiola E, Albuquerque DC, Corbalán R, Ramos A, Bhatt DL, Steg PG, REACH Latin America Collaborative Group. Atherothrombotic disease, traditional risk factors, and 4-year mortality in a Latin American population: the REACH registry. Clin Cardiol. 2012;35(8):451–7.
62. Reynoso-Noverón N, Mehta R, Almeda-Valdes P, Rojas-Martinez R, Villalpando S, Hernández-Ávila M, Aguilar-Salinas CA. Estimated incidence of cardiovascular complications related to type 2 diabetes in Mexico using the UKPDS outcome model and a population-based survey. Cardiovasc Diabetol. 2011;10(1):1.
63. Barquera S, Campos-Nonato I, Aguilar-Salinas C, Lopez-Ridaura R, Arredondo A, Rivera-Dommarco J. Diabetes in Mexico: cost and management of diabetes and its complications and challenges for health policy. Glob Health. 2013;9:3.
64. Strengthening health systems: the role and promise of policy and systems research. Geneva, Alliance for Health Policy and Systems Research, 2004. Available at: http://www.who.int/alliance-hpsr/resources/Strengthening_complet.pdf.
65. Atun R, de Andrade LO, Almeida G, Cotlear D, Dmytraczenko T, Frenz P, Garcia P, Gómez-Dantés O, Knaul FM, Muntaner C, de Paula JB, Rígoli F, Serrate PC, Wagstaff A. Health-system reform and universal health coverage in Latin America. Lancet. 2015;385(9974):1230–47.
66. Barcelo A, Luciani S, Agurto I, Orduñez P, Tasca R, Sued O. Improving chronic illness care through integrated health services delivery networks. Washington, DC: PAHO HQ Library; 2012. PAHO.
67. Barceló A, Cafiero E, de Boer M, Mesa AE, Lopez MG, Jiménez RA, Esqueda AL, Martinez JA, Holguin EM, Meiners M, Bonfil GM, Ramirez SN, Flores EP, Robles S. Using collaborative learning to improve diabetes care and outcomes: the VIDA project. Prim Care Diabetes. 2010;4(3):145–53.
68. Córdova-Villalobos JA, Barriguete-Meléndez JA, Lara-Esqueda A, Barquera S, Rosas-Peralta M, Hernández-Avila M, de León-May ME, Aguilar-Salinas CA. Chronic non-communicable diseases in Mexico: epidemiologic synopsis and integral prevention. Salud Publica Mex. 2008;50(5):419–27.
69. http://www.oment.uanl.mx. Accessed Nov 16 2015.
70. Glassman A, Gaziano TA, Bouillon Buendia CP, Guanais de Aguiar FC. Confronting the chronic disease burden in Latin America and the Caribbean. Health Aff (Millwood). 2010;29(12):2142–8.
71. Arredondo A, De Icaza E. The cost of diabetes in Latin America: evidence from Mexico. Value Health. 2011;14(5 Suppl 1):S85–8.
72. Seuring T, Archangelidi O, Suhrcke M. The economic costs of type 2 diabetes: a global systematic review. Pharmacoeconomics. 2015;33(8):811–31.
73. Gonzalez L, Caporale JE, Elgart JF, Gagliardino JJ. The burden of diabetes in Argentina. Glob J Health Sci. 2014;7(3):124–33.
74. Lopez Stewart G, Tambascia M, Rosas Guzmán J, Etchegoyen F, Ortega Carrión J, Artemenko S. Control of type 2 diabetes mellitus among general practitioners in nine countries of Latin America. Rev Panam Salud Publica. 2007;22(1):12–20.
75. Legetic B, Cecchini M. Applying modeling to improve health and economic policy decisions in the

Americas: the case of noncommunicable diseases. Washington, DC: PAHO; 2015.
76. Commendatore V, Dieuzeide G, Faingold C, Fuente G, Lujan D, Aschner P, Lapertosa S, Villena J, Elgart J, Gagliardino JJ, DIFAR Academic Committee. Registry of people with diabetes in three Latin American countries: a suitable approach to evaluate the quality of health care provided to people with type 2 diabetes. Int J Clin Pract. 2013;67(12):1261–6.
77. Gakidou E, Mallinger L, Abbott-Klafter J, Guerrero R, Villalpando S, Ridaura RL, Aekplakorn W, Naghavi M, Lim S, Lozano R, Murray CJ. Management of diabetes and associated cardiovascular risk factors in seven countries: a comparison of data from national health examination surveys. Bull World Health Organ. 2011;89(3):172–83.
78. Mendivil CO, Márquez-Rodríguez E, Angel ID, Paz G, Rodríguez C, Almada J, Szyskowsky O. Comparative effectiveness of vildagliptin in combination with other oral anti-diabetes agents in usual-care conditions: the EDGE-Latin America study. Curr Med Res Opin. 2014;30(9):1769–76.
79. Reich D, Patterson N, Campbell D, Tandon A, Mazieres S, Ray N, Parra MV, Rojas W, Duque C, Mesa N, García L, Triana O, Blair S, Maestre A, Dib J, Bravi C, Bailliet G, Corach D, Hünemeier T, Bortolini M, Salzano FM, Petzl-Erler M, Acuña-Alonzo V, Aguilar-Salinas CA, Canizales-Quinteros S. Reconstructing native American population history. Nature. 2012;488:370–4.
80. Sarlio-Lähteenkorva S, Winkler J. Could a sugar tax help combat obesity? BMJ. 2015;351:h4047. doi:10.1136/bmj.h4047.
81. Jelalian E, Foster G, Sato A, Berlin K, McDermott C, Sundal D. Treatment adherence and facilitator characteristics in a community based pediatric weight control intervention. Int J Behav Nutr Phys Act. 2014;11:17.
82. Hamlin R. Front of pack nutrition labelling, nutrition, quality and consumer choices. Curr Nutr Rep. 2015;4:323–9.
83. Becerra JM, Reis RS, Frank LD, et al. Transport and health: a look at three Latin American cities. Cad Saude Publica. 2013;29(4):654–66.
84. Available at http://www.salud.gob.mx. Accesssed 16 Nov 2015.
85. Available at http://www.alad-latinoamerica.org.
86. Available at http://www.anmm.org.mx/publicaciones/CAnivANM150/L15-Acciones-para-enfrentar-a-la-diabetes.pdf.
87. Available at http://www.eulachealth.eu/es/.
88. Available at http://www.gacd.org.
89. Available at http://www.paho.org/carmen.
90. Available at: https://funprecal.wordpress.com.
91. Hernandez-Jimenez S, Garcia-Ulloa C, Mehta R, Aguilar-Salinas CA, Kershenobich-Stalnikowitz D. Innovative models for the empowerment of patients with type 2 diabetes: the CAIPaDi program. Recent Pat Endocr Metab Immune Drug Discov. 2014;8(3):202–9.
92. Tricco AC, Ivers NM, Grimshaw JM, Moher D, Turner L, Galipeau J, Halperin I, Vachon B, Ramsay T, Manns B, Tonelli M, Shojania K. Effectiveness of quality improvement strategies on the management of diabetes: a systematic review and meta-analysis. Lancet. 2012;379(9833):2252–61.
93. Villalpando S, Shamah-Levy T, Rojas R, Aguilar-Salinas CA. Trends for type 2 diabetes and other cardiovascular risk factors in Mexico from 1993–2006. Salud Pública Méx. 2010;52(supl1):S72–9.

Diabetes in the Caribbean

8

Michael S. Boyne

Introduction

The Caribbean, also referred to historically as the West Indies, consists of the Caribbean Sea, its islands and the surrounding coasts. This large geopolitical area is bordered by the Gulf of Mexico to the northwest, by the Northern Atlantic Ocean to the northeast and by the coastline of South America in the south. There are over 700 islands, islets and cays stretching over 4000 km containing a large melting pot of nations and cultures. The climate is mostly tropical, although it is subtropical in the north, but is undergoing significant climate change at present.

Prior to European immigration in the late 1400s, the population was estimated to be nearly a million indigenous people (e.g. the Kalinago, also known as Caribs, and the Arawaks such as the Taíno). These Amerindians were wiped out by disease and genocide although a few remain in the Eastern Caribbean. The influence of the European powers, along with the importation of Africans as slaves, followed by Chinese and Indian indentured labourers, as well as Middle Eastern merchants, has ensured that the Caribbean has diverse ethnic populations. There are English-speaking (Anglophone) as well as Spanish-, Dutch- and French-speaking countries (Table 8.1), and there are differences in their cultures also. The majority of Caribbean people have West African ancestry as a remnant of the African slave trade and therefore self-identify as black. Mixed-race and European peoples of Dutch, English, French, Italian and Portuguese ancestry make up a minority. Genetic admixture studies showed rates of 10–15 % for non-African ancestry [1]. Politically, most of the Anglophone countries have formed a socio-economic bloc called the Caribbean Community (CARICOM). There is moderate geographical mobility, and so several millions live outside of the Caribbean, mostly in the USA, Canada and the UK.

The total regional population was 41.9 million in 2014. According to the World Bank, the median per capita income was $8995 in 2014 (http://data.worldbank.org/region/LAC), but the range is wide as countries vary from low to high income (Table 8.1). Tourism is a major source of income for many Caribbean nations as the region has a high literacy rate, tropical weather and relative political stability.

Life expectancy has been increasing over several decades. It increased by 5 years between 1990 and 2013 [2], and it is now 74 years for men and 77 years for women according to the Pan American Health Organisation (PAHO) (http://www.paho.org/hq/index). Hence, the Caribbean

M.S. Boyne, MD, FRCPC
Tropical Metabolism Research Unit, Tropical Medicine Research Institute, The University of the West Indies, Mona, Kingston 7, Jamaica
e-mail: michael.boyne@uwimona.edu.jm

S. Dagogo-Jack (ed.), *Diabetes Mellitus in Developing Countries and Underserved Communities*,
DOI 10.1007/978-3-319-41559-8_8

Table 8.1 Populations of Caribbean countries, some of their developmental indicators, and age-adjusted diabetes prevalence among adults age 20–79 years in 2013

Country	Income level	Population (2014)	Life expectancy at birth (years)	GNI per capita in 2014 (USD)	Age-adjusted prevalence (%)
Dutch speaking					
Aruba	HI	103,400	75	24,990	13.6
Curacao	HI	155,900	77	–	14.5
Sint Maarten	HI	37,660	76	–	14.2
Suriname	UMI	538,200	71	9470	11.1
English speaking					
Anguilla	–	14,100	–	–	12.6
Antigua and Barbuda	HI	90,900	76	13,360	13.3
Bahamas	HI	383,100	75	20,980	14.2
Barbados	HI	283,400	75	14,960	12.4
Belize	UMI	351,700	74	4350	15.9
Bermuda	HI	65,180	81	106,140	12.8
British Virgin Islands	–	28,100	–	–	12.6
Cayman Islands	HI	59,170	–	–	14.3
Dominica	UMI	72,340	77	7070	10.9
Grenada	UMI	106,300	73	7850	9.4
Guyana	LMI	763,900	66	4170	15.9
Jamaica	UMI	2.721 million	73	5220	10.4
Montserrat					
St Kitts and Nevis	HI	54,940	71	14,490	13.0
St Lucia	UMI	183,600	75	7080	8.2
St Vincent and Grenadines	UMI	109,400	73	6560	10.0
Trinidad and Tobago	HI	1.354 million	70	15,550	13.0
Turks and Caicos Islands	HI	33,740	–	–	–
US Virgin Islands	HI	104,200	80	13,660	12.1
French speaking					
Haiti	LI	10.57 million	63	820	6.7
Martinique	HI	386,500	–	–	14.3
Guadeloupe	HI	403,750	79	–	6.3
St Martin	HI	31,530	79	–	–
Spanish speaking					
Cuba	UMI	11.38 million	79	5880	8.1
Dominican Republic	UMI	10.41 million	73	6030	11.4
Puerto Rico	HI	3.548 million	79	19,310	13.0

1. Data obtained from the World Bank (data.world.bank.org/country accessed on Nov 29, 2015)
2. Gross national income (GNI) per capita was calculated by the World Bank Atlas method converted to current US dollars, divided by the midyear population
3. Diabetes prevalence rates from the International Diabetes Federation (http://www.idf.org/diabetesatlas accessed on Nov 27, 2015) that were estimated by logistic regression models to produce smoothed age-specific prevalence rates for adults aged 20–79 years for 2013. This allows for direct country-to-country comparisons
4. Income level can be high income (HI), upper-middle income (UMI), lower-middle income (LMI) or low income (LI)

is rapidly ageing region. Simultaneously, infant and child mortality has fallen.

Coupled with these demographic changes, the Caribbean is undergoing a rapid nutritional and epidemiologic transition like many regions of the world [3]. In the 1940s, the most common causes of morbidity and mortality were infections. However, over the past 40 years, communicable diseases account for less than 10 % of the total mortality. Atherosclerotic complications, i.e. coronary artery disease and stroke, are now the leading cause of mortality (accounting for ~7 out of 10 deaths), and diabetes is the third reported cause in several countries. At the same time, several Caribbean countries have a double burden of infectious diseases (especially HIV/AIDS and newly emerging diseases such as chikungunya) and non-communicable chronic diseases (NCDs), which are assuming epidemic proportions contributing to morbidity and mortality [4].

Classification and Unique Aspects of the Pathophysiology of Type 1 and Type 2 Diabetes in the Region

Type 1A

Exposure to human *enteroviruses* has been implicated as an environmental factor that could trigger and accelerate the autoimmunity leading to type 1A diabetes. In Cuban studies, the presence of *enterovirus* RNA in sera from newly diagnosed patients with type 1 diabetes was significantly higher than in healthy controls (27 % vs. 3 %) [5, 6]. Also, *enterovirus* RNA was detected in sera of first-degree relatives of islet cell antibody-positive patients compared to healthy controls (16 % vs. 0 %). Molecular mimicry or the hygiene hypothesis are plausible explanations for these phenomena similar to other populations and regions.

The human T lymphotropic virus type 1 (HTLV-I) virus is endemic in the Caribbean with a prevalence of 2–5 % [7]. While endocrine disorders such as hypercalcaemia have been reported with HTLV-I, there is relatively little data about hyperglycaemia. One study [8] found a higher than expected seroprevalence of HTLV-I in Jamaicans with type 1 diabetes (i.e. 17 %). However, this initial finding is insufficient to prove a causal association and needs further study. Interestingly, HTLV-I virions use the glucose transporter type 1 (GLUT1) to infect CD4(+) lymphocytes [9].

Type 2 Diabetes

Role of Lifestyle Factors

Obesity is rising in the Caribbean as part of the global pandemic. The evidence for its role as a pathophysiologic driver of incident diabetes is overwhelming, and this is true also for the Caribbean. The population-attributable risk of body mass index for incident diabetes in the Caribbean is 66 %, and it is 80 % for waist/hip ratio, highlighting the role of adiposity [10]. The International Collaborative Study on Hypertension in Blacks (ICSHIB), which was an ecological study on the burden of NCDs in the African Diaspora, showed that the prevalence of obesity increased progressively from West Africa to the Caribbean and then to North America [11–13]. This geographical gradient in obesity also parallels the gradient in the per capita gross national product supporting a nutritional transition as the cause. Also worrisome is that the rates of annual weight increase in Jamaicans (1.37 kg/year) are significantly greater than African Americans (0.52 kg/year) and Nigerians (0.31 kg/year) [14]. Presumably this steep rise in weight gain is due to the effects of rapid cultural changes in a transitional society, and it does not bode well for incident diabetes rates.

Caribbean women have a disproportionate burden of obesity, as approximately one third of Caribbean women were obese and another third were overweight, and these rates are increasing in many countries, such as Barbados and Dominica [11]. Obesity is about half as common in men. This sexual dimorphism for obesity is different to other regions of the world where there is parity, or even greater risk, among men.

The prevalence of diabetes is closely correlated to the BMI and the amount of intra-abdominal fat (as measured by the waist circumference) across the east-to-west gradient of the Diaspora (Figs. 8.1 and 8.2) [15]. The trends in diabetes incidence and mortality paralleled secular changes in obesity. As evidence, obesity rates in Cuba plummeted in the early 1990s driven by an economic crisis, but there was a rebound followed by an overshoot several years later to its current prevalence of ~53 % when the economy and nutrition improved [16]. The population-wide increase in weight was immediately followed by a 116 % increase in diabetes prevalence and 140 % increase in diabetes incidence. A 49 % rise in diabetes mortality followed 6 years later. However, a notable exception is that Indo-Trinidadian men do not have strong correlation of diabetes prevalence with BMI [17], although this may reflect differences in intra-abdominal adipose tissue deposits.

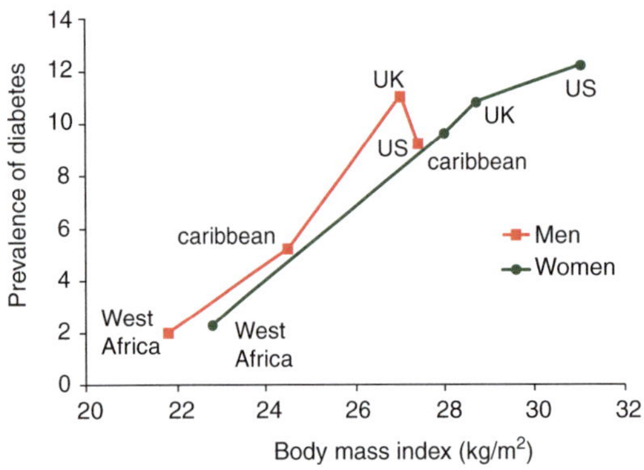

Fig. 8.1 Prevalence of diabetes mellitus (%) in the African Diaspora according to body mass index (Redrawn from data in Ref. [15])

There is a sexual dimorphism in diabetes prevalence as women have higher rates [18]. Although much of the variance is due to the higher prevalence of obesity in women, there is significant residual confounding by other factors, and this area needs more study. Clinical prediction models for diabetes in the Caribbean rely on the predictive ability of obesity using cut points of BMI (≥30 kg/m²) or central obesity (waist circumference >94 cm in men and 80 cm in women) [19, 20]. However, waist circumference is not superior to BMI in Jamaicans in its ability to predict incident diabetes [21]. Other data however suggest that the BMI cut-offs should be lower, i.e. 24.8 kg/m² (men) and 29.3 kg/m² (women). For waist circumference, these would be 88 cm and 84.5 cm for men and women, respectively [21].

Weight gain in Afro-Caribbean people may also be modified by the distribution of fat. Namely, ectopic fat deposits in the liver and within the fascia surrounding the skeletal muscle (i.e. intermuscular adipose tissue or IMAT) may

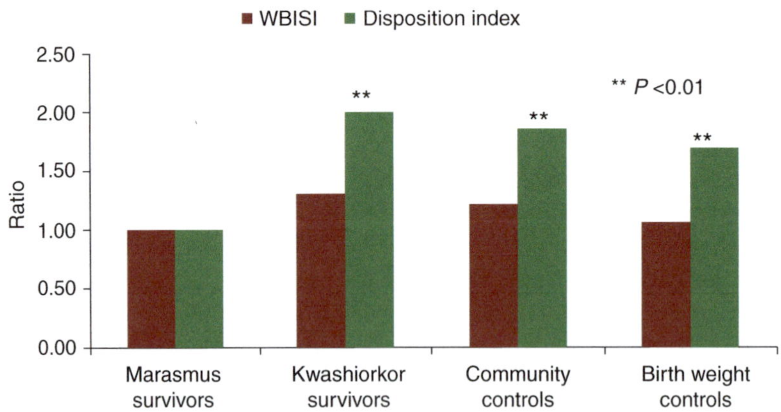

Fig. 8.2 Ratios after age, sex and BMI adjustment of glucose metabolism (WBISI and disposition index) of kwashiorkor survivors, community controls and birth weight controls compared to those of marasmus survivors. Notes: (1) ratios represent the relative differences in each outcome between the kwashiorkor group and controls with the marasmus (comparator) group. (2) Kwashiorkor is a severe acute malnutrition that occurs with moderate wasting (<60 % weight-for-age) and nutritional oedema. (3) Marasmus is a severe acute malnutrition occurring with severe wasting (<60 % weight-for-age) and no oedema. (4) WBISI is the whole-body insulin sensitivity index. (5) Disposition index is derived from oral glucose tolerance testing Data are from Ref. [44]

be independent risk factors for insulin resistance and diabetes. Afro-Caribbean women have large depots of subcutaneous fat and better adiponectin levels than men [22], so the roles of total fat, central adiposity and fat topology remain to be delineated to see if they would explain some of the excess risk of diabetes in Caribbean women. There is a dearth of data about hepatic steatosis in the region. African Americans have greater IMAT compared to Caucasians even after matching for the total body fat and skeletal muscle mass [23]. Afro-Tobagonian men have high amounts of intramuscular fat infiltration as measured by peripheral quantitative CT scan. The degree of IMAT is positively correlated with glycaemia, and this may also be modified by a family history of diabetes. Much of the variability in IMAT may be genetic, as the residual heritability (due to additive genetic effects) was 35 % [24]. IMAT may thus be of equal or greater importance than central adiposity [25]. The ectopic deposition of lipids may be higher in obese Afro-Caribbean women than in obese white women since African-American women have higher rate of fatty acid uptake and higher expression of fatty acid-transporting proteins [26].

Physical activity seems to be declining while sedentarism is increasing as part of the epidemiologic transition. The levels of physical activity in Barbadian young people are comparable to American youth [27], and both are low. There is also sexual dimorphism in physical activity as Caribbean women generally report lower levels of activity. The importance of this is underscored in urban Jamaica where severe or energetic physical activity was uncommon in men, but non-existent in women [28]. The more recent ecological study, Modelling the Epidemiologic Transition (METS), using accelerometry confirmed that moderate-to-vigorous activity only occurred for 12 min daily in Caribbean women and was lower than African populations, but similar to American women [29]. While men had moderate-to-vigorous activity about 10 min more than the women [30], they were still relatively inactive although they remained lean. The protective effect of physical activity for incident diabetes is similar to other populations in a cross-sectional analysis. So, after adjusting for body composition, a one-unit increase in physical activity level (i.e. expending 590–670 kJ or about 20 min of brisk walking daily) was associated with a 20-fold reduction in the risk of diabetes [28].

Role of Developmental Factors

It is well established that low birth weight is associated with the development of NCDs in later life [31, 32]. Birth weight is a crude marker or summation of intrauterine growth, which in turn is determined by genetic factors, maternal body composition, maternal nutrition and placental sufficiency. So, children with low birth weight are more likely to have experienced growth restraint due to intrauterine nutritional restriction or much less commonly, a genetic predisposition to low birth weight [33]. However, the association of birth weight with type 2 diabetes is "J" or "U" shaped, i.e. the prevalence of diabetes is increased in individuals at both extremes of birth weight. The mechanisms underlying this relationship are not clear. However, both beta-cell dysfunction [34, 35] and insulin resistance [34–36] in childhood and adulthood may occur at the extremes of birth weight. Other pathophysiological mechanisms involved in low-birth-weight individuals include hypothalamic-pituitary-adrenal axis activation, visceral adiposity, changes in adipocytokines and altered appetite. Large-for-gestational-age children are more likely to be the offspring of glucose-intolerant mothers. Thus, they experience intrauterine hyperglycaemia causing fuel-mediated teratogenesis, which per se may induce insulin resistance and type 2 diabetes in later life. This was demonstrated in the international Hyperglycemia and Adverse Pregnancy Outcome (HAPO) study which included more than 1200 Afro-Barbadian mothers [37].

Interestingly, fasting glucose was inversely related to birth weight in peri-pubertal Jamaican boys, but directly associated with girls [38]. This sexual dimorphism might be due to girls being intrinsically more insulin resistant as argued by some [39]. However, girls also have an earlier onset of puberty (an insulin-resistant state). Earlier menarche and greater breast development in Jamaican children were associated with higher fasting glucose even after adjusting for current BMI or prior growth rates [40]. In fact, fasting glucose increased by 0.6 mmol/L for each year reduction in the age of menarche.

In Jamaican children, shortness at birth and increased current weight are independent predictors of insulin resistance, as measured by 2-h insulin levels [41] and increased glycosylated haemoglobin levels [42]. However, data from a longitudinal birth cohort showed no relationship of birth size with insulin resistance measured in childhood [38] or in youth [43]. Probably, postnatal growth plays a role in the development of insulin resistance. So, children with faster postnatal growth during childhood (i.e. from ages 2 to 8 years) had greater insulin resistance, as measured by HOMA, in later life [38].

Prenatal factors may play a role in beta-cell dysfunction in later life as seen in animal models. So, greater maternal weight gain in pregnancy and smaller birth size are associated with reduced beta-cell function in youth [43]. This phenomenon is more clearly seen if severe acute malnutrition in infancy also occurs. Namely, if children with low birth weight are weaned early onto low-calorie feeds, they are more likely to develop marasmus (typified by severe wasting, i.e. weight-for-age <60 % but without nutritional oedema). Adult survivors of marasmus have more impaired glucose intolerance (odds ratio 10.9) than age, sex and BMI-matched community controls [44]. They have marked beta-cell dysfunction as measured by an oral disposition index, but were only marginally more insulin resistant.

It is therefore possible that intrauterine growth restriction and/or postnatal undernutrition may impair the development of beta cells during this plastic period of islet development during infancy leading to epigenetic changes that decrease insulin and PDX-1 gene expression. This would result in reduced beta-cell mass and glucose-stimulated insulin secretion in later life. Historically, up to 5 % of Caribbean populations experienced childhood severe acute malnutrition up to the 1950s, and some of these individuals may contribute to the burden of diabetes today. In Jamaican adults, declining beta-cell function is more of a driver of incident glucose tolerance more than worsening insulin resistance [45].

Other developmentally influenced mechanisms can also be in play. Hypothalamic-pituitary-adrenal axis activation by early life events could account for some of the association with glycaemia. Hence, lower birth size and earlier gestational age are associated with higher nocturnal cortisol, which in turn is associated with lower glucose effectiveness in adulthood [46]. Chronic inflammation of adipose tissue has also been implicated. As an example, faster growth in the first 6 months of life is associated with higher serum adiponectin levels in later life [47]. This implies that growth faltering in early infancy may lead to hypoadiponectinaemia in later life, which in turn is associated with insulin resistance and glucose intolerance. Finally, there may be an interaction with socio-economic status, i.e. young adults whose mothers had lower socio-economic status during pregnancy have more adverse outcomes associated with low birth size compared to those from higher status [48]. This may imply the action of other unknown environmental factors and possibly even endocrine disruptors.

The implication of these observations is important for Caribbean people. At present the average birth weight is ~3.1 kg, but there are a significant number of low-birth-weight and macrosomic babies, as well as obese mothers. If these children have growth faltering in early infancy (the first 6 months of life), or rapid growth in late infancy/childhood, they are at an increased risk of type 2 diabetes. Also, when this second generation of women later conceive, their offspring may be exposed to a hyperglycaemic intrauterine environment (and thus be born macrosomic) or experience placental insufficiency (and thus be born small for gestational age). Both conditions would increase the risk of glucose intolerance in the third generation.

Role of Other Metabolic Factors

Other metabolic factors may be involved in the development of type 2 diabetes, such as adipocytokines and oxidative stress. In Caribbean people, hypoadiponectinaemia is associated with incident glucose intolerance (OR ~0.93) [49, 50].

Heritability estimates of adiponectin suggest that genetic factors also influence the interindividual variation in circulating adiponectin levels and therefore the risk of glucose intolerance [51].

While oxidative stress (e.g. lipid peroxides such as isoprostanes) [52] and inflammatory markers (e.g. sialic acid and highly sensitive C-reactive protein) [53] may be involved in diabetic complications in Afro-Caribbean persons, they may not be involved in the pathogenesis of type 2 diabetes [45], but these studies may be underpowered. Similarly, glutathione levels are marginally lower in patients with type 2 diabetes, but are significantly low in diabetic persons with microvascular complications [54].

Chronobiology may play a role in a sex-specific manner. In Caribbean men, insufficient sleep (i.e. <6 h) or excessive sleep (>10 h) was associated with diabetes when adjusted for age, BMI and family history of diabetes (OR of 2.7 and 4.4, respectively). Surprisingly though, in women sleeping less than 6 h was associated with a reduced likelihood of diabetes (OR 0.4) [55].

Atypical Ketosis-Prone Diabetes (AKPD)/Type 1B Diabetes

In 1955, Hugh-Jones published one of the first descriptions of diabetes in the Caribbean where he observed that type 2 diabetes was more common than type 1 diabetes in Jamaica [56]. He also described an unusual variant which he called "J-type" diabetes – "J" standing for Jamaica. In more recent times, there have been other acronyms for J- type such as atypical diabetes, phasic insulin-dependent diabetes, ketosis-prone diabetes, type 3 diabetes, ketosis-prone type 2 diabetes and Flatbush diabetes. This variant was associated with insulin resistance, phasic dependency of insulin and a lean phenotype. It most resembles type 1B diabetes in the WHO classification. It is more common in non-white populations, and marginal nutritional status may play a role in some persons. In the Caribbean, there seems to be fewer cases of AKPD conceivably because improved nutrition in the Caribbean over the past several decades is making undernutrition less common. At present, Caribbean clinics are swamped with classical type 2 cases.

Patients with AKPD have periods in which they are insulin-requiring resulting in ketosis, especially during metabolic stresses, e.g. infections [57]. At other times, their need for insulin decreases such that reasonable glycaemic control can be obtained with only lifestyle modification and/or oral antidiabetic agents. Some persons have insulin resistance and others have experienced malnutrition in childhood [58]. It is conceivable that they may have reduced beta-cell mass and glucose-stimulated insulin secretion due to malnutrition in early life similar to the marasmic child [44]. Their beta cells appear to be sensitive to catabolic conditions leading to transient, decreased glucose-stimulated insulin secretion. The precise metabolic triggers (e.g. glucotoxicity, adipocytokines, non-esterified fatty acids causing lipotoxicity) are not known [59].

APKD may be a heterogeneous collection of different phenotypes with different degrees of impaired beta-cell function and autoimmunity (i.e. anti-GAD_{65} and anti-IA-2 antibodies) [57]. In an African-American series of AKPD which also contained Afro-Caribbean patients, about half had no evidence of autoimmunity (A-) with preserved beta-cell function (β+), while 22 % were A-β-, 17 % were A+β- and 11 % were A+β+ [60]. We do not have comparative data in Caribbean persons, but in one study of diabetes in Caribbean youth, who were not necessarily selected on the basis of having ketosis-prone diabetes, 30 % were A-β+, 41 % were A-β- and 39 % were A+β- or A+β+ [59, 61]. As such, some persons who have less autoimmunity, i.e. antibody negative but with preserved beta-cell reserve, demonstrate a clinical course more in keeping with type 2 diabetes despite having periods of ketosis [62]. Persons with positive autoantibodies tend to eventually need insulin therapy, while persons with preserved beta-cell function may have periods of insulin independence [57].

A few candidate genes have been examined to explain this variant of diabetes, but no genome-wide association studies have been done to date. A missense mutation Gly574Ser in the transcription factor HNF-1α was thought to be a marker of AKPD in African-American children [63]. However, this candidate mutation was not significant in Afro-Caribbean patients [64]. Other investigators working with other ethnic groups found that variants in HNF-1α and HNF-4α are unlikely to be major contributors to the pathogenesis of type 1B diabetes [65], but this is controversial [66].

Maturity-Onset Diabetes of Youth (MODY)

Like most of the world, MODY is rarely seen in the Caribbean. Even though families demonstrating multigenerational inheritance of diabetes and other characteristics consistent with early-onset type 2 diabetes have been identified, evidence of autoimmunity or sequence variants in MODY-1 to MODY-6 genes were absent [67]. Insulin promoter factor-1 (IPF-1) mutations in familial early-onset diabetes mellitus in Trinidadians have been described [68].

Diagnosis of Diabetes and Prediabetes in the Region

Type 2 Diabetes

In the 1950s and 1960s, diabetes was uncommon in the Caribbean with rates <3 % [69–71]. For example, in 1958, the prevalence was 1.4 % after screening 2325 adults for glycosuria in Trinidad [72] and 0.73 % among 958 Jamaican adults [71]. Notably, women with diabetes outnumber men as far back as 1962 in Trinidad [69], even though surprisingly they were not more overweight than the men.

By the mid-1970s, PAHO sounded the alarm for a looming epidemic of diabetes and NCDs in the region [73]. Since then, the prevalence of diabetes has increased significantly, and the Caribbean, like many developing countries, has an epidemic of obesity and diabetes. The International Diabetes Federation (IDF) estimates that the age-adjusted prevalence in 2013 was 9.6 % for the Caribbean which is the second highest in the world after the Middle East and North Africa region. There is some variation in the rates even within countries, depending on the methods used to diagnose diabetes (fasting glucose vs. oral glucose tolerance testing, 1985 WHO diagnostic criteria vs. the 1997 criteria). Table 8.1 also gives a breakdown by country where logistic regression models were used to produce smoothed age-specific prevalence rates for adults aged 20–79 years, which can allow for country-to-country comparisons. Many countries have not carried out national surveys, and their prevalence rates are extrapolated from other Caribbean countries with a similar demographic profile. Clearly it is important for each country to have their data on the burden of disease.

Naturally, incidence rates of diabetes are also high, although there is some difference based on ethnicity. In Jamaica, which is predominantly of African ancestry, the rates are 15 and 20 per 100 person-years for men and women, respectively [21]. However in Trinidad, where approximately 35 % of the population are of Indian ancestry and another 35 % are of African, the incidence of diabetes is higher in Indo-Trinidadians. The rates of Indo-Trinidadian men were 24 per 1000 person-years compared to Afro-Trinidadian men (13 per 1000 person-years) [17]. This was also similar for Indo-Trinidadian women (23 per 1000 person-years) and Afro-Trinidadian women (14 per 1000 person-years) [17]. On account of the high incidence rates, the IDF has been predicted that the prevalence of diabetes in the Caribbean will increase by 37–60 % over the period by 2035. The epidemic is set to continue as there is a significant reservoir of prediabetes. Impaired fasting glucose occurs in ~3 % [74] and impaired glucose tolerance in 13.7 % [10]. Of note, most surveys did not perform oral glucose tolerance testing, so most of the region's estimate by the IDF (13.2 %) is actually extrapolated from one late-1990s Jamaican survey [10]. Remarkably, there are little rural-urban differences [74] although there are differences by income status (lower income having higher prevalence). Undiagnosed diabetes is a heavy burden for the region and will increase the morbidity, mortality and loss of human capital. About 25 % of people with diabetes in the Caribbean are unaware of their status [74, 75].

Youth with Type 2 Diabetes

Although cases of type 2 diabetes have been reported in youth, prevalence data is missing in many countries. Anecdotally, these cases have been increasing with the increasing girth of the region's youth. In the US Virgin Islands, the incidence of type 2 diabetes in youth age ≤19 years rose significantly between 2001 (5.3/100,000) and 2010 (12.5/100,000) giving an age-adjusted annual incidence rates of 9.6 per 100,000 [76]. In Trinidadian schoolchildren, urine screening had a positive predictive value of 65 % for detecting diabetes, and it showed a prevalence of 10·4/100,000 while 7·5/100,000 had IGT [77]. This would, of course, be an underestimate compared to blood screening. In a small Jamaican study, type 2 diabetes occurred in a third of cases of diabetes diagnosed in youth less than age 25 years [78]. Affected youth were more likely to be female, older at diagnosis, obese and have a higher blood pressure when compared to those with type 1 diabetes. However, the strongest predictor of type 2 diabetes was obesity measured by BMI [78].

Type 1 Diabetes

Like many regions, type 1 diabetes is uncommon in the Caribbean. Precise prevalence and incidence data are sparse in many countries, but data exist for Bahamas and the Eastern Caribbean. The prevalence was very high (31/100,000) in Bahamian youth <age 24 years with an incidence rate of 10.1/100,000 in those age 0–14 years [79]. Incident rates are 4–5 per 100,000 person-years in persons with African ancestry in the Eastern Caribbean [80, 81] rising to a peak in the US Virgin Islands (15.3 per 100,000 person-years) [76, 81] which may reflect their higher degree of genetic admixture. The rates show some seasonal variation and a tendency for a secular increase, which augurs for unknown environmental factors being part of the aetiology such as the accelerator hypothesis [80]. About half of patients with type 1 diabetes are type 1A (with anti-GAD_{65} and/or IA-2 antibodies positivity), and half are type 1B (i.e. autoantibody negative) [61].

Gestational Diabetes Mellitus (GDM)

The epidemiologic transition would be expected to increase the risk for gestational diabetes, as well as the number of women who enter pregnancy with type 2 diabetes. About 4–13 % of Jamaican women of child-bearing age have diabetes [10, 74]. There has been an apparent increase in the incidence of GDM in Trinidad. Preliminary data show that from 2005 to 2007, the prevalence of GDM increased from 1.7 to 6.7 % with a mean prevalence of 4.3 % [82]. Unknown genetic factors may play a role. A family history of early-onset autosomal-dominant type 2 diabetes seems to increase the risk of GDM in Jamaican women (12 % vs. 1.5 % in controls, i.e. OR 9.0) which would have implications for screening [83].

Women with prior GDM are at very high risk for incident type 2 diabetes. So, among Trinidadian women with prior gestational diabetes, 62 % develop diabetes and 17 % had IGT within 7 years [84]. These data suggest that 10–18 % of women convert to diabetes per year, and the conversion to IGT occurs in another 3–5 %/year. If confirmed, these rates are extraordinarily high compared to other regions of the world [84].

Genomic Landscape of Diabetes in the Region (Local Data, if Available, or Best Approximation)

With its unique history of migration and colonisation, it is no surprise that the Caribbean is an admixed region. Most persons claim African ancestry, and one study using 28 ancestry informative markers (AIMs) found that 84–90 % had West African ancestry, 10–12 % European ancestry and 0–3 % Native American ancestry [1]. Another study using 416 AIMs found Afro-Barbadians were ~77 % African, 16 % European and 7 % Asian [85]. However, Tobagonians had the lowest rate of admixture (<6 %) [86].

Spanish Caribbean populations may have more Native American ancestry [87], and this may play a role in the development of incident type 1 diabetes in these countries. Genetic susceptibility to type 1 diabetes is determined by a combination of HLA-DQ and DRB1 genes (or a gene in linkage disequilibrium with it). In a Cuban sample, a one-unit change in European admixture proportion was associated with a 5.7-fold risk for type 1 diabetes [88]. The HLA alleles DQA1*0501, *0301 DQB1*0201 and DRB1*0301, *0401 were susceptibility alleles, while DRB1*1501, DQA1*0102/3 and DQB1*0602 were protective. In Afro-Jamaican patients, DRB1*03-DQ2/DRB1*04-DQ8, DRB1*0401-DQ8 and DRB1*0408-DQ8 genotypes increase the risk of type 1 diabetes. The DRB1*1503-DQ6 and DRB1*03-DQA1*0401-DQB1*0402 haplotypes were protective alleles. This pattern in the Jamaicans is different from the protective and predisposing haplotypes on European populations [89]. Clearly more work is needed in this area.

For type 2 diabetes, there have been a few studies utilising a candidate-gene approach as well as genome-wide association studies, although some argue that genetic factors play only a minor role among Caribbean populations [90]. A family history of diabetes in any first-degree relative (parent, sibling) or in a grandparent is associated with a two- to fourfold increased risk of diabetes [10, 91]. A family history of diabetes is probably a summary statement for several interactive related genetic, but there is limited data on specific genetic factors involved in persons of Caribbean origin.

Among the candidate genes, the transcription factor, TCF7L2, which is involved in beta-cell dysfunction, was associated with glucose intolerance in 385 Afro-Caribbean persons living in the UK [92]. This seems persistent among nonmigrant populations as among ~1000 Jamaicans, TCF7L2 was associated with decreased beta-cell function (as measured by HOMA-%B) (unpublished data).

Mutations in the ATP-sensitive potassium channel (KCNJ11) in the beta cell are also associated with impaired glucose-stimulated insulin secretion. The common variant E23K was significantly associated with type 2 diabetes in Indo-Trinidadians (OR = 1.8) along with a few other (novel) missense mutations A94P and R369C and S118L (in an Afro-Trinidadian) [93].

Candidate-gene approaches for insulin resistance have not been very successful. The PC-1 (ENPP1) K121Q polymorphism is not significantly associated (Colin A. McKenzie, personal communication, 2015). Variants in peroxisome proliferator-activated receptor gamma (PPARG), and the obesity-associated gene, FTO, have not been well investigated in Caribbean populations. The Trp64Arg mutation of the beta3-adrenergic receptor has been associated with hyperglycaemia and obesity in women, but not in men [94].

Persons of African ancestry have more fat infiltration of skeletal muscle fat than Europeans. Since this is a heritable polygenic trait, a candidate-gene study examined non-synonymous coding variants in carnitine palmitoyltransferase-1B (CPT1B). CPT1B is an enzyme that regulates skeletal muscle mitochondrial beta oxidation of long-chain fatty acids. The G531L and I66V variants were associated with ectopic fat infiltration in the skeletal muscle among 1774 older men from the population-based Tobago Health Study [95].

Genome-wide association studies by the Genetic Investigation of ANthropometric Trait (GIANT) consortium showed several single nucleotide polymorphisms associated with adiposity. Using the phenotype, waist/hip ratio after adjusting for body mass index, they identified several SNPs (49 loci of which 33 were new), and the effect size was stronger in women among 20 of these SNPs. These SNPs localised to pathways involved in adipogenesis, angiogenesis, transcriptional regulation, white adipose tissue differentiation, insulin resistance, adipose inflammation (including adiponectin) and fat topography in the 14,371 individuals of non-European ancestry, which also included 2437 Afro-Jamaican individuals [96, 97].

Complications of Diabetes in the Region

Health Disparities in Complications

People of African ancestry including Afro-Caribbean populations have lower rates of myocardial infarction compared to Caucasians [98,

99], but conversely stroke [100] and renal failure [101] rates are higher. It is not clear why such disparities exist, but genetic factors [98], coexisting cardiometabolic risk factors [100], access to care and intensity of therapeutic control of risk factors are potential culprits. There is limited data on genetic factors influencing complications in diabetic Caribbean people. Persons of African ancestry have higher systolic blood pressures, but lower triglyceride and total cholesterol levels [99]. Hypertension occurs in 52 % and 35 % of diabetic Jamaican women and men, respectively [10], and there may be less nocturnal dipping of blood pressure [102]. Tobacco use is relatively low in diabetic persons [10] compared to developed countries. As a result, these co-morbid cardiovascular differences may explain some of the higher rates of stroke and renal failure (which are sensitive to blood pressure), and the less atherogenic lipid profile may reduce the risk of coronary artery disease. Notably, youth with diabetes have a more adverse cardiometabolic pattern and thus may be more at risk of complications [103], as was also seen in the SEARCH study.

Mortality and Macroangiopathy (Coronary Heart Disease and Stroke)

The leading cause of death in the Caribbean is ischemic heart disease, and stroke is the second of which diabetes is a major cause [104]. Also, diabetes is the leading causes of disability-adjusted life years. Mortality rates from diabetes have increased dramatically, i.e. 63 % from 1980 to 1990. Diabetes-attributable macrovascular complications are affected by ethnicity. The population-attributable mortality of Indo-Trinidadians is 2.9–6.9 times higher than other ethnic groups [98, 105], and most of this is due to diabetes-induced cardiovascular disease. The age-adjusted death rates due to diabetes in 2000 were 25, 46, 56, 58 and 108 per 100,000 world standard population for Suriname, Bahamas, Barbados, Jamaica and Trinidad, respectively, according to PAHO (Health Statistics for the Americas, 2006 Edition, PAHO). In North America, the rates are less than 16 per 100,000, so these data show significant health disparities. In Barbados, diabetes accounted for an excess mortality of 42 %, and there was a 9 % increase in all-cause mortality for each 1 % increase in A1c [91]. However, there is dearth in data in other Caribbean countries about specific macrovascular complications and their mortality. Cardiovascular disease is present in almost 60 % of hospitalised diabetic Jamaicans and is more frequent among women [106]. Silent MI may occur in a quarter of Guadeloupian patients especially if they have left ventricular hypertrophy [107]. The atrial natriuretic peptide rs5065 (2,238T>C) C allele seems to exert a protective effect (24 % vs. 41 %, OR 0.5) in a relatively small study in Guadeloupe [108].

Diabetes-related mortality is not limited to older age groups, as 38 % of deaths occurred in people under the age of 60 [109, 110]. Mortality in people with type 1 diabetes in the US Virgin Islands is high, as cumulative survival was 98 % at 10 years, but fell to 73 % at 20 years. This high incidence rate of T1D in the US Virgin Islands may be partially responsible for the high mortality rate also seen [111].

Diabetic Foot Disease and Amputations

Diabetic foot disease has major public health consequences for the region. Approximately one of every eight patients in diabetes clinics had a major foot complication (amputation, ulcers, infection). Factors associated with these complications were neuropathy (OR 9.3), high blood pressure (OR 7.9) and longer duration of diabetes (OR 1.32) [112]. Diabetic foot disease accounted for 30 % of admissions in Barbados and 89 % of diabetes-related admissions [113]. In fact, Trinidad uses 0.4 % of their gross domestic product solely to treat patients hospitalised for diabetic foot infections [114].

Amputations for diabetic feet are disturbingly high and are among the highest in the world. Barbados has the most detailed data where the 1-year incidence of lower extremity amputations was 936 per 100,000 populations (557 per 100,000 for minor amputations and 379 per

100,000 for major amputations) [115]. Women had higher amputation rates than those reported for American Indians, and independent risk factors were poor footwear (2.7-fold increased risk), elevated HbA1c (each increase of 1 % led to a 40 % increase in amputations), peripheral neuropathy and peripheral vascular disease [115]. Postamputation mortality rates at 1 and 5 years are 31 % and 56 %, respectively, which are mostly due to sepsis and cardiovascular disease – the highest reported worldwide [116].

Most of these disparities in the Caribbean are probably due to social influences (e.g. inappropriate footwear) and healthcare delivery. However, there may be biological factors. For example, a persistent inflammatory response in diabetic ulcers is mostly due to overproduction of TNFα [117]. This persistent inflammation can be aggravated by low levels of the TNFα-receptor as is seen in persons with the allele, TRAPS P46L. Interestingly, the allele frequency of TRAPS P46L in the Barbadian population was 9.5 %, which is 30 times higher than Caucasian populations, and could contribute to these high amputation rates [118]. It is also possible that haemorheological factors, such as increased plasma viscosity and fibrinogen, may also play a role in the development of the diabetic foot [119].

Retinopathy

Some of the best data are from the Barbados Eye Study which showed that the prevalence of retinopathy was approximately 29 % [120]. Most persons had mild disease while ~8 % had moderate changes, and 1 % had severe retinopathy. Clinically significant macular oedema was found in 9 % of those with diabetes. In the same cohort after 4 years, the incidence was 32 % in those with known diabetes at baseline and 21 % in persons with newly diagnosed diabetes [121]. Clinically significant macular oedema developed in 5 %. This increased to 40 % after 9 years and the incidence of macular oedema was ~9 % [122]. Increased systolic blood pressure was a risk factor, and over 9 years the relative risk was 1.3 for every 10 mmHg increase, while using antihypertensive agents lowered the risk by a half [123]. The risk of retinopathy increased by 30 % for each 1 % increase of A1c [123]. Maculopathy was seen in 48 % of Jamaicans with type 2 diabetes 30 years ago [124] and probably remains as high. In a high-risk clinic, the frequency of diabetic retinopathy was 78 %; 30 % had background retinopathy, and 50 % of the eyes had proliferative retinopathy of which 34 % had tractional retinal detachments [125]. Besides retinopathy, the burden of glaucoma and cataracts is also high [91]. These data clearly demonstrate the need for retinopathy screening glycaemic control and blood pressure control in prevention.

Nephropathy

In a Jamaican diabetes clinic, about 22 % had eGFR <60 ml/min/1.73 m^2, 21 % had moderate albuminuria and 62 % had severe albuminuria [126]. Data from the Caribbean Renal Registry showed that diabetes accounted for ~28 % of the cases of end-stage renal disease [127]. In many countries, diabetic persons of African ancestry have higher rates of nephropathy. One possible explanation is that the increased oxidative stress seen in Afro-Caribbean persons may be involved in increased renal damage [52]. Accordingly, Caribbean patients with microangiopathy have glutathione deficiency that is probably due to reduced synthesis and increased irreversible utilisation by non-glycaemic mechanisms [54]. Nephropathy may also be more common in atypical ketosis-prone diabetes [128] for unclear reasons.

Hyperglycaemic Crises

About 60 % of persons admitted with diabetic ketoacidosis have type 2 diabetes [129]. The prevalence of hyperglycaemic crises in the general diabetic population is unknown. Mortality was 7 % for ketoacidosis, 20 % for hyperosmolar hyperglycaemia and 25 % for persons with the mixed ketoacidosis/hyperosmolar syndrome [129].

Other Complications

Depression was present in 18 % of type 2 diabetic patients, and older age, Indian ancestry, women and co-morbidities were risk factors [130]. There are little or no data on other possible complications of diabetes such as erectile dysfunction, osteopenia, vascular dementia, dental disease and reduced lung function in the Caribbean.

Coordination and Delivery of Diabetes Care Services

Several studies have shown that cardiometabolic control of Caribbean diabetic patients is suboptimal [74] in both private and public sectors [131], although this may be improving [132, 133]. In fact, less than half attain an A1c goal of <7 %, and only a small fraction achieve the trifecta of target A1c, blood pressure and lipids [134]. Patient factors and healthcare system inadequacies probably contributed to these issues. Unfortunately many primary care clinicians are not following any guidelines [135], and, if so, periodic repetition and reinforcement [136] are needed to maintain competency.

Therefore it is no surprise that the loss of human capital and the economic costs to the region are staggering. By one conservative estimate, diabetes costs the English-speaking countries in 2000 US$218.1 million in direct costs, US$812.4 million in indirect costs and US$687 million per capita in direct costs along with 5555 diabetes-related deaths [137]. Diabetes and hypertension cost Bahamas 9.1 % of its GDP, Barbados >5 %, Jamaica 6 % and Trinidad and Tobago 8 %. These data are old and are probably a very conservative underestimate especially with the ageing of the Caribbean and its growing obesity problem. This growing economic burden is borne by individuals and the governments. Many individuals do not have the required financial resources as many have no retirement savings, pension, lack health insurance, and unemployment is high in several middle- and lower-income countries.

As a consequence of this threat to Caribbean health and development, CARICOM proposed that the "The health of the region is the wealth of the region" in their 2001 Nassau Declaration. Subsequently, CARICOM reaffirmed this commitment in the 2007 Declaration of Port of Spain to begin public health initiatives focused against NCDs including diabetes. These initiatives would include primary prevention as well as providing adequate secondary care. They specifically included antitobacco legislation, promoting healthy diets that also include indigenous foods for children, and promote nationwide increases in physical activity and national commissions to coordinate NCD interventions. CARICOM lobbied the United Nations to have a high-level meeting on NCDs which finally occurred in 19–20 September 2011 [138]. This call for a coordinated macroeconomic, multisectoral approach is a credit and desperately needed, although there was no significant funding allocation by CARICOM, which limited the implementation of secondary care. Each nation had to find the resources to achieve the goals. So, more culturally sensitive incentives to promote healthy balanced nutrition, opportunities to incorporate leisure-time physical activities as well as increasing activity during routine daily living are still needed. Many countries adopted socialised, government-subsidised approaches by providing diabetic medications and glucose monitoring supplies. Although many Caribbean countries are small, access to care is still an issue in inner cities, and rural areas are mountainous and many times relatively inaccessible. Some countries have considered mobile clinics to improve access.

There have been some efforts to standardise the clinical care of persons with diabetes. The Caribbean Public Health Agency (CARPHA) is the new single regional public health agency for the Caribbean, established in 2011 by CARICOM and began operation in January 2013. Its predecessor organisation, the Caribbean Health Research Council (CHRC), in partnership with PAHO published clinical guidelines for managing diabetes in the Caribbean primary care setting in 2006. The metabolic target goals were similar to the IDF guidelines although there was a more stringent LDL-cholesterol goal of <1.8 mmol/L. The degree of uptake and implementation appeared to be inadequate by the region's clinicians, and proper multidisciplinary diabetes management teams were not well established in many territories, leading to gaps in holistic care. Newly updated evidence-based guidelines by CARPHA are to be released in 2016 that will try to address areas such as diabetes education, the central role of diabetes self-management and the prevention of diabetic complications. The therapeutic approach will be similar to the ADA/EASD guidelines. CARPHA, along with regional universities, is attempting to establish a structured surveillance system for screening and monitoring of NCDs. Systematic screening for risk factors and strategies aimed at reducing risk factors for obesity and type 2 diabetes among schoolchildren are urgently needed [77, 139].

Non-pharmacological Management

Nutrition

As mentioned, the nutritional transition towards a more Westernised diet has helped to drive the epidemic. Several surveys have shown energy-dense, high-fat, salt are common in the region. Unfortunately, the Caribbean suffers from a lack of trained nutritionists and dietetic professionals. In response to this need, PAHO and the Caribbean Food and Nutrition Institute produced a manual on the nutritional management of obesity, diabetes and hypertension although it is now outdated, especially with the introduction of so many need foodstuffs to the market over the decade.

Encouragingly, Caribbean patients are interested in non-pharmacological management since culturally it is deemed more "natural". However, food security in certain regions poses a threat to this. There is great interest in using locally available foods like sweet potatoes and yams, but the glycaemic indices of these foods were not well documented until more recently (Table 8.2) [140–143]. The mode of cooking can also affect the glycaemic index (GI). Frying and roasting are more popular although these methods increase the GI compared to boiling. Promoting boiling can therefore be an important method for controlling postprandial spikes. In support, a randomised clinical trial showed that incorporating low-intermediate GI indigenous foods into patients' meal planning lowered A1c by 0.84 % and also improved chronic inflammation (hsCRP), homocysteine, HDL-C and triglyceride levels [144].

Table 8.2 Glycaemic indices of some staples commonly eaten in the Caribbean according to their method of cooking/preparation

Food	Boiled	Other Preparation
Cassava	–	94 (baked)
Breadfruit	47	72 (roasted)
Green banana	37	35 (fried)
Ripe plantain	66	90 (fried)
Green plantain	39	40 (fried)
Dasheen	72	–
White yam	75	80 (roasted)
Lucea yam	74	77 (roasted)
Yellow yam	68	80 (roasted)
Negro yam	73	73 (roasted)
Sweet potato	46	76 (fried), 82 (roasted)
Irish potato	59	70 (fried), 83 (baked)
Eddoes	61	–
Pumpkin	66	–
Roti	–	65 (baked)

Data adapted from [142, 143]

Diabetes Education

Diabetes knowledge tends to be poor which affects their care [145–147] but this seems to be slowly improving. Certified diabetes educators are needed although there have been attempts to fill this void over the past decade by the non-profit organisation, Diabetes Educators of the Caribbean. Lay persons in communities trained in diabetes prevention and care can provide an alternative to traditional point of care of access for diabetes management [148]. Using lay diabetes facilitators in Jamaica was associated with an A1c reduction of 0.5 % [149, 150].

Exercise

Physical activity is low especially among women, but there has been increasing interest in recreational physical activity with more gyms, personal trainers, yoga, Pilates and use of public spaces and parks for walking. A randomised trial showed 6 months of hatha yoga exercise or conventional physical therapy improved fasting blood glucose, lipid profile and oxidative stress markers and antioxidant status in Jamaican patients [151].

Nontraditional/Complementary Techniques

There is great interest by patients to use traditional herbs for glycaemic control [152]. Annatto (*Bixa orellana*) [153], bitter yam [154], cashews (*Anacardium occidentale*) [155] and chilli pepper (*Capsicum frutescens* which contains capsaicin) [156] have mild hypoglycaemic activity. Many use guinea hen weed (*Petiveria alliacea*), but it appears to have little hypoglycaemic effect [157]. This area of natural products remains of interest for local research.

Bariatric Surgery

Bariatric surgery is an emerging treatment in the Caribbean but only a very small number of persons have used it. Of these, 85 % had resolution of their diabetes, and 15 % were able to reduce their medication with improvements in quality of life and few complications [158].

Tobacco Cessation

Tobacco use is relatively low in the Caribbean compared to other regions, especially among women. More recently, many countries have passed antitobacco legislation as part of the CARICOM's drive to reduce the impact of NCDs.

Rational Selection of Antidiabetes Medications

The CARPHA and national guidelines emphasise the use of metformin as initial pharmacotherapy. Metformin has been used in the region for more than 40 years and is the most prescribed agent. Sulphonylureas are commonly used because of their low cost although anecdotally there is a significant amount of symptomatic hypoglycaemia among the elderly. Most oral agents and insulins are available in the region, and access is determined by the formulary of the countries. Many clinicians follow the ADA/EASD guidelines, which are incorporated in the updated CARPHA guidelines, and thus use medications (metformin, sulphonylureas, DPP-4 inhibitors, pioglitazone, acarbose, SGLT2 inhibitors, GLP-1 receptor agonists, basal insulin, NPH insulin, regular insulin, rapid-acting insulin analogues) depending on patient factors (cost, risk of hypoglycaemia, co-morbid disease, side effects). In government formularies, metformin, sulphonylureas, acarbose, NPH insulin and regular insulin are used most often.

Translating Primary Prevention of Type 2 Diabetes

Stemming the tide of diabetes requires primary prevention. Of course, this is the most cost-effective strategy, and the rise of NCDs threatens the fragile economies of these island nations. CARPHA instituted the annual Caribbean Wellness Day (CWD) in 2008, in an effort to strengthen public, private and civil society partnerships and to promote multi-country, multisectoral activities in support of wellness [159]. Culturally sensitive initiatives are needed but there are few studies investigating the relationships between the formation of NCD policy and culture [160].

Women

Women need special attention as most studies in the Caribbean identify a higher burden of disease in women as well as poorer glycaemic control. In the many other regions, women are at a similar or lower risk of type 2 diabetes than men, even when obesity is higher in women. This female excess may be due to a much greater excess of obesity and other risk factors in women (e.g. physical activity).

However, there may be other factors involved which need further research. These findings have major implications for preventive policies since gender-sensitive messages are needed [18].

Children and Youth

The burden of cardiometabolic risk starts early and is seen in children. In a recent study [161], about one third of Jamaican adolescents were overweight, the girls were less physically active, over 80 % had ≥3 risk factors for type 2 diabetes and cardiovascular disease and one third had the metabolic syndrome. Thus, interventions are needed to educate children to reduce their risk. A simple measure for risk stratification is the waist circumference. A waist circumference of 82 cm in young men had better sensitivity to identify insulin resistance than the IDF standard of 94 cm (45 % vs. 14 %), but the IDF standard of 80 cm for young women remains a reasonable threshold [162].

Early Life Interventions

If cardiometabolic risk can start during foetal life, it raises the issue of optimising the health of women of child-bearing age. Most specifically, this would involve ensuring a near-normal BMI prior to entering pregnancy. Interventions that start in pregnancy involving physical activity and nutrition may actually be too late in the pathophysiological chain, and thus the effect sizes are likely to be small, if any. However, prevention of excessive weight gain in pregnancy, similar to the Institute of Medicine guidelines, may be useful. Universal screening for gestational diabetes is not present in all countries, and this should also be instituted.

Organising and Conduction Diabetes Research in the Region

The Caribbean Public Health Agency is also responsible for conducting relevant research on public health priorities in the Caribbean (see http://carpha.org/What-We-Do/Research-Training-and-Policy-Development). The mandate of its Research, Training and Policy Development Unit is to promote research for health, advise governments and other stakeholders on research for health, strengthen national and regional health research systems, develop mechanisms to support priority research and promote the sharing of the region's scientific output". Some of its activities include the administration of research grants, the hosting of the annual scientific meetings, the delivery of training workshops along with the production of accompanying manuals (basic and advanced research skills, research ethics, grant writing and monitoring and evaluation) and the promotion of essential national health research. The research agenda is packed as it also includes HIV/AIDS and emerging infectious diseases, but nutrition and NCDs including diabetes are priorities. However, there is no specific set of research priorities for diabetes itself. The region's universities have accelerated their research output for diabetes although each investigator acts independently in determining their research agenda. Investigations into natural products, epidemiological surveys, behavioural studies, developmental origins and complications are more common areas. There is a paucity of clinical trials for the unique needs of the region and this needs expanding.

Future Directions: Unmet Needs, Unanswered Questions, Unquestioned Answers

The preceding description of the state of diabetes in the Caribbean would highlight that there are several areas that need attention in the future. Some are listed below in no particular order of significance:

- Greater efficiencies and synergism of research efforts across the region
- Greater understanding of the role of obesity and fat distribution
- More understanding of the nature of atypical ketosis-prone diabetes and how to effectively intervene

- Expanding foot care and better vascular salvage
- Expanding knowledge about the role of early life factors and possible primary prevention methods appropriate for the region
- Mechanistic understanding of ethnomedicine and relevant clinical studies in promising natural products
- Better systems to collect and track national data about the NCDs and their complications
- Greater development of diabetes team approaches as well as ensuring training of professionals who can be retained in the region as there is significant brain drain by migration to the North
- Useful models of health reform and funding
- Devising mechanisms for improved efficiencies of health delivery
- Gender-sensitive approaches for tailoring public health interventions
- What social re-engineering is necessary for primary prevention
- To understand the interactions between culture and health policy formation
- Health economists are needed to help frame some of the region's data into useful advice for policymakers

References

1. Benn-Torres J, Bonilla C, Robbins CM, Waterman L, Moses TY, Hernandez W, et al. Admixture and population stratification in African Caribbean populations. Ann Hum Genet. 2008;72:90–8.
2. Global, regional, and national age-sex specific all-cause and cause-specific mortality for 240 causes of death, 1990–2013: a systematic analysis for the Global Burden of Disease Study 2013. Lancet. 385:117–71.
3. Wilks R, Bennett F, Forrester T, McFarlane-Anderson N. Chronic diseases: the new epidemic. West Indian Med J. 1998;47 Suppl 4:40–4.
4. Sargeant LA, Wilks RJ, Forrester TE. Chronic diseases – facing a public health challenge. West Indian Med J. 2001;50 Suppl 4:27–31.
5. Sarmiento L, Cubas-Duenas I, Cabrera-Rode E. Evidence of association between type 1 diabetes and exposure to enterovirus in Cuban children and adolescents. MEDICC Rev. 2013;15:29–32.
6. Sarmiento L, Cabrera-Rode E, Lekuleni L, Cuba I, Molina G, Fonseca M, et al. Occurrence of enterovirus RNA in serum of children with newly diagnosed type 1 diabetes and islet cell autoantibody-positive subjects in a population with a low incidence of type 1 diabetes. Autoimmunity. 2007;40:540–5.
7. Bartholomew C, Cleghorn F. Retroviruses in the Caribbean. Bull Pan Am Health Organ. 1989;23:76–80.
8. Smikle MF, Wright-Pascoe R, Barton EN, Dowe G, Gilbert DT, Choo-Kang E, et al. Autoantibodies, human T lymphotropic virus type 1 and type 1 diabetes mellitus in Jamaicans. West Indian Med J. 2002;51:153–6.
9. Costa GC, Azevedo R, Gadelha SR, Kashima SH, Muricy G, Olavarria VN, et al. Polymorphisms at GLUT1 gene are not associated with the development of TSP/HAM in Brazilian HTLV-1 infected individuals and the discovery of a new polymorphism at GLUT1 gene. J Med Virol. 2009;81:552–7.
10. Wilks R, Rotimi C, Bennett F, McFarlane-Anderson N, Kaufman JS, Anderson SG, et al. Diabetes in the Caribbean: results of a population survey from Spanish Town, Jamaica. Diabet Med. 1999;16:875–83.
11. Luke A, Cooper RS, Prewitt TE, Adeyemo AA, Forrester TE. Nutritional consequences of the African diaspora. Annu Rev Nutr. 2001;21:47–71.
12. Luke A, Durazo-Arvizu R, Rotimi C, Prewitt TE, Forrester T, Wilks R, et al. Relation between body mass index and body fat in black population samples from Nigeria, Jamaica, and the United States. Am J Epidemiol. 1997;145:620–8.
13. Cooper R, Rotimi C, Ataman S, McGee D, Osotimehin B, Kadiri S, et al. The prevalence of hypertension in seven populations of west African origin. Am J Public Health. 1997;87:160–8.
14. Durazo-Arvizu RA, Luke A, Cooper RS, Cao G, Dugas L, Adeyemo A, et al. Rapid increases in obesity in Jamaica, compared to Nigeria and the United States. BMC Public Health. 2008;8:133.
15. Cooper RS, Rotimi CN, Kaufman JS, Owoaje EE, Fraser H, Forrester T, et al. Prevalence of NIDDM among populations of the African diaspora. Diabetes Care. 1997;20:343–8.
16. Franco M, Bilal U, Ordunez P, Benet M, Morejon A, Caballero B, et al. Population-wide weight loss and regain in relation to diabetes burden and cardiovascular mortality in Cuba 1980–2010: repeated cross sectional surveys and ecological comparison of secular trends. BMJ. 2013;346:f1515.
17. Miller GJ, Maude GH, Beckles GL. Incidence of hypertension and non-insulin dependent diabetes mellitus and associated risk factors in a rapidly developing Caribbean community: the St James survey, Trinidad. J Epidemiol Community Health. 1996;50:497–504.
18. Sobers-Grannum N, Murphy MM, Nielsen A, Guell C, Samuels TA, Bishop L, et al. Female gender is a social determinant of diabetes in the Caribbean: a systematic review and meta-analysis. PLoS One. 2015;10:e0126799.
19. Sargeant LA, Boyne MS, Bennett FI, Forrester TE, Cooper RS, Wilks RJ. Impaired glucose regulation

in adults in Jamaica: who should have the oral glucose tolerance test? Rev Panam Salud Publica. 2004;16:35–42.
20. El Mabchour A, Delisle H, Vilgrain C, Larco P, Sodjinou R, Batal M. Specific cut-off points for waist circumference and waist-to-height ratio as predictors of cardiometabolic risk in Black subjects: a cross-sectional study in Benin and Haiti. Diabetes Metab Syndr Obes Targets Ther. 2015;8:513–23.
21. Sargeant LA, Bennett FI, Forrester TE, Cooper RS, Wilks RJ. Predicting incident diabetes in Jamaica: the role of anthropometry. Obes Res. 2002;10:792–8.
22. Boyne MS, Bennett NR, Cooper RS, Royal-Thomas TY, Bennett FI, Luke A, et al. Sex-differences in adiponectin levels and body fat distribution: longitudinal observations in Afro-Jamaicans. Diabetes Res Clin Pract. 2010;90:e33–6.
23. Albu JB, Kovera AJ, Allen L, Wainwright M, Berk E, Raja-Khan N, et al. Independent association of insulin resistance with larger amounts of intermuscular adipose tissue and a greater acute insulin response to glucose in African American than in white nondiabetic women. Am J Clin Nutr. 2005; 82:1210–7.
24. Miljkovic-Gacic I, Wang X, Kammerer CM, Gordon CL, Bunker CH, Kuller LH, et al. Fat infiltration in muscle: new evidence for familial clustering and associations with diabetes. Obesity (Silver Spring). 2008;16:1854–60.
25. Miljkovic-Gacic I, Gordon CL, Goodpaster BH, Bunker CH, Patrick AL, Kuller LH, et al. Adipose tissue infiltration in skeletal muscle: age patterns and association with diabetes among men of African ancestry. Am J Clin Nutr. 2008;87:1590–5.
26. Bower JF, Davis JM, Hao E, Barakat HA. Differences in transport of fatty acids and expression of fatty acid transporting proteins in adipose tissue of obese black and white women. Am J Physiol Endocrinol Metab. 2006;290:E87–91.
27. Prochaska JJ, Sallis JF, Griffith B, Douglas J. Physical activity levels of Barbadian youth and comparison to a U.S. sample. Int J Behav Med. 2002;9:360–72.
28. Boyne MS, Gaskin P, Luke A, Wilks RJ, Bennett FI, Younger N, et al. Energetic determinants of glucose tolerance status in Jamaican adults. Eur J Clin Nutr. 2004;58:1666–8.
29. Luke A, Bovet P, Plange-Rhule J, Forrester TE, Lambert EV, Schoeller DA, et al. A mixed ecologic-cohort comparison of physical activity & weight among young adults from five populations of African origin. BMC Public Health. 2014;14:397.
30. Dugas LR, Bovet P, Forrester TE, Lambert EV, Plange-Rhule J, Durazo-Arvizu RA, et al. Comparisons of intensity-duration patterns of physical activity in the US, Jamaica and 3 African countries. BMC Public Health. 2014;14:882.
31. McKeigue PM, Lithell HO, Leon DA. Glucose tolerance and resistance to insulin-stimulated glucose uptake in men aged 70 years in relation to size at birth. Diabetologia. 1998;41:1133–8.
32. McCance DR, Pettitt DJ, Hanson RL, Jacobsson LT, Knowler WC, Bennett PH. Birth weight and non-insulin dependent diabetes: thrifty genotype, thrifty phenotype, or surviving small baby genotype? BMJ. 1994;308:942–5.
33. Gluckman PD, Hanson MA, Cooper C, Thornburg KL. Effect of in utero and early-life conditions on adult health and disease. N Engl J Med. 2008;359: 61–73.
34. Li C, Johnson MS, Goran MI. Effects of low birth weight on insulin resistance syndrome in caucasian and African-American children. Diabetes Care. 2001;24:2035–42.
35. Soto N, Bazaes RA, Pena V, Salazar T, Avila A, Iniguez G, et al. Insulin sensitivity and secretion are related to catch-up growth in small-for-gestational-age infants at age 1 year: results from a prospective cohort. J Clin Endocrinol Metab. 2003;88:3645–50.
36. Crowther NJ, Trusler J, Cameron N, Toman M, Gray IP. Relation between weight gain and beta-cell secretory activity and non-esterified fatty acid production in 7-year-old African children: results from the Birth to Ten study. Diabetologia. 2000;43:978–85.
37. Metzger BE, Lowe LP, Dyer AR, Trimble ER, Chaovarindr U, Coustan DR, et al. Hyperglycemia and adverse pregnancy outcomes. N Engl J Med. 2008;358:1991–2002.
38. Boyne MS, Osmond C, Fraser RA, Reid M, Taylor-Bryan C, Soares-Wynter S, et al. Developmental origins of cardiovascular risk in Jamaican children: the Vulnerable Windows Cohort study. Br J Nutr. 2010; 104:1026–33.
39. Murphy MJ, Metcalf BS, Voss LD, Jeffery AN, Kirkby J, Mallam KM, et al. Girls at five are intrinsically more insulin resistant than boys: the Programming Hypotheses Revisited – The EarlyBird Study (EarlyBird 6). Pediatrics. 2004;113:82–6.
40. Boyne MS, Thame M, Osmond C, Fraser RA, Gabay L, Taylor-Bryan C, et al. The effect of earlier puberty on cardiometabolic risk factors in Afro-Caribbean children. J Pediatr Endocrinol Metab. 2014;27: 453–60.
41. Bennett F, Watson-Brown C, Thame M, Wilks R, Osmond C, Hales N, et al. Shortness at birth is associated with insulin resistance in pre-pubertal Jamaican children. Eur J Clin Nutr. 2002;56: 506–11.
42. Forrester TE, Wilks RJ, Bennett FI, Simeon D, Osmond C, Allen M, et al. Fetal growth and cardiovascular risk factors in Jamaican schoolchildren. BMJ. 1996;312:156–60.
43. Chin-Harty LA, Royal-Thomas T, Thompson DS, Osmond C, Forrester TE, Boyne MS. Role of prenatal factors and postnatal growth on insulin sensitivity and beta-cell function in Afro-Caribbean youth: vulnerable Windows Cohort Study. J Dev Orig Health Dis. 2015;6:S12. (abstract).

44. Francis-Emmanuel PM, Thompson DS, Barnett AT, Osmond C, Byrne CD, Hanson MA, et al. Glucose metabolism in adult survivors of severe acute malnutrition. J Clin Endocrinol Metab. 2014;99:2233–40.
45. Boyne MS, Sargeant LA, Bennett FI, Wilks RJ, Cooper RS, Forrester TE. Isoprostanes, a marker of lipid peroxidation, may not be involved in the development of glucose intolerance. Diabetes Res Clin Pract. 2007;76:149–51.
46. Thompson DS, Ferguson TS, Wilks RJ, Phillips DI, Osmond C, Samms-Vaughan M, et al. Early-life factors are associated with nocturnal cortisol and glucose effectiveness in Afro-Caribbean young adults. Clin Endocrinol (Oxf). 2015;82:352–8.
47. Boyne MS, Thompson DS, Osmond C, Fraser RA, Thame MM, Taylor-Bryan C, et al. The effect of antenatal factors and postnatal growth on serum adiponectin levels in children. J Dev Orig Health Dis. 2013;4:317–23.
48. Ferguson TS, Younger-Coleman NO, Tulloch-Reid MK, Knight-Madden JM, Bennett NR, Samms-Vaughan M, et al. Birth weight and maternal socioeconomic circumstances were inversely related to systolic blood pressure among Afro-Caribbean young adults. J Clin Epidemiol. 2015;68:1002–9.
49. Ezenwaka CE, Kalloo R. Caribbean female patients with type 2 diabetes mellitus have lower serum levels of adiponectin than nondiabetic subjects. Neth J Med. 2005;63:64–9.
50. Bennett NR, Boyne MS, Cooper RS, Royal-Thomas TY, Bennett FI, Luke A, et al. Impact of adiponectin and ghrelin on incident glucose intolerance and on weight change. Clin Endocrinol (Oxf). 2009;70:408–14.
51. Miljkovic-Gacic I, Wang X, Kammerer CM, Bunker CH, Wheeler VW, Patrick AL, et al. Genetic determination of adiponectin and its relationship with body fat topography in multigenerational families of African heritage. Metabolism. 2007;56:234–8.
52. Mehrotra S, Ling KL, Bekele Y, Gerbino E, Earle KA. Lipid hydroperoxide and markers of renal disease susceptibility in African-Caribbean and Caucasian patients with Type 2 diabetes mellitus. Diabet Med. 2001;18:109–15.
53. Nayak BS, Roberts L. Relationship between inflammatory markers, metabolic and anthropometric variables in the Caribbean type 2 diabetic patients with and without microvascular complications. J Inflamm (Lond). 2006;3:17.
54. Lutchmansingh FK, Bennett FI, Badaloo AV, McFarlane-Anderson N, Gordon-Strachan GM, Wright-Pascoe R, et al. Glutathione metabolism in persons with type 2 diabetes. West Indian Med J. 2012;61:24. (abstract).
55. Cumberbatch CG, Younger NO, Ferguson TS, McFarlane SR, Francis DK, Wilks RJ, et al. Reported hours of sleep, diabetes prevalence and glucose control in Jamaican adults: analysis from the Jamaica lifestyle survey 2007–2008. Int J Endocrinol. 2011;716214.
56. Hugh-Jones P. Diabetes in Jamaica. Lancet. 1955;269:891–7.
57. Balasubramanyam A, Nalini R, Hampe CS, Maldonado M. Syndromes of ketosis-prone diabetes mellitus. Endocr Rev. 2008;29:292–302.
58. Morrison EY, Ragoobirsingh D. J type diabetes revisited. J Natl Med Assoc. 1992;84:603–8.
59. Boyne MS. Diabetes in the Caribbean: trouble in paradise. Insulin. 2009;4:94–105.
60. Maldonado M, Hampe CS, Gaur LK, D'Amico S, Iyer D, Hammerle LP, et al. Ketosis-prone diabetes: dissection of a heterogeneous syndrome using an immunogenetic and beta-cell functional classification, prospective analysis, and clinical outcomes. J Clin Endocrinol Metab. 2003;88:5090–8.
61. Tulloch-Reid MK, Boyne MS, Choo-Kang EG, Parkes R, Wright-Pascoe RA, Barton EN, et al. Autoantibodies in Caribbean youth with diabetes mellitus. Hum Antibodies. 2008;17(3–4):57–62.
62. Mauvais-Jarvis F, Sobngwi E, Porcher R, Riveline JP, Kevorkian JP, Vaisse C, et al. Ketosis-prone type 2 diabetes in patients of sub-Saharan African origin: clinical pathophysiology and natural history of beta-cell dysfunction and insulin resistance. Diabetes. 2004;53:645–53.
63. Boutin P, Gresh L, Cisse A, Hara M, Bell G, Babu S, et al. Missense mutation Gly574Ser in the transcription factor HNF-1alpha is a marker of atypical diabetes mellitus in African-American children. Diabetologia. 1999;42:380–1.
64. Mauvais-Jarvis F, Boudou P, Sobngwi E, Riveline JP, Kevorkian JP, Villette JM, et al. The polymorphism Gly574Ser in the transcription factor HNF-1alpha is not a marker of adult-onset ketosis-prone atypical diabetes in Afro-Caribbean patients. Diabetologia. 2003;46:728–9.
65. Aguilera E, Casamitjana R, Ercilla G, Oriola J, Nicoletti F, Gomis R, et al. Clinical characteristics, beta-cell function, HLA class II and mutations in MODY genes in non-paediatric subjects with Type 1 diabetes without pancreatic autoantibodies. Diabet Med: J Br Diabet Assoc. 2005;22:137–43.
66. Stride A, Ellard S, Clark P, Shakespeare L, Salzmann M, Shepherd M, et al. Beta-cell dysfunction, insulin sensitivity, and glycosuria precede diabetes in hepatocyte nuclear factor-1alpha mutation carriers. Diabetes Care. 2005;28:1751–6.
67. Mills JL, Irving RR, Choo-Kang EG, Wright-Pascoe R, McLaughlin W, Mullings AA, et al. Multigenerational inheritance and clinical characteristics of three large pedigrees with early-onset type 2 diabetes in Jamaica. Rev Panam Salud Publ Pan Am J Publ Health. 2010;27:435–41.
68. Cockburn BN, Bermano G, Boodram LL, Teelucksingh S, Tsuchiya T, Mahabir D, et al. Insulin promoter factor-1 mutations and diabetes in Trinidad: identification of a novel diabetes-associated mutation (E224K) in an Indo-Trinidadian family. J Clin Endocrinol Metab. 2004;89:971–8.

69. Pyke DA, Wattley GH. Diabetes in Trinidad. West Indian Med J. 1962;11:22–6.
70. Poon-King T, Henry MV, Rampersad F. Prevalence and natural history of diabetes in Trinidad. Lancet. 1968;291:155–60.
71. Tulloch JA, Johnson HM. A pilot survey of the incidence of diabetes in Jamaica. West Indian Med J. 1958;7:134–6.
72. Wright HB, Taylor B. The incidence of diabetes in a sample of the adult population in South Trinidad. West Indian Med J. 1958;7:123–33.
73. Litvak J. Diabetes mellitus: a challenge for the countries of the region. Bull Pan Am Health Organ. 1975;9:317–24.
74. Cunningham-Myrie C, Younger-Coleman N, Tulloch-Reid M, McFarlane S, Francis D, Ferguson T, et al. Diabetes mellitus in Jamaica: sex differences in burden, risk factors, awareness, treatment and control in a developing country. Tropical Med Int Health: TM IH. 2013;18:1365–78.
75. Ferguson TS, Francis DK, Tulloch-Reid MK, Younger NO, McFarlane SR, Wilks RJ. An update on the burden of cardiovascular disease risk factors in Jamaica: findings from the Jamaica Health and Lifestyle Survey 2007–2008. West Indian Med J. 2011;60:422–8.
76. Washington RE, Orchard TJ, Arena VC, Laporte RE, Tull ES. Incidence of type 1 and type 2 diabetes in youth in the U.S. Virgin Islands, 2001–2010. Pediatr Diabetes. 2013;14:280–7.
77. Batson YA, Teelucksingh S, Maharaj R, Singh V, Balkaran S, Cockburn B. Screening for diabetes in schoolchildren in Trinidad, West Indies. Paediatr Int Child Health. 2013;33:37–41.
78. Tulloch-Reid MK, Boyne MS, Smikle MF, Choo-Kang EG, Parkes RH, Wright-Pascoe RA, et al. Clinical and laboratory features of youth onset type 2 diabetes in Jamaica. West Indian Med J. 2010; 59:131–8.
79. Peter SA, Johnson R, Taylor C, Hanna A, Roberts P, McNeil P, et al. The incidence and prevalence of type-1 diabetes mellitus. J Natl Med Assoc. 2005;97: 250–2.
80. Jordan OW, Lipton RB, Stupnicka E, Cruickshank JK, Fraser HS. Incidence of type I diabetes in people under 30 years of age in Barbados, West Indies, 1982–1991. Diabetes Care. 1994;17:428–31.
81. Tull ES, Jordan OW, Simon L, Laws M, Smith DO, Vanterpool H, et al. Incidence of childhood-onset IDDM in black African-heritage populations in the Caribbean. The Caribbean African Heritage IDDM Study (CAHIS) Group. Diabetes Care. 1997;20: 309–10.
82. Clapperton M, Jarvis J, Mungrue K. Is gestational diabetes mellitus an important contributor to metabolic disorders in Trinidad and tobago? Obstet Gynecol Int. 2009;2009:289329.
83. Irving RR, Mills JL, Choo-Kang EG, Morrison EY, Kulkarni S, Wright-Pascoe R, et al. The burden of gestational diabetes mellitus in Jamaican women with a family history of autosomal dominant type 2 diabetes. Rev Panam Salud Publ Pan Am J Publ Health. 2008;23:85–91.
84. Ali Z, Alexis SD. Occurrence of diabetes mellitus after gestational diabetes mellitus in Trinidad. Diabetes Care. 1990;13:527–9.
85. Murray T, Beaty TH, Mathias RA, Rafaels N, Grant AV, Faruque MU, et al. African and non-African admixture components in African Americans and an African Caribbean population. Genet Epidemiol. 2010;34:561–8.
86. Miljkovic-Gacic I, Ferrell RE, Patrick AL, Kammerer CM, Bunker CH. Estimates of African, European and Native American ancestry in Afro-Caribbean men on the island of Tobago. Hum Hered. 2005;60:129–33.
87. Moreno-Estrada A, Gravel S, Zakharia F, McCauley JL, Byrnes JK, Gignoux CR, et al. Reconstructing the population genetic history of the Caribbean. PLoS Genet. 2013;9:e1003925.
88. Diaz-Horta O, Cintado A, Fernandez-De-Cossio ME, Nazabal M, Ferrer A, Roca J, et al. Relationship of type 1 diabetes to ancestral proportions and HLA DR/DQ alleles in a sample of the admixed Cuban population. Ann Hum Biol. 2010;37:778–88.
89. Heward JM, Mijovic CH, Kelly MA, Morrison E, Barnett AH. HLA-DQ and DRB1 polymorphism and susceptibility to type 1 diabetes in Jamaica. Eur J Immunogenet. 2002;29:47–52.
90. Cruickshank JK, Mbanya JC, Wilks R, Balkau B, McFarlane-Anderson N, Forrester T. Sick genes, sick individuals or sick populations with chronic disease? The emergence of diabetes and high blood pressure in African-origin populations. Int J Epidemiol. 2001;30:111–7.
91. Hennis A, Wu SY, Nemesure B, Li X, Leske MC. Diabetes in a Caribbean population: epidemiological profile and implications. Int J Epidemiol. 2002;31:234–9.
92. Humphries SE, Gable D, Cooper JA, Ireland H, Stephens JW, Hurel SJ, et al. Common variants in the TCF7L2 gene and predisposition to type 2 diabetes in UK European Whites, Indian Asians and Afro-Caribbean men and women. J Mol Med. 2006;84:1005–14.
93. Boodram LG, Miyake K, Hayes MG, Bell GI, Cockburn BN. Association of the KCNJ11 variant E23K with type 2 diabetes in Indo-Trinidadians. West Indian Med J. 2011;60:604–7.
94. McFarlane-Anderson N, Bennett F, Wilks R, Howell S, Newsome C, Cruickshank K, et al. The Trp64Arg mutation of the beta3-adrenergic receptor is associated with hyperglycemia and current body mass index in Jamaican women. Metabolism. 1998;47:617–21.
95. Miljkovic I, Yerges LM, Li H, Gordon CL, Goodpaster BH, Kuller LH, et al. Association of the CPT1B gene with skeletal muscle fat infiltration in Afro-Caribbean men. Obesity. 2009;17: 1396–401.

96. Shungin D, Winkler TW, Croteau-Chonka DC, Ferreira T, Locke AE, Magi R, et al. New genetic loci link adipose and insulin biology to body fat distribution. Nature. 2015;518:187–96.
97. Locke AE, Kahali B, Berndt SI, Justice AE, Pers TH, Day FR, et al. Genetic studies of body mass index yield new insights for obesity biology. Nature. 2015;518:197–206.
98. Beckles GL, Miller GJ, Kirkwood BR, Alexis SD, Carson DC, Byam NT. High total and cardiovascular disease mortality in adults of Indian descent in Trinidad, unexplained by major coronary risk factors. Lancet. 1986;1:1298–301.
99. McKeigue PM, Shah B, Marmot MG. Relation of central obesity and insulin resistance with high diabetes prevalence and cardiovascular risk in South Asians. Lancet. 1991;337:382–6.
100. Chaturvedi N. Ethnic differences in cardiovascular disease. Heart. 2003;89:681–6.
101. Earle KK, Porter KA, Ostberg J, Yudkin JS. Variation in the progression of diabetic nephropathy according to racial origin. Nephrol Dial Transplant. 2001;16:286–90.
102. Chaturvedi N, McKeigue PM, Marmot MG. Resting and ambulatory blood pressure differences in Afro-Caribbeans and Europeans. Hypertension. 1993;22:90–6.
103. Tulloch-Reid MK, Boyne MS, Smikle MF, Choo-Kang EG, Parkes RH, Wright-Pascoe RA, et al. Cardiovascular risk profile in Caribbean youth with diabetes mellitus. West Indian Med J. 2009;58:219–26.
104. Mortality GBD, Causes of Death C. Global, regional, and national age-sex specific all-cause and cause-specific mortality for 240 causes of death, 1990–2013: a systematic analysis for the Global Burden of Disease Study 2013. Lancet. 2015;385:117–71.
105. Miller GJ, Kirkwood BR, Beckles GL, Alexis SD, Carson DC, Byam NT. Adult male all-cause, cardiovascular and cerebrovascular mortality in relation to ethnic group, systolic blood pressure and blood glucose concentration in Trinidad. West Indies Int J Epidemiol. 1988;17:62–9.
106. Ferguson TS, Tulloch-Reid MK, Younger NO, Boyne MS, Wright-Pascoe RA, Elliott VE, et al. Cardiovascular disease among diabetic in-patients at a tertiary hospital in Jamaica. Diab Vasc Dis Res. 2010;7:241–2.
107. Blanchet Deverly A, Amara M, Larifla L, Velayoudom-Cephise FL, Roques F, Kangambega P, et al. Silent myocardial ischaemia and risk factors in a diabetic Afro-Caribbean population. Diabetes Metab. 2011;37:533–9.
108. Larifla L, Maimaitiming S, Velayoudom-Cephise FL, Ferdinand S, Blanchet-Deverly A, Benabdallah S, et al. Association of 2238T>C polymorphism of the atrial natriuretic peptide gene with coronary artery disease in Afro-Caribbeans with type 2 diabetes. Am J Hypertens. 2012;25:524–7.
109. Yisahak SF, Beagley J, Hambleton IR, Narayan KM, Atlas IDFD. Diabetes in North America and the Caribbean: an update. Diabetes Res Clin Pract. 2014;103:223–30.
110. Andrade F. Estimating diabetes and diabetes-free life expectancy in Mexico and seven major cities in Latin America and the Caribbean. Rev Panam Salud Publ Pan Am J Publ Health. 2009;26:9–16.
111. Washington RE, Orchard TJ, Arena VC, LaPorte RE, Secrest AM, Tull ES. All-cause mortality in a population-based type 1 diabetes cohort in the U.S. Virgin Islands. D Diabetes Res Clin Pract. 2014;103:504–9.
112. Ferguson TS, Tulloch-Reid MK, Younger NO, Wright-Pascoe RA, Boyne MS, McFarlane SR, et al. Diabetic foot complications among patients attending a specialist diabetes clinic in Jamaica: prevalence and associated factors. West Indian Med J. 2013;62:216–23.
113. Taylor Jr CG, Krimholtz M, Belgrave KC, Hambleton I, George CN, Rayman G. The extensive inpatient burden of diabetes and diabetes-related foot disease in Barbados. Clin Med. 2014;14:367–70.
114. Cawich SO, Islam S, Hariharan S, Harnarayan P, Budhooram S, Ramsewak S, et al. The economic impact of hospitalization for diabetic foot infections in a Caribbean nation. Permanente J. 2014;18:e101–4.
115. Hennis AJ, Fraser HS, Jonnalagadda R, Fuller J, Chaturvedi N. Explanations for the high risk of diabetes-related amputation in a Caribbean population of black African descent and potential for prevention. Diabetes Care. 2004;27:2636–41.
116. Hambleton IR, Jonnalagadda R, Davis CR, Fraser HS, Chaturvedi N, Hennis AJ. All-cause mortality after diabetes-related amputation in Barbados: a prospective case-control study. Diabetes Care. 2009;32:306–7.
117. Landis RC, Evans BJ, Chaturvedi N, Haskard DO. Persistence of TNFalpha in diabetic wounds. Diabetologia. 2010;53:1537–8.
118. Quimby KR, Greenidge AR, Hennis AJ, Harrison DK, Landis RC. Tumor necrosis factor receptor-associated periodic syndrome P46L and bilateral amputation in diabetes. Rheumatology. 2010;49:2454–5.
119. Vigilance JE, Reid HL. Glycaemic control influences peripheral blood flow and haemorheological variables in patients with diabetes mellitus. Clin Hemorheol Microcirc. 2005;33:337–46.
120. Leske MC, Wu SY, Hyman L, Li X, Hennis A, Connell AM, et al. Diabetic retinopathy in a black population: the Barbados Eye Study. Ophthalmology. 1999;106:1893–9.
121. Leske MC, Wu SY, Hennis A, Nemesure B, Hyman L, Schachat A. Incidence of diabetic retinopathy in the Barbados Eye Studies. Ophthalmology. 2003;110:941–7.
122. Leske MC, Wu SY, Hennis A, Nemesure B, Schachat AP, Hyman L, et al. Nine-year incidence of diabetic retinopathy in the Barbados Eye Studies. Arch Ophthalmol. 2006;124:250–5.

123. Leske MC, Wu SY, Hennis A, Hyman L, Nemesure B, Yang L, et al. Hyperglycemia, blood pressure, and the 9-year incidence of diabetic retinopathy: the Barbados Eye Studies. Ophthalmology. 2005;112: 799–805.
124. Moriarty BJ, Dunn DT, Moriarty AP. Diabetic maculopathy in a Jamaican population. Int Ophthalmol. 1989;13:301–3.
125. Mowatt L. Diabetic retinopathy and its risk factors at the university hospital in Jamaica. Middle East Afr J Ophthalmol. 2013;20:321–6.
126. Ferguson TS, Tulloch-Reid MK, Younger-Coleman NO, Wright-Pascoe RA, Boyne MS, Soyibo AK, et al. Prevalence of chronic kidney disease among patients attending a specialist diabetes clinic in Jamaica. West Indian Med J. 2015;64:201.
127. Soyibo AK, Barton EN. Report from the Caribbean renal registry, 2006. West Indian Med J. 2007;56: 355–63.
128. Ragoobirsingh D, Bennett F, Morrison EY. Kidney function in phasic insulin dependent diabetes mellitus in Jamaica. West Indian Med J. 1997;46:22–4.
129. Chung ST, Perue GG, Johnson A, Younger N, Hoo CS, Pascoe RW, et al. Predictors of hyperglycaemic crises and their associated mortality in Jamaica. Diabetes Res Clin Pract. 2006;73:184–90.
130. Frederick FT, Maharajh HD. Prevalence of depression in type 2 diabetic patients in Trinidad and Tobago. West Indian Med J. 2013;62:628–31.
131. Wilks RJ, Sargeant LA, Gulliford MC, Reid ME, Forrester TE. Management of diabetes mellitus in three settings in Jamaica. Rev Panam Salud Publica. 2001;9:65–72.
132. Mahabir D, Gulliford MC. Changing patterns of primary care for diabetes in Trinidad and Tobago over 10 years. Diabet Med. 2005;22:619–24.
133. Apparico N, Clerk N, Henry G, Seale J, Sealy R, Ward S, et al. How well controlled are our type 2 diabetic patients in 2002? An observational study in North and Central Trinidad. Diabetes Res Clin Pract. 2007;75:301–5.
134. Forde H, Marshall M, Cohall D, Nielsen AL. Assessing predictors for sustainable management of type 2 diabetes using evidence-based guidelines in public primary care in a predominantly Afro-Caribbean population. Ethn Dis. 2014;24:469–74.
135. Adams OP, Carter AO. Are primary care practitioners in Barbados following diabetes guidelines? – a chart audit with comparison between public and private care sectors. BMC Res Notes. 2011;4:199.
136. Adams OP, Carter AO. Diabetes and hypertension guidelines and the primary health care practitioner in Barbados: knowledge, attitudes, practices and barriers – a focus group study. BMC Fam Pract. 2010;11:96.
137. Barcelo A, Aedo C, Rajpathak S, Robles S. The cost of diabetes in Latin America and the Caribbean. Bull World Health Organ. 2003;81:19–27.
138. Hassell T, Hennis A. The road to the United Nations High Level Meeting on chronic non-communicable diseases. West Indian Med J. 2011;60:384–6.
139. Batson YA, Teelucksingh S, Maharaj RG, Cockburn BN. A cross-sectional study to determine the prevalence of obesity and other risk factors for type 2 diabetes among school children in Trinidad, West Indies. Paediatr Int Child Health. 2014;34:178–83.
140. Bahado-Singh PS, Riley CK, Wheatley AO, Lowe HI. Relationship between processing method and the glycemic indices of ten sweet potato (Ipomoea batatas) cultivars commonly consumed in Jamaica. J Nutr Metab. 2011;2011:584832.
141. Riley CK, Bahado-Singh PS, Wheatley AO, Ahmad MH, Asemota HN. Relationship between the physicochemical properties of starches and the glycemic indices of some Jamaican yams (Dioscorea spp.). Mol Nutr Food Res. 2008;52:1372–6.
142. Bahado-Singh PS, Wheatley AO, Ahmad MH, Morrison EY, Asemota HN. Food processing methods influence the glycaemic indices of some commonly eaten West Indian carbohydrate-rich foods. Br J Nutr. 2006;96:476–81.
143. Ramdath DD, Isaacs RL, Teelucksingh S, Wolever TM. Glycaemic index of selected staples commonly eaten in the Caribbean and the effects of boiling v. crushing. Br J Nutr. 2004;91:971–7.
144. Bahado-Singh PS, Wheatley AO, Osagie AU, Boyne MS, Morrison EYS, Ahmad MH, et al. Low to intermediate-glycemic-index Caribbean foods reduce glycemia, cardiovascular and inflammatory markers in overweight persons with type 2 diabetes. Curr Res Nutr Food Sci. 2015;3:36–45.
145. Wint YB, Duff EM, McFarlane-Anderson N, O'Connor A, Bailey EY, Wright-Pascoe RA. Knowledge, motivation and barriers to diabetes control in adults in Jamaica. West Indian Med J. 2006;55:330–3.
146. Babwah F, Baksh S, Blake L, Cupid-Thuesday J, Hosein I, Sookhai A, et al. The role of gender in compliance and attendance at an outpatient clinic for type 2 diabetes mellitus in Trinidad. Rev Panam Salud Publ Pan Am J Publ Health. 2006;19:79–84.
147. Adams OP, Carter AO. Knowledge, attitudes, practices, and barriers reported by patients receiving diabetes and hypertension primary health care in Barbados: a focus group study. BMC Fam Pract. 2011;12:135.
148. Morrison E, Haye I, Amarakoon K, Whitbourne F, Kirlew J, Less L, et al. An interim report of an intervention strategy for diabetes care in Jamaica. West Indian Med J. 2001;50 Suppl 1:55–9.
149. Less LA, Ragoorbirsingh D, Morrison EY, Boyne M, Johnson P. Assessment of a community based Intervention for diabetes control in adults with type 2 diabetes mellitus in three parishes in Jamaica: participant were assigned to interventions using random allocations. West Indian Med J. 2008;57 Suppl 1:39.
150. Less LA, Ragoobirsingh D, Morrison EY, Boyne M, Johnson PA. A preliminary report on an assessment of a community-based intervention for diabetes control in adults with type 2 diabetes. Fam Pract. 2010;27 Suppl 1:i46–52.

151. Gordon LA, Morrison EY, McGrowder DA, Young R, Fraser YT, Zamora EM, et al. Effect of exercise therapy on lipid profile and oxidative stress indicators in patients with type 2 diabetes. BMC Complement Altern Med. 2008;8:21.
152. Picking D, Younger N, Mitchell S, Delgoda R. The prevalence of herbal medicine home use and concomitant use with pharmaceutical medicines in Jamaica. J Ethnopharmacol. 2011;137:305–11.
153. Russell KR, Omoruyi FO, Pascoe KO, Morrison EY. Hypoglycaemic activity of Bixa orellana extract in the dog. Methods Find Exp Clin Pharmacol. 2008;30:301–5.
154. McAnuff MA, Harding WW, Omoruyi FO, Jacobs H, Morrison EY, Asemota HN. Hypoglycemic effects of steroidal sapogenins isolated from Jamaican bitter yam, Dioscorea polygonoides. Food Chem Toxicol: Int J Published Br Ind Biol Res Assoc. 2005;43:1667–72.
155. Alexander-Lindo RL, Morrison EY, Nair MG. Hypoglycaemic effect of stigmast-4-en-3-one and its corresponding alcohol from the bark of Anacardium occidentale (cashew). Phytother Res: PTR. 2004;18:403–7.
156. Tolan I, Ragoobirsingh D, Morrison EY. Isolation and purification of the hypoglycaemic principle present in Capsicum frutescens. Phytother Res: PTR. 2004;18:95–6.
157. Christie SL, Levy A. Evaluation of the hypoglycaemic activity of Petiveria alliacea (Guinea Hen Weed) extracts in normoglycaemic and diabetic rat models. West Indian Med J. 2013;62:685–91.
158. Dan D, Harnanan D, Singh Y, Hariharan S, Naraynsingh V, Teelucksingh S. Effects of bariatric surgery on type-2 diabetes mellitus in a Caribbean setting. Int J Surg. 2011;9:386–91.
159. Samuels TA, Fraser H. Caribbean Wellness Day: mobilizing a region for chronic noncommunicable disease prevention and control. Rev Panam Salud Publ Pan Am J Publ Health. 2010;28:472–9.
160. Samuels TA, Guell C, Legetic B, Unwin N. Policy initiatives, culture and the prevention and control of chronic non-communicable diseases (NCDs) in the Caribbean. Ethn Health. 2012;17:631–49.
161. Barrett SC, Huffman FG, Johnson P, Campa A, Magnus M, Ragoobirsingh D. A cross-sectional study of Jamaican adolescents' risk for type 2 diabetes and cardiovascular diseases. BMJ Open. 2013;3:e002817.
162. Tulloch-Reid MK, Ferguson TS, Younger NO, Van den Broeck J, Boyne MS, Knight-Madden JM, et al. Appropriate waist circumference cut points for identifying insulin resistance in black youth: a cross sectional analysis of the 1986 Jamaica birth cohort. Diabetol Metab Syndr. 2010;2:68.

Diabetes in Indigenous Australians and Other Underserved Communities in Australia

9

Stephen Colagiuri

Introduction

Australia's population has just reached 24 million which is relatively small for its large land mass. The population is diverse with over one in four being born overseas and includes a unique Indigenous population which has lived here for thousands of years. It is well recognized that diabetes and other chronic diseases are overrepresented in these diverse groups. This review examines aspects of diabetes prevalence and care in three population groups in Australia in which health outcomes are of particular concern and are a significant source of disadvantage:

- Australia's Indigenous population of Aboriginal and Torres Strait Islander people
- People from culturally and linguistically diverse backgrounds
- People living in rural and remote areas

Diabetes in Australia

It is estimated that more than 1.2 million Australians are living with diabetes based on data from three sources [1]: the National Diabetes Services Scheme (NDSS) [2], the Australian Health Survey (National Health Measures Survey, 2011–2013) [3], and the AusDiab study (1999–2000) [4]. The Australian Health Survey found that using HbA1c (glycated hemoglobin ≥6.5 %) as the measure, 5.4 % of the population over the age of 18 had diabetes, which translates to almost 1 million people [3]. Using fasting plasma glucose ≥7.0 mmol/l as the measure, 5.1 % of Australians aged 18 years and over had diabetes. The majority were people known to have diabetes with approximately one newly diagnosed case of diabetes for every four already diagnosed cases. Diabetes was more common in men than women (6.3 % compared with 3.9 %) for both known diabetes (4.9 % compared with 3.4 %) and newly diagnosed diabetes (1.4 % compared with 0.4 %) [3].

The 1999–2000 AusDiab (Australian Diabetes and Obesity Lifestyle) study used an oral glucose tolerance test (OGTT) to estimate that 7.5 % of Australians over the age of 25 had diabetes, which equates to approximately 1.2 million people [4]. A similar estimate comes from the NDSS, a government-funded national scheme which provides registrants with subsidized consumables for self-monitoring blood glucose, insulin needles, and insulin pump consumables. The NDSS has registered 1.2 million people with diabetes and registers over 250 people every day [2].

However, it is likely that all three sources underestimate the total number of people affected

S. Colagiuri, MD
Boden Institute of Obesity, Nutrition and Exercise, University of Sydney, Sydney, NSW, Australia
e-mail: stephen.colagiuri@sydney.edu.au

S. Dagogo-Jack (ed.), *Diabetes Mellitus in Developing Countries and Underserved Communities*, DOI 10.1007/978-3-319-41559-8_9

by diabetes. The Australian Health Survey did not perform an OGTT. The AusDiab study was conducted over 15 years ago, and during this time, there has been a considerable increase in the proportion of people who are overweight and obese. Both these studies excluded children. Registration with the NDSS is voluntary, and it is likely that a number of people with diabetes are not registered.

While the contribution of many chronic diseases to the national burden of disability is decreasing, the diabetes burden continues to increase and is predicted to become the largest contributor to disability-adjusted life years by 2017 [5]. In 2011, diabetes was the underlying cause of 3 % of all deaths and an underlying or associated cause of 10 % of all deaths in Australia [6]. There are a significant number of diabetes-related complications, including heart attacks, strokes, limb amputations, blindness, kidney failure, nerve damage, and depression. It is estimated that annually there are 840,000 hospitalizations for diabetes, 3500 people having dialysis due to diabetes, and 3500 lower-limb amputations due to diabetes [7].

Diabetes impacts the individual, their family, and society in general. People with diagnosed diabetes (approximately 5 % of Australians) account for 12 % of total health care costs in Australia. For type 1 diabetes, total direct costs amount to a minimum of A$570 million per annum: A$4669 annually for a person with no complications, rising to A$16,698 per annum once complications develop [8]. Type 2 diabetes costs at least A$14.6 billion annually, 42 % of which is attributed to direct medical costs. These costs are projected to increase to A$30 billion by 2025 [9]. The cost pattern is similar in people with type 2 diabetes with the annual cost increasing from A$3500 for people without diabetes complications to A$9600 for people with complications [9]. Australia is fortunate in having the NDSS to offset some of these costs.

In addition to diabetes, intermediate hyperglycemia ("prediabetes") is also common. The AusDiab study found that 16.4 % of adults over the age of 25 (approximately 2.5 million people) had prediabetes based on a standard 2 h OGTT [4]. More recent data from the Australian Health Survey reported prediabetes in 4.0 % of adults diagnosed on the basis of a fasting plasma glucose of 6.1–6.9 mmol/l and 6.0 % based on an HbA1c of 6.0–6.4 %. These data highlight the underestimation of prediabetes when using tests which do not specifically identify impaired glucose tolerance (IGT) [3].

The greatest risk factor for diabetes is obesity. In 2011–2012, 63 % of Australians aged 18 years and over were overweight or obese, comprised of 35 % overweight and 28 % obese. The prevalence of overweight and obesity has increased in Australia over time, from 56 % in 1995 to 61 % in 2007–2008. Overweight and obesity vary with age, with 74.9 % of people aged 65–74 years being overweight or obese compared with 36.4 % of people aged 18–24 years. More men were overweight or obese than women (70 % vs. 56 %). However, looking at only those people who were obese, rates are the same for men and women (both 28 %). The proportion of people who are obese has increased across all age groups over time, up from 19 % in 1995 to 28 % in 2011–2012. Between 1995 and 2011–2012, average weight increased 3.9 kg in men and 4.1 kg in women. Rates of overweight and obesity in children and adolescents aged 5–17 have remained stable at 25 % [10].

Australia's Indigenous People

The term "Indigenous Australians" refers to the Aboriginal and Torres Strait Islander people of Australia, descended from groups that existed in Australia and surrounding islands prior to European colonization in the late eighteenth century. The time of arrival of the first Indigenous Australians is at least 40,000 years ago and may even date back as far as 125,000 years. There is great diversity among different Indigenous communities and societies in Australia, each with its own mixture of cultures, customs, and languages.

The Indigenous population of Aboriginal and Torres Strait Islanders make up approximately 3 % of the entire population. The age profile of Australia's Indigenous and non-Indigenous populations is considerably different with a larger proportion of young people and a smaller proportion of older people (4 % vs. 15 % aged 65 and over) among Indigenous Australians [11].

Life expectancy at birth for Indigenous Australians in the period 2010–2012 was 69.1 years for males and 73.7 years for females compared with 79.7 years for males and 83.1 years for females for non-Indigenous Australians – a gap of 10.6 years for males and 9.5 years for females [12]. Between 2005–2007 and 2010–2012, life expectancy at birth for Indigenous males increased from 67.5 to 69.1 years and from 73.1 to 73.7 years for Indigenous females [13].

In 2009–2013, the age-standardized mortality rate for Indigenous Australians was 985 per 100,000, 1.7 times higher than the 585 per 100,000 for non-Indigenous Australians. The rate ratio was highest for the 35–44 years age group where the Indigenous mortality rate was 4.2 times that of the non-Indigenous rate [14].

Although there have been some improvements, the overall health status of Indigenous Australians remains a concern. Smoking rates have declined from 51 % to 44 % between 2002 and 2012–2013 for Indigenous Australians aged 15 and over but remain high with a current 25 percentage point gap between Indigenous and non-Indigenous Australians. Smoking during pregnancy remains high at 50 %. Low birth weight rate for babies born to Indigenous mothers is twice that of non-Indigenous mothers (11 % compared with 5 %). It is estimated that 51 % of low birth weight births to Indigenous mothers is attributable to smoking, compared with 19 % for non-Indigenous Australian mothers. If smoking rates for Indigenous pregnant women were the same as for other Australian mothers, it is estimated that the proportion of low birth weight babies could be reduced by 26 % [14].

Diabetes in Indigenous Australians

Prevalence

The burden of diabetes is not shared equally in Australia, and no group is more severely affected than Australia's Indigenous population which has higher rates of diabetes, significant premature mortality, and high rates of complications, especially cardiovascular and renal disease. In addition, the diabetes burden is increased in populations living in rural and remote areas of Australia [14].

The 2012–2013 National Aboriginal and Torres Strait Islander Health Measures Survey is the largest biomedical survey ever conducted in Indigenous Australians and included some 3300 individuals aged 18 years and over across Australia. In addition to collecting data on self-reported diabetes, it included measurement of fasting plasma glucose and glycated hemoglobin. The survey showed that 11.1 % of Indigenous adults had diabetes – 9.6 % with previously diagnosed diabetes and 1.5 % with newly diagnosed diabetes, indicating approximately one newly diagnosed case for every six diagnosed cases. After taking age differences into account, Indigenous people were more than three times as likely as non-Indigenous people to have diabetes – 3.6 times more likely to have known diabetes and twice as likely to have newly diagnosed diabetes. Indigenous women were significantly more likely than men to have diabetes [15].

Diabetes prevalence among Indigenous people increased with age. Rates were especially high among those aged 55 years and over, with around one in every three people in this age group having diabetes (34.5 %), compared with 12 % among non-Indigenous Australians, a gap of 22 percentage points [15] (Fig. 9.1).

Although this overall age pattern was similar to non-Indigenous Australians, diabetes tended to occur earlier. The prevalence of diabetes for Indigenous people aged 35–44 years was 9.0 % which is similar to that for non-Indigenous people aged 55–64 years (8.2 %). Similarly, the prevalence for those aged 45–54 years was 17.8 %, similar to that for those aged 65–74 in the non-Indigenous population (15.0 %). This pattern was apparent for both known diabetes and newly diagnosed diabetes [15].

Minges et al. performed a systematic review of diabetes prevalence in Indigenous Australians prior to the 2012–2013 Australian Aboriginal and Torres Strait Islander Health Survey [16].

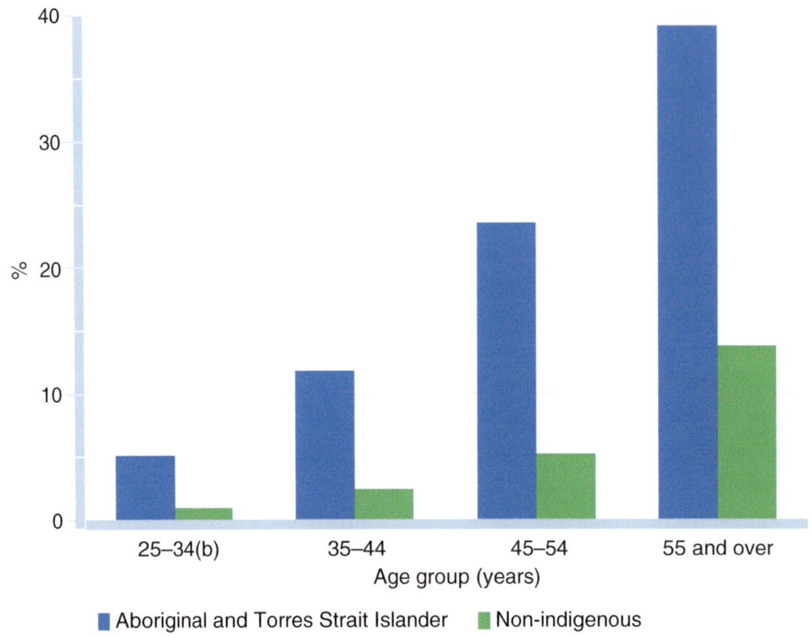

Fig. 9.1 Diabetes or high blood sugar levels by Indigenous status and age (Sources: 2012–2013 Australian Aboriginal and Torres Strait Islander Health Survey and 2011–2012 Australian Health Survey)

Among 24 studies, sample sizes varied from 152 to 29,687 participants, with 71 % of studies having a sample size over 500 people. The mean sample study age ranged from 21 to 51 years. Eighteen studies included blood testing with 14 using WHO diagnostic criteria and 4 the ADA criteria, while 25 % presented self-reported data and 13 % used medical records. The prevalence estimates of diabetes ranged from 3.5 % to 33.1 %. Even when only considering the 16 studies with a mean sample age of 30–40 years, the diabetes prevalence still varied between 6.5 % and 26.2 %. Consequently, the authors were unable to establish a true single prevalence estimate due to the marked heterogeneity of the data. These differences may have been the result of major differences in the Indigenous populations, the Indigenous communities, or in the way studies were conducted.

The most recent study which included 2 h OGTT testing was the DRUID (Diabetes and Related conditions in Urban Indigenous people in the Darwin region) study [17] which included 861 people aged 15 years or older. The overall prevalence of diabetes was 19.4 %. There was a sharp rise in diabetes prevalence with age with 31.7 % of those aged 35 years and over and 52.4 % of those 55 years and over having diabetes. Of the people with diabetes, 48 (28.7 %) were newly diagnosed of whom 24 (50 %) would not have been diagnosed without an OGTT.

The Australian Health Survey reported that 4.7 % of the Indigenous population had impaired fasting glucose (IFG) indicating an increased risk for future diabetes. After taking age differences into account, Indigenous people were nearly twice as likely to be at high risk of diabetes compared with non-Indigenous Australians. The prevalence of IFG increased with age with 7.5 % of those aged 55 and over having IFG [3]. The review by Minges et al. included five studies which reported an IGT prevalence of 4.7–21.1 % [16]. With the exception of one study, there was a greater prevalence of diabetes than IGT. IFG was only assessed in one study of an island population in the top end of Australia and reported a prevalence of 5.1 %. The DRUID study [17] reported a prevalence for IGT of 12 %. In contrast to diabetes, both IGT and IFG remained relatively stable in the age groups above 25.

Type 2 Diabetes in Young People

Craig et al. determined the incidence of type 2 diabetes in young people <19 years old and their characteristics in the Indigenous group in a prospective population-based study. From 2001 to 2006, there were 128 incident cases of type 2 diabetes (62 boys, 66 girls). The median age at diagnosis was 14.5 years (interquartile range, 13.0–16.4), and 90 % were overweight or obese (BMI >85th percentile for age). Mean annual incidence was 2.5/100,000 person-years (95 % CI, 2.1–3.0) in 10–18-year-olds. Of the ethnic groups represented, white Australian comprised 29 %, Indigenous 22 %, Asian 22 %, North African/Middle Eastern 12 %, and Maori/Polynesian/Melanesian 10 %. The incidence of type 2 diabetes was significantly higher in the Indigenous compared with the non-Indigenous group (incidence rate ratio, 6.1; 95 % CI, 3.9–9.7; $P<0.001$), but incidence rates of type 1 diabetes were similar (15.5 vs. 21.4/100,000, respectively). Type 2 diabetes accounted for 11 % of incident cases of diabetes in 10–18-year-olds [18].

Type 2 diabetes among Indigenous children and adolescents appears to be increasing in incidence, and the burden is much greater than that experienced by non-Indigenous young people [19]. Indigenous children and adolescents with type 2 diabetes typically have a family history of type 2 diabetes and are overweight or obese and may have signs of hyperinsulinism such as acanthosis nigricans [20]. Onset of type 2 diabetes is usually during early adolescence, and patients are often asymptomatic at presentation. Data on comorbidities at diagnosis are lacking and may be a reflection of poor screening.

There is evidence that young-onset type 2 diabetes is a more lethal phenotype of diabetes and is associated with a greater mortality, more diabetes complications, and unfavorable cardiovascular disease risk factors when compared with type 1 diabetes. Long-term clinical outcomes and survival in young-onset type 2 diabetes were compared with type 1 diabetes with a similar age of onset using an ambulatory diabetes center database. Outcomes in 354 people with type 2 diabetes with age of onset between 15 and 30 years were compared with 470 type 1 diabetes subjects with similar age of onset. The median observation period was similar at 21.4 (interquartile range, 14–30.7) and 23.4 (15.7–32.4) years for the type 2 and the type 1 diabetes cohorts, respectively. A significant mortality excess was noted in the type 2 diabetes subjects compared with the type 1 diabetes subjects (11 vs. 6.8 %, $P=0.03$), with an increased hazard for death (hazard ratio, 2.0 [95 % CI 1.2–3.2], $P=0.003$). Death in the type 2 diabetes subjects occurred after a significantly shorter disease duration (26.9 [18.1–36.0] vs. 36.5 [24.4–45.4] years, $P=0.01$) and at a relatively young age, and there were more cardiovascular deaths (50 vs. 30 %, $P<0.05$). Despite equivalent glycemic control and shorter disease duration, the prevalence of albuminuria and less favorable cardiovascular risk factors was greater in the type 2 diabetes subjects and neuropathy scores, and macrovascular complications were also increased [21].

Risk Factors for Diabetes

Obesity

The National Aboriginal and Torres Strait Islander Health Survey showed that four in every ten (39.8 %) Indigenous persons were obese, and these obese individuals were around seven times more likely than normal weight or underweight individuals to have diabetes (17.2 % compared with 2.4 %) [15].

Daniel et al. reported the risk of having IGT and diabetes relative to body mass index (BMI) among 2626 aboriginal men and women aged 15–94 years. The population was divided into five strata of BMI (<22, 22–24.9, 25–29.9, 30–34.9, and ≥35 kg/m^2). The prevalence of IGT and diabetes, respectively, adjusted for age and BMI, was 13.9 % and 14.2 % among men and 15.7 % and 15.2 % among women. Odds ratios (95 % CI) for IGT and diabetes for increasing BMI strata ≥22 kg/m^2 ranged from 1.7 (1.0–2.9) to 5.1 (2.4–10.5) for IGT and from 2.0 (1.2–3.5) to 6.1 (3.3–11.1) for diabetes. For IGT and diabetes, across genders, the population-attributable risk percentages (95 % CI) for BMI ≥22 kg/m^2 were 34.1 % (26.2–41.9 %) for IGT and 46.4 % (38.5–54.5 %) for diabetes [22].

The DRUID study reported the association between various indices of obesity and diabetes after adjusting for age. Among males, the odds ratios for diabetes in the highest quartile compared to the lowest quartile were 10.4 (95 % CI 1.2–90.6) for WHR, 6.0 (1.2–29.6) for waist circumference, and 2.0 (0.6–6.3) for BMI. Among females, the corresponding odds ratios were WHR 25.9 (6.0–112.0), waist circumference 7.5 (2.9–19.2), and BMI 4.8 (2.1–10.8) [17].

Low Birth Weight

Child health, and especially low birth weight, is considered an important factor in the development of diabetes. In 2011, the low birth weight rate for babies born to Indigenous mothers was twice the rate for those with a non-Indigenous mother (13 % compared with 6 %) and was significantly higher in remote areas (15 %) than in non-remote areas (12 %) [23]. Despite these high rates, there has been a significant 9 % decline in low birth weight rates between 2000 and 2011 in Indigenous mothers.

A major factor in low birth weight is smoking. Fifty percent of Indigenous women smoked during pregnancy in 2011, four times the rate for non-Indigenous women, and 51 % of low birth weight births to Indigenous mothers has been attributed to smoking, compared with 19 % for non-Indigenous mothers. After adjusting for age differences and other factors, it is estimated that if the smoking rate for Indigenous pregnant women was the same as for other Australian mothers, the proportion of low birth weight babies could be reduced by 26 % [14].

Social Determinants

There remains a significant gap between Indigenous and non-Indigenous Australians in several parameters which can impact health. These include education attainment rates, employment, household incomes (43 % of Indigenous adults were in the lowest quintile compared with 17 % of non-Indigenous adults), and homelessness [14].

Genetic Studies

There have been a limited number of gene-related studies including studies on diabetes susceptibility genes in Indigenous Australians [24]. Busfield et al. studied an Indigenous Australian community with a phenotype characterized by severe insulin resistance. A genome-wide scan for type 2 diabetes susceptibility genes in a large multi-generation pedigree from this community identified a region of significant positive linkage with type 2 diabetes on chromosome 2q with several candidate genes identified in the region [25]. Another genome-wide analysis found peaks on chromosomes 1 and 21. On chromosome 1, the gene had a strong association with type 2 diabetes, hyperlipidemia, and blood pressure in type 2 diabetes in European populations. The gene with a strong association with type 2 diabetes on chromosome 21 is involved with regulating insulin [26]. Further studies are required to replicate these findings in other Indigenous and international populations.

Gestational Diabetes

Ishak and Petocz investigated the prevalence, trends, and risk factors of gestational diabetes mellitus (GDM) in Indigenous Australians compared with the non-Indigenous population in a retrospective population analysis of 230,011 deliveries from an administrative database in the state of South Australia between 1988 and 1999. The age-standardized GDM rate for Indigenous mothers was more than 2.5 times higher than that for non-Indigenous mothers (4.3 vs. 1.8 %) with no significant trend changes over the time period of the study [27]. However, a more recent systematic review of diabetes in pregnancy included 11 studies which reported prevalence of GDM in Indigenous Australians. The overall rate of GDM was higher at 8.4 % compared with 2–5 % worldwide [28].

People Living in Rural and Remote Areas

Australia's population is largely concentrated in the east and southeast of the country, and most Australians live in capital cities with the majority living in major cities (71 %), 18 % in inner regional areas, 9 % in outer regional areas, 1.4% in remote areas, and 1% in very remote areas. The proportion living in major cities has increased over the past decade, while the population in very remote areas has fallen [29].

Health outcomes, such as higher rates of death, are worse outside of major cities related to differences in access to services, risk factors, and the remote environment, although it is not possible to apportion the generally poorer health outcomes outside major cities to these factors [30]. With respect to health services, there are lower rates of some hospital surgical procedures, lower rates of primary care physician consultation, and generally higher rates of hospital admission in regional and remote areas than in major cities. There are also significant differences in interregional health behavior and risk factors. People in regional and remote areas are more likely than their urban counterparts to be a daily smoker (outer regional and remote 22 % and inner regional 18 % compared with 15 % in major cities), be overweight or obese (70 % and 69 % compared with 60 %), be insufficiently active (60 % and 63 % compared with 54 %), drink alcohol in harmful quantities (24 % and 21 % compared with 19 %), and have high blood cholesterol (37 % and 38 % compared with 31 %) [31]. In addition, over half of outer regional, remote, and very remote residents live in areas classified as the lowest socioeconomic status compared with around one-quarter of people in major cities and 77 % in very remote areas.

Another contributing factor to the health status of people living in rural and remote areas is the higher proportion of Indigenous people and their generally poorer health outcomes. Most Indigenous Australians live in urban areas – 35 % in major cities, 22 % in each of inner and outer regional areas, and the remaining 21 % in either remote or very remote areas. Nevertheless, they make up a relatively large proportion of the population living in remote areas of Australia – 45 % of all people living in very remote areas and 16 % living in remote areas [30].

Overall, death rates increase with increasing remoteness. In 2012, the age-standardized rate was highest in very remote areas (840 per 100,000 population), followed by remote (670 per 100,000 population), outer regional (640 per 100,000 population), inner regional (610 per 100,000 population), and major cities (550 per 100,000 population) [31]. Death rates in regional and remote areas are between 10 % and 70 % as high as in major cities. Cardiovascular diseases are responsible for nearly a third of the elevated male death rates outside major cities. Male death rates from diabetes are 1.3 times as high in inner regional areas and 3.7 times as high in very remote areas compared with major cities [31].

In 2010, 5.4 % of all deaths that year were attributed to diabetes and causes related to diabetes, although as is well known this will be an underestimate. Diabetes-related death rate was 55 % higher among males than females (39 deaths per 100,000 males and 25 deaths per 100,000 females) [32]. Death rate from diabetes-related causes increased with increasing remoteness – 28 deaths per 100,000 population among people living in major cities, 32 deaths per 100,000 population among people living in inner regional areas, and 43 deaths per 100,000 population among people living in outer regional, remote, and very remote areas.

Diabetes prevalence is also linked with region of residence. Overall in Australia, the age-standardized prevalence of diabetes in 2011–2012 was 4.2 %. Rates of diabetes were 3.9 % in major cities and 4.9 % in outer regional and remote areas [3].

The situation is worse for Indigenous people living in remote areas with around one in five (20.8 %) having diabetes compared with around one in ten people in non-remote areas (9.4 %). This difference is particularly pronounced for newly diagnosed diabetes, which was five times as high in remote areas than in non-remote areas (4.8 % compared with 0.9 %) [3]. In addition, Indigenous adults in remote areas are less likely to have their diabetes effectively managed (25.1 % compared with 43.5 %) and two and a half times more likely to have chronic kidney disease (33.6 % compared with 13.1 %).

People from Culturally and Linguistically Diverse Backgrounds

Around 28 % of Australia's population was born overseas with migration from more than 200 countries around the world [33]. The proportion of the population born overseas has grown steadily from one in ten (10 %) in 1947. Between 2004 and 2014, Australia's overseas-born population increased from 4.8 million to 6.6 million people. The largest proportion was born in the United Kingdom (5.2 %) followed by New Zealand (2.6 %), China (excluding Hong Kong) (1.9 %), India (1.7 %), the Philippines (1 %), Vietnam (1.0 %), Italy (0.9 %), South Africa (0.8 %), Malaysia (0.7 %), and Germany (0.5 %) [33]. The relative proportion of Australian residents born overseas is changing with a decrease in those born in the United Kingdom and an increase in those born in New Zealand, China, and India. Of overseas-born Australians, the biggest proportion come from Northwest Europe (including the United Kingdom) (25 %) followed by Southeast Asia (14 %), Southern and Eastern Europe (12 %), Oceania (including New Zealand) (12 %), Northeast Asia (12 %), and Southern and Central Asia (10 %). This increase in cultural diversity has implications for health services and the demographics of health in Australia [30].

Culturally and linguistically diverse (CALD) communities in Australia experience both significant health disparities and a lack of access to services. A systematic review of the literature on the effectiveness of culturally appropriate interventions to manage or prevent chronic disease in CALD communities found that the health of Australia's CALD population is poor in comparison to the general population. Hospital admissions for CALD people were more than double, particularly for chronic and disabling conditions, such as diabetes, traumatic injury, heart and kidney disease, and respiratory problems [34].

The prevalence of type 2 diabetes varies by ethnicity and socioeconomic status (SES), and migrants experience a disproportionate burden of disease compared with locally born groups. Abouzeid et al. compared the prevalence odds of type 2 diabetes among immigrant groups in the Australian state of Victoria with Australian-born residents. The overall prevalence of diagnosed type 2 diabetes in Victoria was 4.1 % in men and 3.5 % in women [35]. Of those with type 2 diabetes, over one in five born in Oceania and in Southern and Central Asia were aged under 50 years. For both men and women, odds of type 2 diabetes were higher for all migrant groups than the Australian-born reference population. After adjusting for age and SES, odds were 6.3 and 7.2 times higher for men and women born in the Pacific Islands, respectively, and 5.2 and 5.0 times higher for men and women born in Southern and Central Asia, respectively. However, compared with Australian-born people, age- and SES-adjusted prevalence odds were significantly increased across all groups for males and females including Oceania (2.6 and 3.0), Northwest Europe (1.5 and 1.7), Southern and Eastern Europe (2.0 and 2.4), North Africa and the Middle East (4.0 and 4.7), Southeast Asia (3.1 and 4.0), Northeast Asia (1.9 and 2.6), Southern and Central Asia (5.2 and 5.0), America (2.0 and 2.4), and sub-Saharan Africa (2.7 and 3.1). These sociocultural differences have implications for health service planning and delivery, policy, and preventive efforts in Australia.

Gestational diabetes is a particular problem in mothers from different ethnic groups. A computerized database of all births ($n=956{,}738$) between 1995 and 2005 in the Australian state of New South Wales was used to examine the association between sociodemographic characteristics and the occurrence of gestational diabetes [36]. Between 1995 and 2005, the prevalence of GDM increased by 45 %, from 3.0 % to 4.4 %. Women born in South Asia had the highest adjusted odds ratio of any region (4.22 [95 % CI 4.01–4.44]) relative to women born in Australia. However, all regions showed increased adjusted odds – Northeast and Southeast Asia 3.24 (3.16–3.34), Europe and North America 1.21 (1.16–1.26), Middle East and North Africa 2.40 (2.30–2.51), Pacific 2.94 (2.78–3.11), other Africa 1.62 (1.46–1.80), and Caribbean, Central, and South America 1.82 (1.65–2.01).

The rate of progression from GDM to developing postpartum abnormal glucose tolerance is greater in certain ethnic groups. In a prospective study of 101 women who had GDM, ethnicity was a major risk factor for the development of diabetes during a mean follow-up of 5.5 years [37]. South Asian women had a significantly higher risk of developing abnormal glucose tolerance (69 %) than women of all other ethnicities.

The prevalence of diabetes and impaired glucose tolerance was also very high among other groups – Southeast and East Asian (41 %), Middle Eastern (44 %), South European backgrounds (42 %), and Australian-born women (39 %).

Differences in the clinical characteristics and outcomes of women with GDM from various ethnic groups have also been reported. Wong reported a retrospective review of 827 women with GDM from five ethnic groups (Southeast Asian, South Asian, Middle Eastern, Anglo-European, and Pacific Islander). Southeast Asians had the lowest BMI and lowest need for insulin therapy and their offspring had the lowest rate of macrosomia and lowest birth weight. In contrast, women from Pacific Islands had the highest BMI and greatest need for insulin therapy, and their offspring had the highest birth weights. This study highlighted the significant differences in clinical characteristics of women with GDM [38].

Diabetes Management

In general, information on diabetes management and rates of complications in Australia are less well documented than epidemiological data. While there are some data for Indigenous Australians, there are few specific data for the other two groups included in this review.

Indigenous Australians have evidence of poorer glycemic and metabolic control and high rates of diabetes complications and cardiovascular mortality.

In the National Aboriginal and Torres Strait Islander Health Measures Survey, the following goals on the optimal management in those with known diabetes were assessed:

- Fasting blood glucose between 6.0 and 8.0 mmol/L
- HbA1c levels less than or equal to 7.0 %
- Total cholesterol less than 4.0 mmol/L
- HDL cholesterol greater than or equal to 1.0 mmol/L
- LDL cholesterol less than 2.0 mmol/L
- Non-HDL cholesterol less than 2.5 mmol/L
- Triglycerides less than 2.0 mmol/L
- Albumin/creatinine ratio less than 3.5 mg/mmol for women and less than 2.5 mg/mmol for men
- Urinary albumin excretion less than 20 mg/L
- Blood pressure less than or equal to 130/80 mmHg
- "Normal" body mass index (i.e., a BMI score of between 18.5 and 24.9)
- Nonsmoker

In 2012–2013, around two in five (38.9 %) Indigenous Australian adults with known diabetes had an HbA1c result of 7.0 % or less. Overall, Indigenous women were more likely than men to achieve this result (47.0 % compared with 28.1 %). Indigenous people with known diabetes were less likely than their non-Indigenous counterparts to have an HbA1c of 7.0 % or less (38.9 % compared with 55.9 %) [15].

Just over half (56.9 %) met the management target for triglycerides and 44.4 % met the target for albumin/creatinine ratio (ACR). However, Indigenous people with diabetes were less likely than non-Indigenous people to meet these targets, particularly for ACR (44.4 % compared with 71.0 %) [15].

Two of the most common problems in Indigenous people are cardiovascular (CVD) and kidney disease. CVD risk factors are prevalent. The DRUID study found that while people with diabetes had a greater number of CVD risk factors than those without diabetes, these risk factors were relatively common in young people (aged <35 years) without diabetes with almost half (45 %) having at least two risk factors and only 18 % having none [17]. Six in ten (60.5 %) Indigenous people with diabetes had lower than normal levels of HDL cholesterol compared with 32.9 % of those without diabetes (Fig. 9.2). They were also around twice as likely to have high triglycerides (45.1 % compared with 20.7 %). A quarter (25.0 %) had high cholesterol, but only around one in ten (9.1 %) of this group were aware they had it [15]. Many Indigenous people with diabetes also had signs of other chronic conditions. Around half (53.1 %) had signs of chronic kidney disease, significantly higher than the corresponding rate in the non-Indigenous population (32.5 %) [15].

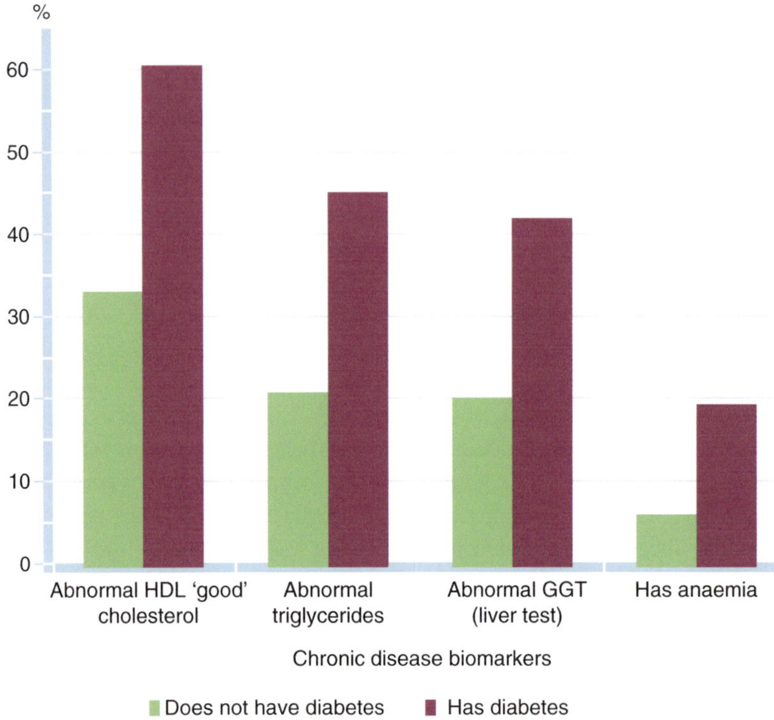

Fig. 9.2 Selected chronic disease biomarkers in Indigenous subjects with and without diabetes (Source: 2012–2013 Australian Aboriginal and Torres Strait Islander Health Survey Biomedical Results)

Thomas et al. examined the management of 144 Indigenous people with type 2 diabetes in Australian primary care compared with that in non-Indigenous patients presenting consecutively to the same medical practitioner ($n=449$). Indigenous Australians had high rates of micro- and macrovascular disease with 60 % having an abnormal ACR compared to 33 % of non-Indigenous patients ($p<0.01$). In addition, they were more likely to have established macrovascular disease (adjusted odds ratio 2.7). This excess in complications was associated with poor glycemic control, with an HbA1c ≥8.0 %, observed in 55 % of all Indigenous patients, despite the similar frequency of use of oral antidiabetic agents and insulin. Smoking was more common in Indigenous patients (38 % vs. 10 %, $p<0.01$). However, the achievement of LDL and blood pressure targets was the same or better in Indigenous patients. This cross-sectional study confirmed aboriginal ethnicity as a powerful risk factor for microvascular and macrovascular disease [39].

Davis et al. used data from the observational Fremantle Diabetes Study to examine disparities in the nature and management of type 2 diabetes between Indigenous Australians and Anglo-Celt patients in an urban Australian community [40]. Data from the Fremantle Diabetes Study collected from 1993 to 1996 (phase I) and from 2008 to 2011 (phase II) were analyzed. Indigenous participants were younger at entry and, at diabetes diagnosis, were less likely to be educated beyond primary level and more likely to be smokers. HbA1c decreased in both groups over time (Indigenous median 9.6 % [interquartile range 7.8–10.7 %] to 8.4 % [6.6–10.6 %] vs. Anglo-Celt median 7.1 % [6.2–8.4 %] to 6.7 % [6.2–7.5 %]), but the gap persisted. Indigenous patients were more likely to have microvascular disease in both phases. The prevalence of peripheral arterial disease (ankle-brachial index <0.90 or lower-extremity amputation) increased in Indigenous but decreased in Anglo-Celt participants.

While renal disease is common in Indigenous Australians, there is considerable regional variation in the incidence of end-stage renal disease (ESRD). Cass and colleagues reviewed information on 719 Indigenous ESRD patients who commenced treatment in Australia during 1993–1998 using data from the Australian and New Zealand

Dialysis and Transplant Registry who started ESRD treatment. Standardized ESRD incidence among Indigenous Australians was highest in remote regions, where it was up to 30 times the national incidence for all Australians. In urban regions, the standardized incidence was much lower, but remained significantly higher than the national incidence. Forty-eight percent of Indigenous ESRD patients came from regions without dialysis or transplant facilities and 16.3 % from regions with only satellite dialysis facilities. Because of the location of treatment centers, there is inequitable access to ESRD treatment services for a significant proportion of Indigenous patients [41].

A number of attempts have been made to improve clinical systems for addressing the gap in care of Indigenous Australians with diabetes. McDermott and colleagues assessed changes in clinical indicators of adults diagnosed with diabetes using audits of clinical records of Torres Strait Islander adults on diabetes registers in 21 primary care clinics. Over a 6-year period, the number of adults included on the diabetes register increased from 555 in 1999 to 1024 in 2005. Mean weight increased from 86.8 to 95.6 kg, and mean HbA1c level remained unchanged at about 9 %, but the proportion with HbA1c level <7 % increased from 18.4 % to 26.1 % and the proportion with BP <140/90 mmHg increased from 40.3 % to 66.8 %. This study showed that some improvements can be achieved by introducing clinical systems, but important clinical parameters such as weight gain and hyperglycemia remain a challenge [42].

The effectiveness of a systematic treatment program to modify renal and cardiovascular disease in an Indigenous Australian community from the Tiwi Islands with high rates of renal failure and cardiovascular deaths was reported by Hoy et al. [43]. Adults with blood pressure ≥140/90, with diabetes and ACR ≥3.4 g/mol, or with progressive overt albuminuria were offered the intervention which included attempts to achieve blood pressure goals and improve control of blood glucose and lipid levels and health education. Two hundred fifty-eight people enrolled in the program, and 118 had complete data for 2 years of treatment. In these 118, blood pressures fell significantly, while ACR and GFR stabilized. Rates of the combined end points of renal failure and natural death per 100 person-years were 2.9 for the treatment group (95 % CI, 1.7–4.6) and 4.8 for the historical control group (95 % CI, 3.3–7.0). After adjustment for baseline ACR category, the relative risk of the treatment group versus the control group for these combined end points was 0.47 (95 % CI, 0.25–0.86; $P=0.013$). Treatment benefit was especially marked in people with overt albuminuria or hypertension and in people without diabetes. The estimates of benefit were supported by a fall in community rates of death and renal failure.

Point of care testing (POCT) for HbA1c and urine ACR is increasingly available in Indigenous communities under the auspices of the Quality Assurance for Aboriginal Medical Services (QAAMS) Program. Shephard et al. evaluated the QAAMS Program and assessed satisfaction with POCT for HbA1c and urine ACR in a medical service in a remote area of Northern Australia for Indigenous people with type 2 diabetes [44]. Both doctors and patients reported that the immediacy of POCT had contributed positively to the identification and management of diabetes, improved doctor-patient relationship, and facilitated compliance and self-motivation to control diabetes. At the end of the 12 months, there was a statistically significant drop in HbA1c from 9.3 % to 8.6 % ($P=0.003$) with an improvement in the percentage of patients controlling their diabetes.

The addition of HbA1c as a diagnostic criterion for diabetes has simplified algorithms for testing and detecting undiagnosed diabetes. POCT for HbA1c in this context has particular advantages in Indigenous communities. Marley and colleagues compared the Australian glucose-based algorithm [45] with an HbA1c-based algorithm applied in a remote Australian Aboriginal community. The HbA1c-based algorithm used an initial POCT HbA1c assessment followed by laboratory HbA1c assay if needed. Participants were significantly more likely to receive a definitive result within 7 days and to be diagnosed with diabetes using the HbA1c algorithm than with the glucose-based protocol. The study also highlighted the increased likelihood of follow-up with HbA1c testing; only 42 % of participants with an equivocal glucose result underwent an OGTT as recommended by the Australian guideline [46].

Conclusions

Like other countries around the world, Australia is experiencing a steady increase in the number of people with diabetes which is placing a considerable burden on individuals, their families, and the whole society. The impact on Indigenous Australians is particularly heavy with diabetes prevalence rates, threefold higher than non-Indigenous Australians. Indigenous Australians also have increased rates of complications, especially renal. Two other groups also experience significant disadvantage – people from culturally and linguistically diverse backgrounds and people living in rural and remote areas. While epidemiological data are available for these groups, information on diabetes management and rates of complications are less well documented. While some programs are being implemented to improve quality of care and outcomes, an increased effort is needed to reduce the care gap in these groups compared with other Australians.

There are many gaps in our knowledge of diabetes in these populations and unmet needs with respect to prevention, care, and treatment. Future research will be needed to address these gaps and reduce the disparity between these groups and other Australians.

References

1. Australian National Diabetes Strategy 2016-2020. http://www.health.gov.au/internet/main/publishing.nsf/Content/nds-2016-2020.
2. National Diabetes Service Scheme (NDSS). Data snapshots. 2014. [Online]. Available: http://www.ndss.com.au/en/Research/Data-Snapshots/.
3. Australian Bureau of Statistics (ABS). Australian health survey – biomedical results for chronic diseases. 2011–12. Available: http://www.abs.gov.au/australianhealthsurvey.
4. Dunstan DW, Zimmet PZ, Welborn TA, et al. The rising prevalence of diabetes and impaired glucose tolerance: the Australian diabetes, obesity and lifestyle study. Diabetes Care. 2002;25:829–34.
5. Australia Institute of Health and Welfare Australia's Health. Australia's health series no 12. Cat no. AUS 122. Canberra: AIHW; 2010.
6. Australian Institute of Health and Welfare (AIHW). Causes of death. 2013. [Online]. Available: http://www.aihw.gov.au/deaths/causes-of-death/.
7. Australian Institute of Health and Welfare (AIHW). Diabetes: Australian facts 2008. Canberra: Diabetes Series; 2008.
8. Colagiuri S, Brnabic A, Gomez M, et al. DiabCo$t Australia: assessing the burden of type 1 diabetes in Australia. Canberra: Diabetes Australia; 2009.
9. Lee CM, Colagiuri R, Magliano DJ, et al. The cost of diabetes in Adults in Australia. Diabetes Res Clin Pract. 2013;99(3):385–904.
10. Australian Bureau of Statistics. http://www.abs.gov.au/ausstats/abs@.nsf/Lookup/by%20Subject/4338.0~2011-13~Main%20Features~Overweight%20and%20obesity~10007.
11. ABS. Projected population, Aboriginal and Torres Strait Islander Australians, Australia, states and territories, 2011–2026. ABS cat. no. 3238.0. Canberra: ABS; 2014.
12. ABS. Life tables for Aboriginal and Torres Strait Islander Australians, 2010–2012. ABS cat. no. 3302.0.55.003. Canberra: ABS; 2013.
13. AIHW. Mortality and life expectancy of Indigenous Australians 2008 to 2012. Cat. no. IHW 140. Canberra: AIHW; 2014.
14. AIHW. Aboriginal and Torres Strait Islander health performance framework 2014 report: detailed analyses. 2015. Cat. no. IHW 167. http://www.aihw.gov.au/publication.
15. ABS. Australian Aboriginal and Torres Strait Islander Health Survey: biomedical results, 2012-13. 2014. Cat. no. 4727.0.55.003.
16. Minges KE, Zimmet P, Magliano DJ, et al. Diabetes prevalence and determinants in Indigenous Australian populations: a systematic review. Diabetes Res Clin Pract. 2011;93(2):139–49.
17. O'Dea K, Cunningham J, Maple-Brown L, Weeramanthri T, Shaw J, Dunbar T, et al. Diabetes and cardiovascular risk factors in urban Indigenous adults: results from the DRUID study. Diabetes Res Clin Pract. 2008;80:483–9.
18. Craig ME, Femia G, Broyda V, et al. Type 2 diabetes in Indigenous and non-Indigenous children and adolescents in New South Wales. Med J Aust. 2007;186:497–9.
19. Azzopardi P, Brown AD, Zimmet P, Fahy RE, Dent GA, Kelly MJ, Kranzusch K, Maple-Brown LJ, Nossar V, Silink M, Sinha AK, Stone ML. Type 2 diabetes in young Indigenous Australians in rural and remote areas: diagnosis, screening, management and prevention. Med J Aust. 2012;197:32–6.

20. Sinha A, O'Rourke S, Yarker J, et al. Type 2 diabetes in children and adolescents in the Indigenous communities of Far North Queensland. Diabetes Res Clin Pract. 2000;50(Supplement 1):126.
21. Constantino MI, Molyneaux L, Limacher-Gisler F, Al-Saeed A, Luo C, Wu T, Twigg TM, Yue DK, Wong J. Long-term complications and mortality in young-onset diabetes type 2 diabetes is more hazardous and lethal than type 1 diabetes. Diabetes Care. 2013;36: 3863–9.
22. Daniel M, Rowley KG, McDermott R, O'Dea K. Diabetes and impaired glucose tolerance in Aboriginal Australians: prevalence and risk. Diabetes Res Clin Pract. 2002;57:23–33.
23. Australian Institute of Health and Welfare. Birthweight of babies born to Indigenous mothers. Cat. no. IHW 138. Canberra: AIHW; 2014.
24. Kowal EE. Genetic research in Indigenous health: significant progress, substantial challenges. Med J Aust. 2012;197:19–20.
25. Busfield F, Duffy DL, Kesting JB, Walker SM, Lovelock PK, Good D, Tate H, Watego D, Marczak M, Hayman N, Shaw JTE. A genomewide search for type 2 diabetes–susceptibility gene in indigenous Australians. Am J Hum Genet. 2002;70: 349–57.
26. Kowal E, Anderson I. Genetic research in Aboriginal and Torres Strait Islander communities: continuing the discussion. Lowitja Institute. 2012. www.lowitja.org.au/lowitja-institute-publishing.
27. Ishak M, Petocz P. Gestational diabetes among Aboriginal Australians: prevalence, time trend and comparisons with non-Aboriginal Australians. Ethn Dis. 2003;13:55–60.
28. Porter C, Skinner T, Ellis I. The current state of Indigenous and Aboriginal women with diabetes in pregnancy: a systematic review. Diabetes Res Clin Pract. 2012;98:209–22.
29. ABS. Regional population growth, Australia, 2013–14, ABS cat. no. 3218.0. Canberra: ABS; 2015.
30. Australian Institute of Health and Welfare. Australia's welfare 2015. Australia's welfare series no. 12. Cat. no. AUS 189. Canberra: AIHW; 2015.
31. ABS Australian Institute of Health and Welfare. 2010. A snapshot of men's health in regional and remote Australia. Rural health series no. 11. Cat. no. PHE 120. Canberra: AIHW. http://www.aihw.gov.au/rural-health-publications/.
32. Australian Institute Health and Welfare (AIHW). http://www.aihw.gov.au/diabetes-indicators/deaths/.
33. ABS. Migration, Australia, 2013–14. ABS cat. no. 3412.0. Canberra: ABS; 2015.
34. Henderson S, Kendall E, See L. The effectiveness of culturally appropriate interventions to manage or prevent chronic disease in culturally and linguistically diverse communities: a systematic literature review. Health Soc Care Community. 2011;19(3):225–49.
35. Abouzeid M, Philpot B, Janus ED, Coates MJ, Dunbar JA. Type 2 diabetes prevalence varies by socioeconomic status within and between migrant groups: analysis and implications for Australia. BMC Public Health. 2013;13:252–60.
36. Anna V, Van der Ploeg HP, Cheung WN, Huxley RR, Bauman AE. Sociodemographic correlates of the increasing trend in prevalence of gestational diabetes mellitus in a large population of women between 1995 and 2005. Diabetes Care. 2008;31:2288–93.
37. Girgis CM, Gunton JE, Cheung NW. The influence of ethnicity on the development of type 2 diabetes mellitus in women with gestational diabetes: a prospective study and review of the literature. ISRN Endocrinol. 2012;2012:3416381; 1–7.
38. Wong VW. Gestational diabetes mellitus in five ethnic groups: a comparison of their clinical characteristics. Diabet Med. 2012;29:366–71.
39. Thomas M, Weekes AJ, Thomas MC. The management of diabetes in indigenous Australians from primary care. BMC Public Health. 2007;7:303–11.
40. Davis TM, Hunt K, McAullay D, Chubb SA, Sillars BA, Bruce DG, Davis WA. Continuing disparities in cardiovascular risk factors and complications between aboriginal and Anglo-Celt Australians with type 2 diabetes: the Fremantle Diabetes Study. Diabetes Care. 2012;35:2005–11.
41. Cass A, Cunningham J, Wang Z, Hoy W. Regional variation in the incidence of end-stage renal disease in Indigenous Australians. Med J Aust. 2001;175:24–7.
42. McDermott RA, McCulloch BG, Campbell SK, Young DM. Diabetes in the Torres Strait Islands of Australia: better clinical systems but significant increase in weight and other risk conditions among adults, 1999–2005. Med J Aust. 2007;186:505–8.
43. Hoy WE, Baker PR, Kelly AM, Wang Z. Reducing premature death and renal failure in Australian Aboriginals. A community-based cardiovascular and renal protective program. Med J Aust. 2000;172: 473–8.
44. Shephard MD. Cultural and clinical effectiveness of the 'QAAMS' point-of-care testing model for diabetes management in Australian Aboriginal medical services. Clin Biochem Rev. 2006;27(3):161–70.
45. Marley JV, Oh MS, Hadgraft NT. Using glycated haemoglobin testing to simplify diabetes screening in remote Aboriginal Australian health care settings. Med J Aust. 2105;204:28–32.
46. Colagiuri S, Davies D, Girgis S, Colagiuri R. National evidence based guideline for case detection and diagnosis of type 2 diabetes. Canberra: Diabetes Australia, NHMRC; 2009. http://www.nhmrc.gov.au/guidelines/publications/di17. Accessed Dec 2015.

Diabetes Among Māori and Other Ethnic Groups in New Zealand

10

Evan Atlantis, Grace Joshy, Margaret Williams, and David Simmons

Unique Aspects of Diabetes in New Zealand

New Zealand, known by the indigenous people (Māori) as Aotearoa, is in the South Pacific to the West of Australia. With a land mass of 270,500 km^2 over two major islands (North and South Islands), the population was estimated in 2015 to be 4,637,847. In the 2013 census, 74.0 % identified with one or more European identities, 14.9 % (598,605 people) identified as Māori, 11.8 % identified as Asian and 7.4 % identified as Pacific peoples [1]. European New Zealanders are predominantly of British descent arriving from the mid-nineteenth century. Māori are Polynesians who arrived mainly between 800 and 1200 AD. Pacific peoples largely started arriving in the 1960s and are mainly Polynesians from Samoa, Tonga, Cook Islands, Niue and Tokelau Islands. Asians are from across the continent and first arrived in the nineteenth century, with more rapid increases in immigration in the 1990s. Although Māori and other minority groups are distributed across the country, the ethnic mix differs depending on location, with Auckland (population 1.4 million) recognised as the city with the largest Polynesian population in the world (approximately 32 %).

E. Atlantis, PhD
Western Sydney University,
Campbelltown, NSW, Australia
e-mail: e.atlantis@westernsydney.edu.au

G. Joshy, PhD
Australian National University,
Canberra, ACT, Australia
e-mail: Grace.Joshy@anu.edu.au

M. Williams, PhD
Auckland University of Technology,
Auckland, New Zealand
e-mail: marwilli@aut.ac.nz

D. Simmons, FRACP, FRCP, MD (✉)
School of Medicine, Western Sydney University,
Locked Bag 1797, Penrith,
NSW NSW 2751, Australia
e-mail: Da.Simmons@westernsydney.edu.au

Māori Perspective on Health and Research

Historically, mainstream health services and research models have not always benefitted indigenous peoples, including Māori [2–5]. The information collected was led by health professionals (including researchers) who may have perpetuated colonial values, while the true complexities of Māori values, belief systems and customs were often not reported accurately [3, 6].

Since the 1960s, in Aotearoa, New Zealand, there has clearly been a shift in the way non-indigenous health professionals, researchers and academics have positioned themselves and their work in relation to working with Māori [2, 4–9]. An important starting point includes bicultural

S. Dagogo-Jack (ed.), *Diabetes Mellitus in Developing Countries and Underserved Communities*,
DOI 10.1007/978-3-319-41559-8_10

strategies developed between Māori and non-Māori. These strategies are unique to Aotearoa, New Zealand, because they are an active response from the Crown (Government) towards the Treaty of Waitangi, signed in 1840 [12]. It is about honouring of the Treaty through the acknowledgement and application of the principles–partnership, participation and protection [5, 9–12]. Evans and Paewai [13] provided definitions of each principle as follows:

(a) *Partnership*. Māori and non-Māori are all citizens of New Zealand; Māori are also afforded tangata whenua (people of the land) status and, as such, might identify with a whānau (extended family), hapu (subtribe) or iwi (tribal group).
(b) *Protection*. This applies to the principle of self-determination and rights to traditional properties or taonga (treasures) such as culture, land, language and all that is deemed important, including self-determination in matters affecting personal well-being such as health, welfare, educational policies and legislation.
(c) *Participation*. The recognition that Māori, as individuals and equal partners, should be afforded equal access and participation in society's benefits.

These principles provide a framework for identifying Māori ethical and practice issues in terms of the rights, roles and responsibilities for health professionals, researchers and Māori communities in Aotearoa, New Zealand.

The dynamics of Māori usually infer whānau (family) or groups to compete, while individuals cooperate within the whānau (extended families). Such dynamics emphasise the sense of inclusiveness where people usually feel part of a whānau (family), hapu (subtribe) or iwi (tribes/people) [14–16]. In contrast, some health professionals, researchers and academics report that mainstream (New Zealand European) perspectives have a bias towards autonomy rather than towards affiliation and a sense of community within a group [7]. Fundamentally, the collaborative and collective methods of learning associated with Māori traditions, values and customs would be useful within learning environments for Māori [2, 4, 17]. The use of kaupapa Māori research concepts may also be helpful for those living with chronic health diseases, such as type 2 diabetes, in acquiring knowledge and understanding and then engaging in activities around health and well-being. For the individual newly diagnosed with type 2 diabetes, managing their blood glucose concentration through increased physical activity and consumption of nutritious food is a priority. The following are concepts often associated with kaupapa Māori styles of learning that encompasses collecting and sharing information with individuals actively involved in education and/or research projects [6, 17]:

- Tino rangatiratanga (relative autonomy/self-determination of Māori culture).
- Taonga tuku iho (cultural aspirations) – the treasures from the ancestors include cultural aspirations Māori hold for their children and messages that guide our/their relationships and interaction patterns.
- Ako (reciprocal learning) literally meaning to teach and to learn – the teacher or health professional does not have to be the fountain of all knowledge.
- Kia piki ake i nga raruraru o te kainga (mediation of socioeconomic and home difficulties).
- Whānau primary concept (a cultural preference) that contains both values (cultural aspirations) and social processes (cultural practices).
- Kaupapa, the collective vision principle.

Māori research ethics guidelines and academic bodies in health (e.g. New Zealand Research Health Council and Nga Pae o te Maramatanga) can now be sourced for learning and sharing information about best practice in the delivery of health services and research with indigenous people, in particular, Māori [5, 16, 19]. Such knowledge advocates for equal sharing of power and control through the processes of reciprocity and feedback as a partnership principle. It also requires consolidation that Māori exist in a cultural dynamic that is collective and/or cooperative [2, 4, 5, 8, 9, 18]. Overall, the goal of the kaupapa Māori research approach is to improve the Hauora (health and well-being) of each individual within and for the whānau (family), in this instance for those living with type 2 diabetes. Essentially the core of kaupapa Māori is the catch cry 'to be Māori is the norm' where the research approach is for/with/by Māori and it does not exclude or reject mainstream or other indigenous cultures [2, 4, 17, 19].

Diabetes in Aotearoa, New Zealand

The high type 2 diabetes (T2D) prevalence among Māori was first reported in 1962 [20]. Immigrants from the nearby Tokelau Islands were subsequently shown to have an increasing prevalence of T2D compared with those remaining on the Islands [21]. Work was commenced in South Auckland, an area with large Māori, Pacific and Asian communities, in the 1990s [22] to obtain diabetes epidemiological data linked with a range of diabetes preventative strategies to inform a comprehensive diabetes management and prevention strategy. A local plan (the first such plan published globally) was developed and reviewed in 2000, showing progress in some areas but not others [23]. By 2006, subsequent data showed that the national epidemic of diabetes was continuing unabated and now included Asians [24].

Since 2006, a number of new publications have emerged, reporting the prevalence of diabetes and its complications. The impression is that the diabetes epidemic continues to make inroads in spite of a range of policies to reduce the obesity epidemic and improve diabetes care. There remain few studies describing molecular biological differences between Polynesians and Europeans. This chapter will describe an updated review on diabetes and its complications among Māori, Pacific people and Asian vs. European ethnic groups in New Zealand.

Objectives

This review sought to provide an updated report on the epidemiology of diabetes including prevalence, risk factors for complications and severe outcomes (e.g. hospitalisation, death) in Māori and other ethnic groups in New Zealand.

Methods

Eligibility Criteria

Population

This review considered studies in indigenous and underserved ethnic groups (Māori, Pacific [namely, Samoa, Cook Islands, Tonga, Fiji, Niue, Samoa, and Solomon Islands], South Asian [namely, Bangladesh, India, Sri Lanka, and Nepal] and other Asian ethnic groups) with or without comparison with European ethnic groups in New Zealand.

Study Type

This review considered non-experimental (observational) study designs including before and after studies, prospective and retrospective cohort studies, case control studies and cross-sectional studies for inclusion.

Outcomes

This review considered studies that reported on one or more of the following outcomes: incidence or prevalence of any type of diabetes (type 1 diabetes [T1D], T2D or gestational diabetes mellitus [GDM]), biological (namely, pre-diabetes, metabolic syndrome, obesity) and lifestyle (namely, smoking, physical inactivity, and poor diet) risk factors for diabetes; and health (mortality and morbidity (namely, complications)).

Search Strategy and Information Sources

The search strategy aimed to find both peer-reviewed published studies and current reports by the New Zealand Ministry of Health. A two-step search strategy was utilised in this review. An initial search of electronic databases (MEDLINE/PubMed, EMBASE, Scopus and CINAHL) and the New Zealand Ministry of Health website was undertaken using identified keywords and index terms (see Appendix 1). Next, the reference list of all identified reports and articles was searched for additional studies.

Studies in English published after 2004 were considered for inclusion in this review. Where possible, efforts were made to contact authors for missing information.

Data Collection

Data were extracted from papers included in the review independently by two reviewers using data extraction tools developed for this review. The data extracted included specific details about the study design, participants and setting and outcomes.

Data Synthesis

Since statistical pooling was not possible because of the diverse types of studies reviewed, the findings were presented in narrative form, including tables to aid in data presentation where appropriate.

Results

Figure 10.1 presents a flow diagram summarising the identification of studies included for review. Our search strategy identified 292 citations after duplicates were removed. Of these, 246 citations were excluded after the first screening of titles and/or abstracts for inclusion and exclusion criteria, leaving 46 citations for a second full text screening. After further assessment, 12 citations were excluded leaving 34 observational studies for final inclusion in the review.

Descriptive Data Synthesis

Table 10.1 presents study characteristics of 34 studies included for review, which were published in years ranging from 2005 to 2015 [25–60]. Studies were heterogeneous for age, ethnicity and screening/diagnostic characteristics. For instance, case definition of diabetes using HbA1c diagnostic cutoffs was varied across studies between ≥6.5 and >7.0 %, and from 5.7–6.4 % to >6.0 % for pre-diabetes (Table 10.1). Only one study used the oral glucose tolerance test (OGTT) in a population-based sample [57]. Similarly, pre-existing diabetes has been identified through self-report, primary care/general practice records, hospital chart review and data linkage between pharmaceuticals and/or laboratory investigations and hospital admissions/national administrative datasets. Study populations were identified/recruited using various methods including community screening, clinic databases and population based health databases (Table 10.1).

Table 10.2 shows the prevalence of diabetes and pre-diabetes. The prevalence of known diabetes was estimated to be 2.2–5.0 % among Europeans vs. 7.0–12.2 % among Māori, 8.9–38 % among Pacific people and 9.1–37.1 % among Asians. The prevalence of diabetes including known diabetes and undiagnosed diabetes by HbA1c screening ranged from 1.1 to 6.1 % among Europeans but 3.3 to 9.8 % among Māori, 5.3–15.4 % among Pacific peoples and 4.3–9.3 % among Asians. Undiagnosed diabetes alone ranged from 0.4 to 1.1 % among Europeans but 3.6–6.5 % among Māori, 4.6–8.1 % among Pacific people and 7.4–7.5 % among Asians. No consistent gender differences were found.

Three studies (South Auckland, Waikato and Auckland) described the prevalence of diagnosed diabetes [34, 47, 55] in patients who had been hospitalised with an acute cardiovascular event (mean ages 60, 68 and 15+ years, respectively). The prevalence among Māori, Pacific and Asians was approximately double that of European New Zealanders (23.3–39.2 % vs. 11.3–18.1 %). One, a nationwide study among people with a mood and anxiety disorder, aged ≥16 years, again showed the greater prevalence of known diabetes among Māori and Pacific peoples over Europeans (8.0–11.3 % vs. 3.6 %) [38].

A key theme is that within each study, the prevalence of diabetes is generally highest in Pacific people and then Māori, who generally have a prevalence approximately twice that of Europeans. Asians also have a high prevalence generally between (but sometimes below or

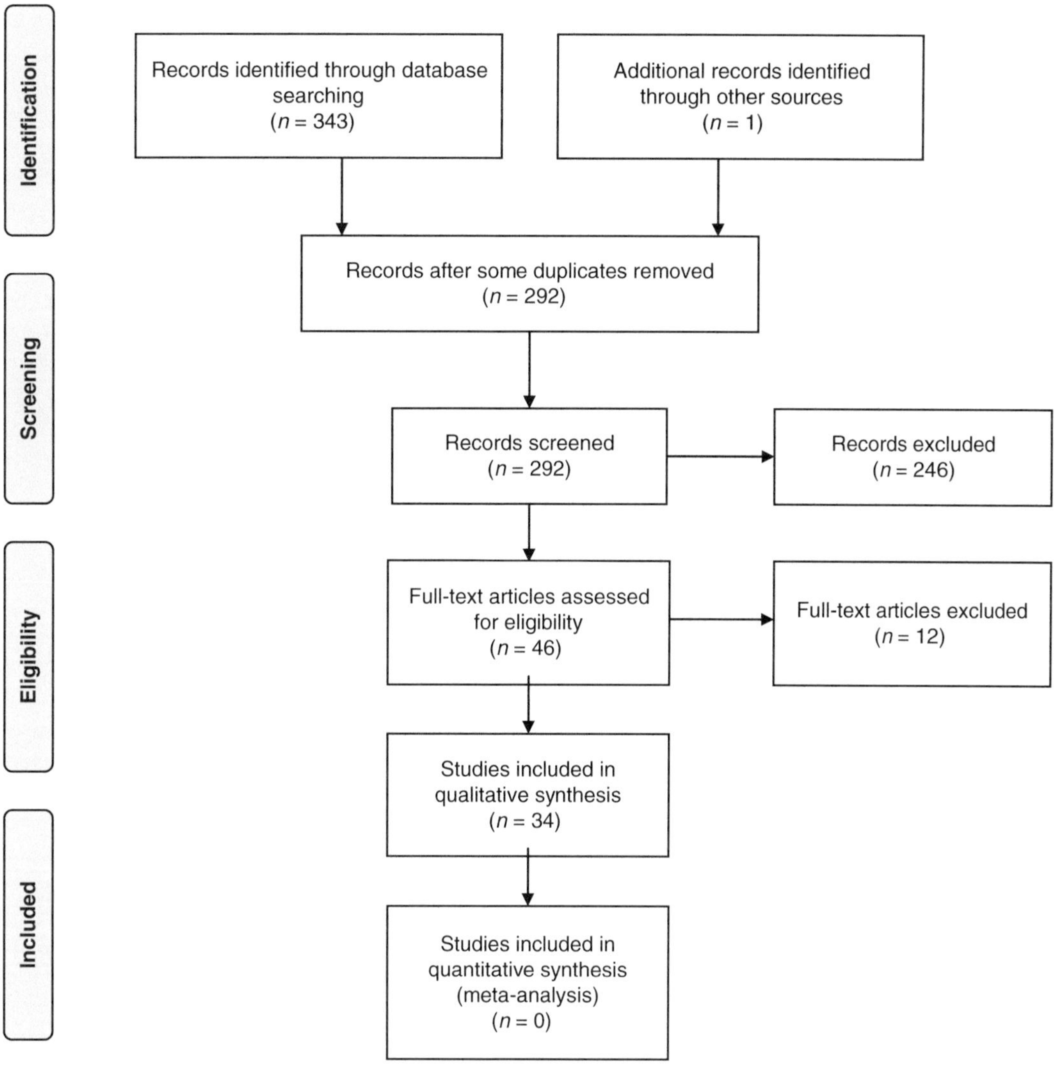

Fig. 10.1 PRISMA 2009 Flow Diagram for systematic review of publications since 2006, when the last review was undertaken

above) Māori and Pacific people. These odds ratios are consistent with the 2013/2014 New Zealand Health Survey.

There are few studies of pre-diabetes. Two, a national study and a South Auckland study [29, 32], using HbA1c of 5.7–6.4 % and 6.1–7.0 % as diagnostic criteria, respectively, found that the prevalence of HbA1c defined pre-diabetes was approximately sixfold higher among non-Europeans than Europeans (12.8–19.9 % vs. 2.1–2.5 %, respectively). Similarly, high prevalence estimates for impaired glucose tolerance and/or impaired fasting glucose were reported among Māori in the Waikato region [57].

Table 10.3 shows the prevalence of risk factors for complications among people with diabetes by ethnic group. Across the data sources from primary care (including the national 'Get Checked' data) to a mixture of primary care and hospitals and from both national, Waikato, South Auckland, West Auckland and South Island studies, Māori, Pacific people and Asians are more likely to have poor glucose control than Europeans. European and Māori patients with type 1 diabetes were more

Table 10.1 Characteristics of observational studies reviewed

Study identification	Study design (follow-up)	Participants and setting	Outcomes (measures, units)
Agban et al. (2008) [25]	Cross-sectional (baseline and 2 years from cohort study)	*Sample size:* N = 7782 *Age (years):* range in mean from 56 to 68 *Gender:* male 42 % *Ethnicity:* European, Māori, Pacific, Asian (Indian), other Asian, Other (Middle Eastern, Latin American/Hispanic and African) *Eligibility criteria*: T2D patients who had undertaken an annual review in 2002 or 2003, and had a follow-up review 2 years later *Setting:* nationwide data from primary health care reviews of patients with T2D collated within 15 primary care organisations or diabetes trusts	*Baseline and 2 years for all outcomes* Poor glycaemic control prevalence (HbA1c >8 %, %) HBP prevalence (>130/80, %) Obesity prevalence (measured BMI ≥30 for European, Asian, Indian and 'Other'; BMI ≥32 for Māori and Pacific, %) Current smoker prevalence (self-report, %),
Brian et al. (2010) [26]	Population-based cross-sectional survey using multistage cluster random sampling	*Sample size:* N = 1381 (73 %) *Age (years):* ≥40 *Gender:* NR *Ethnicity:* Fijian *Eligibility criteria*: HbA1c and visual acuity were measured *Setting:* Diabetic eye disease was assessed using 90-dioptre lens dilated funduscopy	HbA1c and visual acuity measured Mean HbA1c (9.9 ± 2.3 %) Vision threat occurred in at least one eye of 11.5 %. Diabetes (predominantly maculopathy) caused pinhole acuity <6/18, <6/60 and <3/60 for 3.8 %, 1.1 % and 0.7 % of eyes, respectively. No person was bilaterally blind (<6/60) due to diabetes, but 2.3 % (all on oral antiglycaemics alone) were 6/60 bilaterally. Compared with recent diabetes diagnosis, diagnosis >10 years ago was predictive of any (odds ratio [OR] 8.13; 95 % confidence interval [CI] 3.28–20.21; $P<0.001$) and vision-threatening (OR 5.25; 95 % CI 1.71–16.12; $P=0.004$) eye disease. Although 80.6 % claimed regular general diabetes checkups, only 36.5 % recalled previous dilated ocular examination. Four eyes had received laser treatment

Table 10.1 (continued)

Study identification	Study design (follow-up)	Participants and setting	Outcomes (measures, units)
Brewer et al. (2008) [27]	Cross-sectional (baseline from cohort study) and prospective cohort and (median 2 years)	*Sample size: N*=47,904 (408 with prior diagnosis of diabetes) *Age (years)*: ≥0 *Gender*: male 44 % *Ethnicity*: European/other, Māori, Pacific, Asian (unspecified) *Eligibility criteria*: participants in a Hepatitis Foundation screening campaign for hepatitis B (1999–2001) *Setting*: lower half of the North Island of NZ	Diabetes prevalence (HbA1c ≥7 %, %) All-cause mortality (data linkage, HR with 95 % CI)
Chan et al. (2015) [28]	Retrospective cohort (from 2004 to 2010)	*Sample size: N*=1,475,347 *Age (years)*: ≥0 *Gender*: male 48 % *Ethnicity*: European/other, Māori, Pacific, Asian (Indian), Chinese, other Asian *Eligibility criteria*: residents who had utilised publicly funded health services in NZ and lived in Auckland in 2010 *Setting:* Auckland metropolitan region, linked data between a laboratory repository and national administrative datasets for District Health Boards	Age-standardised diabetes prevalence (dysglycaemia by modified ADA and WHO criteria, %)
Coppell et al. (2013) [29]	Cross-sectional	*Sample size: N*=4721 *Age (years)*: ≥15 *Gender*: NR *Eligibility criteria*: NR *Ethnicity*: European/Other (Asian, Middle Eastern, Latin American and African), Māori, Pacific *Setting*: nationwide, 2008/2009 New Zealand Adult Nutrition Survey	Diabetes prevalence (self-report diagnosed or HbA1c ≥6.5 %, %) Pre-diabetes prevalence (HbA1c 5.7–6.4 %, %)
Elley et al. (2008) [30]	Cross-sectional	*Sample size: N*=29,179 *Age (years)*: range in mean from 56 to 68 *Gender*: NR *Eligibility criteria*: T2D *Ethnicity*: European, Māori, Pacific, Asian (Indian), Other Asian, Other *Setting*: nationwide linked hospital records and data obtained from primary health care reviews of patients with T2D	Poor glycaemic control prevalence (HbA1c >8 %, %) HBP prevalence (>130/80, %) Obesity prevalence (measured BMI ≥30, %) Albuminuria prevalence (ACR ≥2.5 for men; ≥3.5 for women, %) Current smoker (self-report, %), 5-year CVD risk prevalence (Framingham risk score ≥15 %, %)

(continued)

Table 10.1 (continued)

Study identification	Study design (follow-up)	Participants and setting	Outcomes (measures, units)
Elley et al. (2010) [31]	Prospective cohort (median 3.9 years)	*Sample size: N*=36,127 *Age (years)*: median 59 *Gender*: male 49 % *Eligibility criteria*: T2D without previous CVD *Ethnicity*: European, Māori, Pacific, Asian (Indian), East Asian, Other (Middle Eastern, Latin American/Hispanic, African, and others) *Setting*: nationwide linked hospital records and data obtained from primary health care reviews of patients with T2D	Fatal or nonfatal CVD incidence (data linkage using ICD-9 and ICD-10 codes, HR with 95 %CI)
Ellison et al. (2005) [32]	Cross-sectional	*Sample size: N*=50,819 *Age (years):* >20 *Gender:* male 44.6 % *Ethnicity:* European, Māori, Samoan, Cook Island, Asian (Indian), Chinese *Eligibility criteria:* none specified *Setting:* South Auckland. Screening programme to detect elevated fasting hyperglycaemia using HbA1c	Diabetes prevalence (HbA1c >7 %, %) Pre-diabetes or diabetes prevalence (HbA1c >6 %, %)
Faatoese et al. (2011) [33]	Cross-sectional	*Sample size: N*=252 *Age (years):* range 20–64 *Gender:* male 40 % *Ethnicity:* Māori *Eligibility criteria:* Māori descent *Setting:* community screening for CVD risk factors in Wairoa	T2D prevalence (prior diagnosis by medical records, %)
Feigin et al. (2006) [34]	Cross-sectional	*Sample size: N* = 1423 *Age (years):* ≥15 *Gender:* Male 47 % *Ethnicity:* European, Māori/Pacific, Asian/other (unspecified) *Eligibility criteria:* first-ever cases of stroke 2002–2003 *Setting:* Auckland population-based register	Diabetes (doctor diagnosed by self-report, %)
Frederikson and Jacobs (2008) [35]	Cross-sectional (baseline from cohort study)	*Sample size: N*=11,977 *Age (years):* range 7–100 *Gender:* Male 52 % *Ethnicity:* European, Māori, Pacific (Samoan, Cook Island Māori, Tongan, Niuean), Asian (Indian), Chinese, Other *Eligibility criteria:* all records of first screening visits 2002–2005 for people with diabetes *Setting:* Wellington regional retinal screening programme for people with diabetes	Maculopathy prevalence (clinical retinopathy screening, %)

Table 10.1 (continued)

Study identification	Study design (follow-up)	Participants and setting	Outcomes (measures, units)
Grey et al. [36]	Cross-sectional	*Sample size:* N = 10,301 *Age (years):* range 35–74 *Gender:* male 52 % *Ethnicity:* Pacific (Samoans, Tongan, Cook Island Māori, Niuean) Other Pacific (including Tokelauan) *Eligibility criteria:* none specified (Fijian excluded) *Setting:* primary care practices in nine Primary Health Organisations in Auckland and Northland	Diabetes prevalence (electronic medical records, %)
Ihaka et al. (2012) [37]	Cross-sectional	*Sample size:* N = 53 *Age (years):* ≥18 *Gender:* men 53 % *Ethnicity:* Māori *Eligibility criteria:* Māori with diabetes who had not received a national diabetes assessment for >12 months and had undetected pedal pulses, absence of sensation, previous history of peripheral vascular disease, or ulceration and no below-knee amputation *Setting:* Waitemata district, Auckland 2007–2008	Classification of foot risk status (podiatric practitioners category ≥2, %) Obesity, hypertension, dyslipidaemia and retinopathy prevalence (self-report, %)
Jackson et al. (2009) [38]	Retrospective cohort (from 1996 to 2007)	*Sample size:* N = 45,970 *Age (years):* ≥0 *Gender:* NR *Ethnicity:* European/other, Māori, Pacific, Asian (Indian), Chinese, Other Asian *Eligibility criteria:* public hospital discharge with any mention of T1D or T2D from 1996 to 2007 *Setting:* counties Manukau National Minimum Dataset, 2007	Hospital admissions for people with diagnosed diabetes (hospital records, %)
Jeffreys et al. (2005) [39]	Prospective cohort (13 years)	*Sample size:* N = 74,847 *Age (years):* ≥25 *Gender:* male 50 % *Ethnicity:* European/other (non-Māori/non-Pacific), Māori, Pacific *Eligibility criteria:* hospital discharge diagnosis of diabetes between 1988 and 2001 *Setting:* record linkage study of national hospital discharge records to death records	All-cause mortality (data linkage hospital discharge to death records, %)

(continued)

Table 10.1 (continued)

Study identification	Study design (follow-up)	Participants and setting	Outcomes (measures, units)
Joshy et al. (2009) [40]	Retrospective cohort (from 2003 to 2006)	*Sample size: N*=7900 *Age (years):* NR *Gender:* male % NR *Ethnicity:* European, Māori *Eligibility criteria:* renal complication-free adult diabetes patients registered with Waikato regional diabetes service, diagnosed with diabetes before 2003 *Setting:* Waikato District Health Board region	Hospital renal admission (hospital records, HR with 95 % CI) Start dialysis or kidney transplantation (hospital records, HR with 95 % CI) Death from renal disease (data linkage to death records, HR with 95 % CI)
Joshy et al. (2009) [41]	Cross-sectional	*Sample size: N*=45,500 *Age (years):* NR *Gender:* Male % NR *Ethnicity:* European, Māori, Pacific, Asian *Eligibility criteria:* all patients registered with the practices as of 1 July 2007 *Setting:* 10 Rotorua General Practice Group practices	Age-standardised diabetes prevalence (medical records, %)
Joshy et al. (2009) [42]	Cross-sectional	*Sample size: N*=1819 *Age (years):* ≥18 *Gender:* Male 49 % *Ethnicity:* European, Māori, Pacific, Asian *Eligibility criteria:* all patients with diabetes registered with the practices as of 1 July 2007 *Setting:* 10 Rotorua General Practice Group practices	CKD prevalence (eGFR<60, %) Microalbuminuria prevalence (ACR 2.5–29.9 for men; 3.5–29.9 for women, %) Albuminuria prevalence (ACR ≥30, %)
Joshy et al. (2010) [43]	Retrospective cohort (from 2003 to 2007)	*Sample size: N*=9043 *Age (years):* ≥18 *Gender:* male 50 % *Ethnicity:* European, Māori *Eligibility criteria:* diabetes patients registered with the Waikato Regional Diabetes Service database before 2008, diagnosed before 2003 and alive as of 2003 *Setting:* Waikato region	Age-standardised, all-cause mortality rate (data linkage,/100,000 person-years)

Table 10.1 (continued)

Study identification	Study design (follow-up)	Participants and setting	Outcomes (measures, units)
Kenealy et al. (2008) [44]	Cross-sectional (baseline from cohort) and prospective cohort (median 2.4 years)	*Sample size:* $N=48{,}444$ *Age (years):* range in mean 53–66 *Gender:* male 49 % *Ethnicity:* European, Māori, Pacific, Asian (Indian), East Asian, Other (Middle Eastern, Latin American/Hispanic, African, others) *Eligibility criteria:* T2D and no previous CVD *Setting:* people with T2D who attended at least one diabetes annual review in primary health care as part of a national programme from 2000 to 2005; forms the NZ Diabetes Cohort Study	Fatal/nonfatal CVD incidence (data linkage to hospital/mortality data, HR with 95 %) Microalbuminuria prevalence (ACR ≥2.5 for men; ≥3.5 for women, %) Macroalbuminuria prevalence (ACR >30, %) Current smoker prevalence (self-report, %) Poor glycaemic control prevalence (HbA1c ≥10 %, %)
Kenealy et al. (2012) [45]	Cross-sectional	*Sample size:* 65,171 *Age (years):* median 65 *Gender:* male 51 % *Ethnicity:* European, Māori, Pacific, Asian (Indian), East Asian, Other (Middle Eastern, Latin American/Hispanic, African, others) *Eligibility criteria:* adults in primary care with T2D, not on renal replacement therapy *Setting:* T2D who had attended at least one diabetes annual review in primary health care as part of a national programme between 2000 and 2006 in New Zealand; forms the NZ Diabetes Cohort Study	Microalbuminuria prevalence (ACR >2.5 men, 3.5 women to <30, %) Macroalbuninuria prevalence (ACR 30–<100, %) Advanced albuminuria prevalence (ACR ≥100, %)
Kerr et al. (2006) [46]	Cross-sectional (baseline from cohort) and prospective cohort (mean 3.8 years)	*Sample size:* $N=4193$ *Age (years):* range in mean 55–60 *Gender:* Male 49 % *Ethnicity:* European, Māori, Pacific, Asian, Other *Eligibility criteria:* T2D Hospital admission for MI or CCF from 1999 to 2001 *Setting:* the study population included 4193 individuals with T2D from South Auckland who participated in a primary care audit from 1994 to 1999	Mortality (data linkage, HR with 95% CI) Smoking prevalence (self-report, %)

(continued)

Table 10.1 (continued)

Study identification	Study design (follow-up)	Participants and setting	Outcomes (measures, units)
Kerr et al. (2008) [47]	Cross-sectional	*Sample size:* $N=973$ *Age (years):* mean 60 *Gender:* Male 75 % *Ethnicity:* European/other, Māori, Pacific, Asian *Eligibility criteria:* patients admitted for acute CV event *Setting:* patients presenting to Middlemore Hospital Coronary Care Unit with an acute CVD event from July 2004 to June 2006. CVD risk factor data was electronically collected using acute PREDICT	T2D prevalence (diagnosed, %)
Kolt et al. (2007) [48]	Cross-sectional	*Sample size:* 112 *Age (years):* mean 66 *Gender:* male 45 % *Ethnicity:* Asian (India, Sri Lanka, Pakistan, Fiji) *Eligibility criteria:* NR *Setting:* Auckland-based Asian Indian community organisations	Diabetes prevalence (self-report, %)
Lawrenson et al. (2009) [49]	Cross-sectional	*Sample size:* $N=26{,}096$ *Age (years):* ≥20 *Gender:* NR *Ethnicity:* European, Māori, Asian *Eligibility criteria:* aged ≥20 years with T2D *Setting:* Hamilton general practice register linked to Waikato regional diabetes service register	Poor glycaemic control prevalence (HbA1c >8 %, OR with 95% CI)
Lim et al. (2008) [50]	Cross-sectional	*Sample size:* 180 *Age (years):* mean 54 *Gender:* male 44 % *Ethnicity:* Māori *Eligibility criteria:* household members with at least one Māori resident, or Māori with past GDM or aged ≥23 years with 2 parents with known diabetes *Setting:* newly diagnosed with diabetes during a community screening programme, Te Wai o Rona Diabetes Prevention Strategy	Poor glycaemic control prevalence (HbA1c ≥8.0 %, %) HBP prevalence (treated hypertension or ≥130/85, %) Central obesity prevalence (waist circumference >102 cm for men, >88 cm for women, %) Metabolic syndrome prevalence, (ATPIII criteria, %) Current prevalence (self-report, %) Microalbuminuria prevalence (ACR 2.5–29.9 for men, 3.5–29.9 for women, %) Albuminuria prevalence (ACR ≥30, %) CKD prevalence (eGFR <60, %) Retinopathy prevalence (microaneurysms ≥5, %)

Table 10.1 (continued)

Study identification	Study design (follow-up)	Participants and setting	Outcomes (measures, units)
New Zealand Ministry of Health (2013/2014) [51]	Cross-sectional	*Sample size:* $N = 13{,}309$ *Age (years)*: ≥15 *Gender*: men and women, the proportion is not noted *Eligibility criteria*: resident population aged ≥15 years living in permanent dwellings, aged-care facilities or student accommodation *Ethnicity*: European/Other, Māori, Pacific, Asian *Setting*: nationwide, New Zealand Health Survey	Diabetes prevalence (self-report, adjusted rate ratios [for age, gender, ethnicity])
Robinson et al. (2006) [52]	Cross-sectional	*Sample size:* 5917 *Age (years):* mean 60 *Gender:* male 50 % *Ethnicity:* European, Māori, Pacific, Asian (Indian), Other Asian, Other *Eligibility criteria:* patients with diabetes *Setting:* external audit of general practice diabetes care carried out in South and West Auckland by the Diabetes Care Support Service	Poor glycaemic control prevalence (HbA1c >8.0 %, %) Albuminuria prevalence (ACR ≥2.5 for men; ≥3.5 for women, %) Current smoker prevalence (self-report, %) Obesity prevalence (BMI >30, %) HBP prevalence (systolic >140, %) At-risk feet (by clinical review, %) Dyslipidaemia prevalence (TC:HDL ratio>4.5)
Robinson et al. (2015) [53]	Cross-sectional (baseline from cohort) and prospective cohort (median 7.14 years)	*Sample size:* $N = 62{,}002$ *Age (years):* range in mean 55–66 *Gender:* male 49 % *Ethnicity:* European/other, Māori, Pacific, Asian (Indian subcontinent or Fijian Indians), other Asian (Southeast Asian, Chinese) *Eligibility criteria:* T2D *Setting:* nationwide	Microalbuminuria prevalence (ACR ≥2.5 for men or ≥ 3.5 for women, and < 30 for both, %) Macroalbuminuria prevalence (ACR ≥30, %) Lower limb amputation incidence (linked hospital records ICD codes, rate/1000 person years)
Scott et al. (2006) [54]	Cross-sectional	*Sample size:* 1251 *Age (years):* <26 *Gender:* male 50 % *Ethnicity:* Māori/Pacific Islanders, Europeans, Others *Eligibility criteria:* attended a diabetes centre at least once in the previous 3 years, any person with diabetes born after 1 January 1978 *Setting:* 12 paediatric hospital and adult hospitals across NZ and forms the all-NZ young person's diabetes audit, 2003–2004	Microalbuminuria prevalence (ACR >2.5 for males; >3.5 for females, %)

(continued)

Table 10.1 (continued)

Study identification	Study design (follow-up)	Participants and setting	Outcomes (measures, units)
Scott et al. (2007) [55]	Cross-sectional (baseline from retrospective cohort)	*Sample size:* 4408 *Age (years):* mean 68 *Gender:* male 65 % *Ethnicity:* European, Māori *Eligibility criteria:* hospital discharge diagnosis of all with acute coronary syndromes from 1999 to 2002 *Setting:* Waikato hospital, Hamilton	Diabetes prevalence (chart review, %)
Scott et al. (2008) [56]	Cross-sectional	*Sample size:* $N=12{,}992$ *Age (years):* ≥16 *Gender:* male 41 % *Ethnicity:* European/other, Māori, Pacific *Eligibility criteria:* subsample with any 12-month mood and anxiety disorder prevalence (CIDI 3.0/DSM-IV) for diabetes prevalence and subsample with diabetes for mental disorder prevalence *Setting:* nationwide	Diabetes prevalence (self-report, %) Any 12-month mood and anxiety disorder prevalence (CIDI 3.0/DSM-IV, %)
Simmons et al. (2009) [57]	Cross-sectional	*Sample size:* 3784 *Age (years):* ≥28 *Gender:* male 36 % *Ethnicity:* Māori *Eligibility criteria:* nonpregnant adult Māori *Setting:* all Māori residents within the boundaries of the Waikato District Health Board and the tribal area of Ngati Tuwharetoa in the neighbouring Lakes District Health Board	Undiagnosed diabetes, IGT, and IFG age-standardised prevalence (OGTT 1998 WHO criteria, % with 95 %CI)
Smith et al. (2010) [58]	Cross-sectional	*Sample size:* 1.4 million *Age (years):* ≥0 *Gender:* male 46 % *Ethnicity:* European/other, Māori, Pacific, Asian *Eligibility criteria:* health events recorded between January 2006 and December 2007 for those alive *Setting:* records of subsidy claims for pharmaceuticals and laboratory investigations were linked to records in a national hospital admissions database to 'reconstruct' populations of four District Health Boards – Counties Manukau, Northland, Waitemata and Auckland	Diabetes age-standardised prevalence (data linkage records ICD-10-AM system, %) Age-standardised proportion of diabetes cases ≥1 medical/surgical hospital admissions in 2007 (data linkage records, %)

Table 10.1 (continued)

Study identification	Study design (follow-up)	Participants and setting	Outcomes (measures, units)
Tomlin et al. (2006) [59]	Cross-sectional	*Sample size:* 13,281 *Age (years):* ≥0 *Gender:* Male 52 % *Ethnicity:* European, Māori/Pacific *Eligibility criteria:* any diabetes *Setting:* data were collected from all 242 practices participating in the South Link Get Checked programme, every practice in the South Island outside Christchurch city (the main urban centre) and 14 practices within Christchurch	Poor glycaemic control prevalence (HbA1c >9.0 %, %) Microalbuminuria prevalence (ACR >2.5 for males; >3.5 for females, %) High Cholesterol prevalence (≥6.0, %) Smoking prevalence (self-report, %)

T1D type diabetes, *T2D* type 2 diabetes, *HbA1c* glycated haemoglobin, *BMI* body mass index, *NR* not reported, *ADA* American Diabetes Association, *WHO* World Health Organization, *ACR* albumin creatinine ratio, *CVD* cardio vascular disease, *ICD* International Classification of Diseases, *ATPIII* Adult Treatment Panel, *IFG* impaired fasting glucose, *IGT* impaired glucose tolerance, *OGTT* oral glucose tolerance test, *HR* hazard ratio, *OR* odds ratio, *CKD* chronic kidney disease, *eGFR* estimated glomerular filtration rate, *TC* total cholesterol *HDL* high-density lipoprotein, *NZ* New Zealand, *CIDI* Composite International Diagnostic Interview, *DSM* Diagnostic and Statistical Manual of Mental Disorders

Table 10.2 Prevalence of diabetes and pre-diabetes

	Gender	European	Māori	Pacific	Asian
Diabetes prevalence and key features					
Brewer et al. (2008) [27] HbA1c screening/prior diagnosis; age 56–68 years		1.1	3.3	5.3	4.3
Chan et al. (2015) [28][a] Prior diagnosis; age 0+ years	Male	3.0	8.2	11.4	10.8
	Female	2.2	7.0	11.6	9.3
Coppell et al. (2013) [29] HbA1c screening/prior diagnosis; age 15+ years		6.1	9.8	15.4	
Ellison et al. (2005) [32][a] HbA1c screening; age >20 years	Male	1.0	4.8	8.1 (Cook Island Māori) 5.1 (Samoan)	7.5
	Female	0.4	3.6	4.6 (Cook Island Māori) 5.4 (Samoan)	7.4
Faatoese et al. (2011) [33] Prior diagnosis; age 20–64 years	Male		11.8		
	Female		10.0		
Feigin et al. (2006) [34] Prior diagnosis; age 15+ years; post stroke		11.3	31.4		23.3
Grey et al. (2010) [36] Prior diagnosis; age 35–74 years	Male			25–37 26 (Other Pacific)	
	Female			29–38 32 (Other Pacific)	

(continued)

Table 10.2 (continued)

	Gender	European	Māori	Pacific	Asian
Joshy et al. (2009) [41] Prior diagnosis; age not specified		3.1	7.0	8.9	6.7
Kerr et al. (2008) [46] Prior diagnosis; age 60 years; post-acute CVD		18.1	31.5	39.2	33.0
Kolt et al. (2007) [48] Prior diagnosis; age 66 years	Male				34.0
	Female				37.1
New Zealand Ministry of Health (2013/2014) [51] Prior diagnosis; age 15+ years: rate ratio's			2.0 (vs. non-Māori)	2.8 (vs. non-Pacific)	1.8 (vs. non-Asian)
Scott et al. (2007) [55] Prior diagnosis; age 68 years; post-acute CVD		17.5	33.0		
Scott et al. (2008) [56] Prior diagnosis; age 16+ years; mental health		3.6	8.0	11.3	
Simmons et al. (2009) [57] Undiagnosed by OGTT; 28+ years	Male		6.5		
	Female		4.2		
Smith et al. (2010) [58] Prior diagnosis; age 0+ years; subsidy claims	Male	5.0	12.2	13.9	11.3
	Female	4.0	10.6	15.0	9.1
Pre-diabetes prevalence					
Coppell et al. (2013) [29]		18.1	20.5	24.0	
Ellison et al. (2005) [32]	Male	2.5	14.7	19.9 (Cook Island Māori) 12.8 (Samoan)	18.3
	Female	2.1	12.8	15.0 (Cook Island Māori) 13.3 (Samoan)	13.3
Simmons et al. (2009) [57]	Male		5.4 (IFG) 8.5 (IGT)		
	Female		3.0 (IFG) 9.7 (IGT)		

[a]Denotes studies which reported data for additional ethnic minority groups not presented

likely to have poor glucose control than those with type 2 diabetes in the South Island [59].

Other complication risk factors were more variable between ethnic groups. Māori and Pacific people with known diabetes were more likely to be obese (60.7–76 %) than Europeans (43.8–46.6 %) or Asians (24.9–28.4 %). The prevalence of obesity among Māori with newly diagnosed diabetes in a diabetes prevention programme in the Waikato was particularly high (90.0 %) [50]. Current smoking was higher among Māori across studies (25.0–34.9 %) than Pacific people (15.8–17.8 %), Europeans (8.5–19.9 %) and Asians (5.8–7.7 %). High blood pressure was consistently lowest among Asians (17.5–52 %). However, the prevalence of high blood pressure was higher among Māori and Pacific people than Europeans in one national study [25] but lower in

Table 10.3 Prevalence or risk of clinical and lifestyle risk factors for complications and mortality in people with diabetes

	Gender	European	Māori	Pacific	Asian
Poor glycaemic control					
Agban et al. (2008) (baseline) [25][a]		23.6	46.6	68.4	40.2
Agban et al. (2008) [25] (2 years)[a]		23.1	44.4	51.9	31.7
Elley et al. (2008) [30]		23	43	50	36
Kenealy et al. (2012) [45]		6	19	27	12
Lawrenson et al. (2009) [49]		1 (reference)	OR 1.78 (95 %CI: 1.33,2.39)		OR 1.53 (95 %CI: 1.33,1.76)
Lim et al. (2008) [50]			34.4		
Robinson et al. (2006) [52][a]		22.7	49.5	55.7	44.9
Tomlin et al. (2006) [59]		30.7 (T1D) 10.4 (T2D)	51.1 (T1D) 26.0 (T2D)		
High blood pressure					
Agban et al. (2008) [25] (baseline)		27.8	39.8	34.7	27.4
Agban et al. (2008) [25] (2 years)		23.1	30.5	26.2	17.5
Elley et al. (2008) [30]		67	65	61	52
Ihaka et al. (2012) [37]			49		
Lim et al. (2008) [50]			89.4		
Robinson et al., (2006) [52][a]		32.6	27.6	23.7	24.0
CVD risk/poor metabolic control[b]					
Elley et al. (2008) [30]		29.6	30.1	18.5	19.6
Ihaka et al. (2012) [37]			55		
Lim et al. (2008) [50]			89.4		
Robinson et al. (2006) [52][a]		27.3	46.3	35.4	34.8
Tomlin et al. (2006) [59]		19.8 (T1D) 28.9 (T2D)	17.1 (T1D) 31.8 (T2D)		
Obesity					
Agban et al. (2008) [25] (baseline)		45.1	62.2	62.8	28.4
Agban et al. (2008) [25] (2 years)		43.8	60.7	60.8	25.3
Elley et al. (2008) [30]		46	73	73	25
Ihaka et al. (2012) [37]			62		
Lim et al. (2008) [50]			90.0		
Robinson et al. (2006) [52][a]		46.6	76.0	73.7	24.9
Current smoker					
Agban et al. (2008) [25] (baseline)		8.5	28.0	16.5	5.8
Agban et al. (2008) [25] (2 years)		7.8	25.7	14.4	4.2
Elley et al. (2008) [30]		9.6	27.0	16.6	6.1
Ihaka et al. (2012) [37]			25		
Kenealy et al. (2008) [44]		11	31	17	6

(continued)

Table 10.3 (continued)

	Gender	European	Māori	Pacific	Asian
Kenealy et al. (2012) [45]		10.0	28.3	15.8	6.2
Kerr et al. (2006) [46]		11.0	26.9		
Lim et al. (2008) [50]			30.6		
Robinson et al. (2006) [52][a]		13.1	34.9	17.8	7.7
Tomlin et al. (2006) [59]		19.9 (T2D) 10.9 (T2D)	25.5 (T1D) 27.5 (T2D)		
Depression/anxiety					
Scott et al. (2008) [56]		9.3 (depression) 17.5 (anxiety)	16.5 (depression) 23.5 (anxiety)	9.6 (depression) 22.5 (anxiety)	

[a]Denotes studies which reported data for additional ethnic minority groups not presented
[b]Includes metabolic syndrome, dyslipidaemia and CVD risk

one national and one South/West Auckland/study (27.6–65 % vs. 23.7–61 % vs. 23.1–67 % Māori, Pacific, Europeans, respectively [30, 52]. Generally Europeans had lesser CVD risk than Māori, but other inter-ethnic group comparisons were variable. In one study [56], comorbid depression and anxiety in people with diabetes were higher among Māori compared with European or Pacific ethnic groups.

One study compared risk factor prevalence in 2002 and among the same patients 2 years later in primary care [25]. All risk factors improved to a greater or lesser extent, but the degree varied by ethnic group. The greatest improvements in glycaemia occurred in Pacific people and Asians, and the least improvements in blood pressure occurred in the Māori and Europeans. There was limited change in smoking or obesity across ethnic groups. There remained a very high prevalence of risk factors across all ethnic groups.

Table 10.4 shows the prevalence of diabetes complications and mortality in the studies reviewed. One study showed that Māori people had a substantially increased risk (hazard ratio was 25) of starting dialysis or having transplant therapy compared with Europeans [40]. Rates of microalbuminuria (28.4–39.0 %) and macroalbuminura (9–58.2 %) were highest among Māori in primary care, secondary care and in both T1D and T2D compared with Europeans (17–24.9 % and 3.5–6 % respectively), Pacific people (31–32.1 % and 9.1–17.0 %) and Asians (23–24.1 % and 4.1–7.0 %). While the rate of microalbuminuria was similar among Māori who were newly diagnosed as those with known diabetes, albuminuria rates were lower (but already higher at European rates) [50].

Other complications have been less commonly studied. There are only two recent studies of eye disease: one of maculopathy in those with known diabetes, with the highest prevalence among Pacific people and similar prevalence between Europeans, Māori and Asians [35]. The other showed a very low rate of retinopathy at diagnosis among Māori in the Waikato [50]. Foot complications were most common among Māori, followed by Europeans, Pacific people and then Asians [53]. Cardiovascular event rates were 23–30 % higher among Māori than Europeans in two national samples [30, 44], but not significantly higher among Pacific people. Asian cardiovascular event rates were 6 % (nonsignificant) to 29 % higher than Europeans.

Hospitalisation and mortality are integrated measures of a range of diabetes, both comorbid and psychosocial characteristics. Hospitalisation is also substantially higher among Māori than Europeans and Pacific people (who experience roughly similar rates) whose hospitalisation rates are higher than Asians. Standardised mortality rates are significantly higher among Māori than Europeans. However, mortality rates are lower among Pacific people than Europeans. Mortality risk for Asians vs. Europeans was not statistically significant in the three studies reviewed (Table 10.4).

Table 10.4 Prevalence of diabetes-related complications, risk or rate of CVD/mortality

	Gender	European	Māori	Pacific	Asian
Renal complications					
Elley et al. (2008) [30] (albuminuria)[a]		27	49	49	30
Joshy et al. (2009) (start dialysis or transplant)		1 (reference)	HR 25.2 (95 % CI: 10.7,59.7)		
Joshy et al. (2009) (CKD)	Male	25.7	17.9		
	Female	26.2	20.3		
Joshy et al. (2009) (microalbuminuria)	Male	24.1	39.0		
	Female	18.9	28.4		
Joshy et al. (2009) (albuminuria)	Male	5.8	19.2		
	Female	6.0	14.8		
Kenealy et al. (2008) [44] (microalbuminuria)[a]		20	32	31	23
Kenealy et al. (2008) [44] (macroalbuminuria)[a]		4	14	15	5
Kenealy et al. (2012) [45] (microalbuminuria)[a]		22.9	32.8	32.1	24.1
Kenealy et al. (2012) [45] (macroalbuminuria)[a]		3.5	9.0	9.1	4.1
Kenealy et al. (2012) [45] (advanced albuminuria)[a]		1.7	8.1	7.8	2.2
Lim et al. (2008) [50] (microalbuminuria)			29.6		
Lim et al. (2008) [50] (macroalbuminuria)			7.7		
Lim et al. (2008) [50] (CKD)			5.6		
Robinson et al. (2006) [52] (albuminuria)[a]		27.4	55.2	50.4	36.6
Robinson et al., (2015) [53] (microalbuminuria)[a]		23	33	31	23
Robinson et al., (2015) [53] (macroalbuminuria)[a]		5	17	17	7
Scott et al. (2006) [54] (microalbuminuria)[a]		17	43.8 (Māori/Pacific)		
Tomlin et al. (2006) [59]	Male	27.8 (T1D) 35.1 (T2D)	33.3 (T1D) 58.2 (T2D)		
	Female	24.8 (T1D) 26.0 (T2D)	47.6 (T1D) 42.2 (T2D)		
Eye complications					
Frederikson and Jacobs (2008) [35][a]		12	11	16 (Samoan) 14 (Cook Island Māori) 19 (Tongan)	13
Lim et al. (2008) [50]			1.9		
Foot complications					
Ihaka et al. (2012) [37]			100		
Robinson et al. (2015) [53][a]		2.13/1000	3.48/1000	1.70/1000	0.68/1000

(continued)

Table 10.4 (continued)

	Gender	European	Māori	Pacific	Asian
Hospital admissions					
Jackson et al. (2009) [38][a]		19	24	18	13
Joshy et al. (2009)		1 (reference)	HR 7.0 (95 %CI: 4.6,10.6)		
Smith et al. (2010)		27	37	25	21
CVD events/mortality					
Brewer et al. (2008) [27] (ref. HbA1c 4.0–<5.0 %)		HR 2.56 (95 %CI: 0.71,9.19)	HR 2.71 (95 %CI: 1.90,3.85)	HR 0.53 (95 %CI: 0.161.75)	HR 1.70 (95 %CI: 0.10,29.73)
Elley et al. (2010) [31]		1 (reference)	HR 1.23 (95 %CI: 1.14,1.32)	HR 1.07 (95 %CI: 0.99,1.15)	HR 1.29 (95 %CI: 1.14,1.46)
Jeffreys et al. (2005) [33] (ref. not hospitalised diabetes)		SMR 2.99 (95 %CI: 2.93,3.04)	SMR 3.44 (95 %CI: 3.30,3.58)	SMR 2.23 (95 %CI: 2.06,2.41)	
		SMR 2.98 (95 %CI: 2.93,3.04)	SMR 3.80 (95 %CI: 3.64,3.97)	SMR 2.41 (95 %CI: 2.21,2.61)	
Joshy et al. (2009)		1 (reference)	HR 4.1 (95 %CI: 1.5,11.4)		
Joshy et al. (2010)	Male	551/100,000	1012/100,000		
	Female	491/100,000	808/100,000		
Kenealy et al. [44]		1 (reference)	HR 1.30 (95 %CI: 1.19,1.41)	HR 1.04 (95 %CI: 0.95,1.13)	HR 1.06 (95 %CI: 0.91,1.24)

[a]Denotes studies which reported data for additional ethnic minority groups not presented

Discussion

The results of this review show that the burden of diabetes and related complications remains greater among Māori and other non-European ethnic groups as shown in our previous reviews in 2000 and 2006 [22, 24]. The prevalence of known diabetes among those aged ≥30 years in South Auckland in the early 1990s was 4.2 % in Europeans, 7.9 % among Māori and 5.5 % among Pacific people [42] with approximately 33–50 % undiagnosed [6, 43, 61]. Decades later, these rates have approximately doubled. Glycaemic control remains poorer among non-European groups and many of the other complications and risk factors are especially common among Māori. Renal complications rates, particularly microalbuminuria and macroalbuminuria, remain substantially higher among Māori. Conversely, the low prevalence of retinopathy at diagnosis among Waikato Māori [32] suggests that screening for diabetes in that area may have had a positive impact on early case finding and management for prevention of diabetes-related complications. Despite this, the increased burden of diabetes among Māori/Pacific rates and Asians compared with Europeans has continued to rise and is now one of New Zealand's most serious health issues, which should inform the new national diabetes plan in New Zealand.

Diabetes-Related Policy

Since the last review [24], diabetes-related policy has positively changed for quality of care, screening and prevention. For those with diabetes, the Ministry of Health funded a national programme ('Get Checked') in 2001 that paid general practitioners to undertake a diabetes annual review that could provide the clinical assessments to inform the next steps in the management plan of each participating patient. An evaluation in 2007 [62] reported that many Primary Health Organisations (PHOs), especially those with larger Māori and Pacific Island people's populations, had identified barriers to these population groups using the programme and had put in place initiatives to address these barriers. From the numbers and coverage rates reported by DHBs, it appears that these initiatives were more successful with Pacific peoples. Although the numbers of Māori accessing the programme were increasing, the coverage rates continued to fall short of the target rate set by District Health Boards (DHBs). In 2008, poor retention in Get Checked was shown [63] such that in 2005/2006, only 6100 (57 %) of the estimated 10,600 diabetes patients enrolled in the Waikato utilised the free check. Younger patients aged <40 years, those of Māori or Asian origin, and those with type 1 diabetes were less likely to be retained in the programme with regular checks. A further review in 2011 [64] demonstrated that the Get Checked programme did not systematically result in improved management or outcomes for people with diabetes. As a result, from July 2012, the 'Get Checked' programme was shelved and was replaced by the 'Diabetes Care Improvement Package' [65]. A key change under the new package was placing the responsibility for coordination of diabetes care in the hands of each DHB, thus allowing DHBs to tailor diabetes care towards their population structure, as opposed to a standard national plan under the 'Get Checked' programme.

Wider guidance for quality care were released by the Ministry of Health in 2014 [66] to complement work from the New Zealand Guidelines Group. A Virtual Diabetes Register (VDR) created from six major databases was established by the Ministry of Health in 2013 [67]. The six data sources were: hospital admissions coded for diabetes, outpatient attendees for diabetes and diabetes retinal screening, prescriptions of specific antidiabetic therapies, laboratory orders for measuring diabetes management and primary health (general practitioner) enrolments. There are no special guidelines for the use of antidiabetes medications among Polynesians.

In 2015, a 5-year plan 'Living Well with Diabetes' [68] was proposed to ensure that all New Zealanders with diabetes, or at risk of developing T2D, had access to high-quality, people-centred health services.

Diabetes Screening

As non-European populations are at greater risk of diabetes, they are theoretically more likely to be screened under the DHB managed health targets programme [69]. This programme was introduced in 2007 but reduced in 2009. One of the targets was that 90 % of the eligible population would have had their cardiovascular risk assessed within the last 5 years (this would include a diabetes test).

Diabetes Prevention and Prevention Research

Strategies to prevent diabetes include the Green Prescription [70] where a prescription of physical activity to a patient is provided. A recent randomised controlled trial among Māori and Europeans with diabetes found that both face-to-face and telephone delivery of the Green Prescription are associated with improvements in both weight and HbA1c [71]. Generally, fewer Māori have participated in the GRx programme [72]. This lower participation may have been due to lower referrals from primary care even when fees, administrative and other barriers have been removed [70].

Wider family-based [73] healthy eating and activity guidelines [73] are also in place. A comprehensive plan for [74] includes 22 initiatives that target interventions for those who are obese, increase support for those at risk of becoming obese and introduce broad strategies to make healthier choices easier. A limited review of obesity (as the main risk factor for type 2 diabetes) prevention strategies over the past 20 years have indicated that key strategies have largely been unimplemented [75]. A key success over these 20 years has been the Energize programme in the

Waikato [76], associated with reductions in childhood obesity. The sister study, Te Wai o Rona: Diabetes Prevention Strategy [77], was associated with reductions in weight among Māori with and without pre-diabetes in a vanguard study, but research funding was not continued after 3 years. The coach-supported structured approach to lifestyle change has recently been shown to successfully limit gestational weight gain across nine European countries [78]. Other prevention studies among Māori (e.g. Ngāti and Healthy) showing initial promise [79] have not progressed.

Future Directions: Unmet Needs, Unanswered Questions, Unquestioned Answers

The focus of this chapter has been the epidemiology of diabetes among Māori and other ethnic communities in New Zealand. In spite of substantial policy initiatives, the prevalence of diabetes, the risk factors for complications, especially poor blood glucose control, and the rates of complications remain substantially higher in these ethnic populations groups compared with European New Zealanders. There have been successful initiatives such as Project Energize, the school based lifestyle programme, with its high acceptability among Māori and Pacific people and has not been extended to too many other areas in the country. The early promise from Te Wai o Rona: Diabetes Prevention Strategy has not been followed up, and diabetes metabolic targets are frequently not met based upon primary care data. Diabetes among all ethnic groups, particularly Māori, remains a major public health menace.

There clearly needs to be more research as to why the gap remains between current diabetes outcomes and what should be possible with a national organisational structure that includes a single payer across primary and secondary care, well-developed primary care including Māori and Pacific health services, a well-trained workforce and a raft of policy initiatives to prevent diabetes and its complications and their wider social determinants. Specific research into the excess renal disease among Māori is urgently needed. Current research into the genetic, intrauterine/foetal determinants of diabetes and its complications should be broadened within a culturally safe framework. More research into appropriate behavioural and self-management interventions, building upon global research but tailoring to local cultural needs, are also crucial for those with diabetes. However, the real need is for more large scale intervention studies, developed to go to scale, that can transform the current diabetes healthcare landscape.

We call on the New Zealand's Ministry of Health to make diabetes prevention and management among ethnic minority groups a national health priority area for urgent action in both diabetes health services development and rollout, and both outcomes and translational research.

Appendix: Database Searching Strategies

Search Outline

Concept	Search terms
Diabetes	Diabetes mellitus, type 1
	Diabetes, gestational
	Diabetes mellitus, type 2
	Diabetes mellitus
New Zealand	New Zealand
Native and unserved ethnic groups	Pacific Islander
	Māori
	Samoa
	Cook Islands
	Polynesia (MESH)
	Tonga
	Fiji
	Niue
	Solomon Islands
	Melanesia (MESH)
	Oceanic Ancestry Group (MESH)
	Southeast Asian
	Bangladesh
	India
	Sri Lanka
	Nepal

Medline Search -8/10/15

1	Diabetes mellitus, type 1 or diabetes, gestational/ or diabetes mellitus, type 2 or diabetes mellitus	158,509
2	Diabetes.ab,ti.	243,850
3	1 or 2	274,256
4	New Zealand	20,180
5	New Zealand.ab,ti.	26,249
6	4 or 5	35,119
7	'Pacific Islander'.ab, ti.	1069
8	Māori.ab, ti.	1680
9	Samoa	220
10	Polynesia	695
11	'Cook Islands'.ab, ti.	88
12	Tonga	141
13	Fiji	437
14	Niue.ab, ti.	26
15	Melanesia	357
16	Solomon Islands.ab, ti.	282
17	Oceanic Ancestry Group	5709
18	Bangladesh	5328
19	India	50,204
20	Sri Lanka	2620
21	Nepal	4202
22	7 or 8 or 9 or 10 or 11 or 12 or 13 or 14 or 15 or 16 or 17 or 18 or 19 or 20 or 21	70,730
23	3 and 6 and 22	220
24	*Limit 23 to yr = '2005 -Current'*	*156*

NB: search terms with/are MESH terms

Scopus Search

TITLE-ABS-KEY ('diabetes') AND TITLE-ABS-KEY ('New Zealand') AND TITLE-ABS-KEY ('Pacific Islander' OR 'Māori' OR 'Samoa' OR 'Cook Islands' OR 'Polynesia' OR 'Tonga' OR 'Fiji' OR 'Niue' OR 'Solomon Islands' OR 'Melanesia' OR 'Ocean Ancestry Group' OR 'Southeast Asian' OR 'Bangladesh' OR 'India' OR 'Sri Lanka' OR 'Nepal') AND PUBYEAR > 2004 AND NOT ALL ('trials') OR ('RCT') OR ALL ('intervention')

Total results: 98

Search date: 12/10/2015

References

1. New Zealand Census. 2013. www.stats.govt.nz. Accessed 2/12/2015.
2. Smith LT, editor. Decolonising methodologies: research and indigenous peoples. Dunedin: University of Otago Press; 1999.
3. Bishop R. Initiating empowering research? N Z J Educ Stud. 1994;29(1):175.
4. Smith LT, editor. Decolonizing methodologies: research and indigenous peoples. 2nd ed. Dunedin: University of Otago Press; 2012.
5. Hudson M, Milne M, Reynolds P, Russell K, Smith B. Te Ara Tika: guidelines for researchers on health research involving Māori. Auckland: Health Research Council of New Zealand; 2010. ISBN 978-9-908700-86-5.
6. Bishop R, Glynn T, editors. Culture counts: changing power relations in education. 1st ed. Palmerston North: Dunmore Press Limited; 1999.
7. Durie MH. The health of indigenous peoples. Br Med J. 2003;326(7388):510–1. Epub 2003/03/08. Eng.
8. Durie MH, editor. Whaiora: Māori Health development. 2nd ed. Auckland: Oxford University Press; 1998.
9. Hudson M, Milne M, Reynolds P, Russell K, Smith B. Te Ara Tika: guidelines for researchers on health research involving Māori. Auckland: Health Research Council of New Zealand; 2008.
10. Durie MH. The treaty of Waitangi and health care. N Z Med J. 1989;102(869):283–5. Epub 1989/06/14. Eng.
11. Durie MH, editor. Te Mana, te kawanatanga: the politics of Māori self-determination. 1st ed. Auckland: Oxford University Press; 1998.
12. Orange C, editor. The treaty of Waitangi. Wellington: Bridget Williams Books Limited; 1987.
13. Evans I, Paewai MK. Functional analysis in a bicultural context. Behav Chang. 1999;16(1):20–36.
14. Thomas DR. Science, values and culture. In: Department Psychology, editor. Understanding culture and ethnicity: patterns and policies in plural societies. Hamilton: University of Waikato; 1995. p. 76–87.
15. Cram F, Smith L, Johnstone W. Mapping the themes of Māori talk about health. New Zealand Med J. 2003;116(1170):1p following U353. Epub 2003/03/28. eng.
16. Mane J. Kaupapa Māori: a community approach. MAI Rev. 2009;3(1):1–9.
17. Smith GH. Māori education: revolution and transformative action. Can J Nativ Educ. 2001;24(1):57–67.
18. Walker R, Amoamo J, editors. Nga tau tohehe: years of anger. Auckland: Penguin; 1987.
19. Came HA. Doing research in Aotearoa: a Pākehā exemplar of applying Te Ara Tika ethical framework. Kōtuitui: N Z J Soc Sci Online. 2013;8(1–2):64–73.
20. Prior IAM. A health survey in a rural Māori community with particular emphasis on the cardiovascular, nutritional and metabolic findings. NZ Med J. 1962;61:333.
21. Ostbye T, Welby TJ, Prior IAM, Salmond CE, Stokes YM. Type 2 (non-insulin-dependent) diabetes mellitus, migration and westernisation: the Tokelau Island Migrant study. Diabetologia. 1989;32:585–90.
22. Simmons D. Diabetes and its complications in New Zealand: an epidemiological perspective. N Z Med J. 2000;113:42–3.
23. Simmons D, Kenealy T, Scott DJ. Implementing the South Auckland Diabetes Plan: barriers and lessons. NZ Med J. 2000;113:364–6.
24. Joshy G, Simmons D. Epidemiology of diabetes in New Zealand: revisit to a changing landscape. N Z Med J. 2006;119(1235):U2003.
25. Agban H, Elley CR, Kenealy T, Robinson E. Trends in the management of risk of diabetes complications in different ethnic groups in New Zealand primary care. Prim Care Diabetes. 2008;2(4):181–6.
26. Brian G, Fischer-Harder K, Sikivou B, Qoqonokana MQ, Szetu J, Ramke J. Diabetic eye disease among adults in Fiji with self-reported diabetes. Clin Exp Ophthalmol. 2010;38(9):867–74.
27. Brewer N, Wright CS, Travier N, et al. A New Zealand linkage study examining the associations between A1C concentration and mortality. Diabetes Care. 2008;31(6):1144–9.
28. Chan WC, Jackson G, Wright CS, et al. The future of population registers: linking routine health datasets to assess a populations' current glycaemic status for quality improvement. BMJ Open. 2014;4(4), e003975.
29. Coppell KJ, Mann JI, Williams SM, et al. Prevalence of diagnosed and undiagnosed diabetes and prediabetes in New Zealand: findings from the 2008/09 Audit Nutrition Survey. NZ Med J. 2013;126(1370):23.42.
30. Elley CR, Kenealy T, Robinson E, et al. Cardiovascular risk management of different ethnic groups with type 2 diabetes in primary care in New Zealand. Diabetes Res Clin Pact. 2008;79(3):468–73.

31. Elley CR, Robinson E, Kenealy T, Bramley D, Drury PL. Derivation and validation of a new cardiovascular risk score for people with type 2 diabetes: the New Zealand Diabetes Cohort Study. Diabetes Care. 2010;33(6):1347–52.
32. Ellison TL, Elliott R, Moyes SA. HbA1c screening for undiagnosed diabetes in New Zealand. Diabetes Metab Res Rev. 2005;21(1):65–70.
33. Faatoese AF, Pitama SG, Gillies TW, et al. Community screening for cardiovascular risk factors and levels of treatment in a rural Māori cohort. Aust NZ J Publ Health. 2011;35(6):517–23.
34. Feigin V, Carter K, Hackett M, et al. Ethnic disparities in incidence of stroke subtypes: Auckland Regional Community Stroke Study, 2002–2003. Lancet Neurol. 2006;5(2):130–9.
35. Fredrikson LG, Jacobs RJ. Diabetes eye screening in the Wellington region of New Zealand: characteristics of the enrolled population (2002–2005). NZ Med J. 2008;121(1270):21–34.
36. Grey C, Wells S, Ridell, et al. A comparative analysis of cardiovascular disease risk profiles of five Pacific ethnic groups assessed in New Zealand primary care practice: PREDICT CVD-13. NZ Med J. 2010;123(1325):41–52.
37. Ihaka B, Bayley A, Rome K. Foot problems in Maori with diabetes. NZ Med J. 2012;125(1360):48–56.
38. Jackson G, Orr Walker B, Smith J, Papa D, Field A. Hospital admissions for people with diagnosed diabetes: challenges for diabetes prevention and management programmes. NZ Med J. 2009;122(1288):13–21.
39. Jeffreys M, Wright C, Mannetje A, Huang K, Pearce N. Ethnic differences in cause specific mortality among hospitalised patients with diabetes: a linkage study in New Zealand. J Epidemiol Community Health. 2005;59(11):961–6.
40. Joshy G, Dunn P, Fisher M, Lawrenson R. Ethnic differences in the natural progression of nephropathy among diabetes patients in New Zealand: hospital admission rate for renal complications, and incidence of end-stage renal disease and renal death. Diabetologia. 2009;52(8):1474–8.
41. Joshy G, Porter T, Le Lievre C, Lane J, Williams M, Lawrenson R. Prevalence of diabetes in New Zealand general practice: the influence of ethnicity and social deprivation. J Epidemiol Coummunity Health. 2009;63(5):386–90.
42. Joshy G, Porter T, Le Lievre C, Lane J, Williams M, Lawrenson R. Implications of using estimated glomerular filtration rate (GFR) in a multi ethnic population of diabetes patients in general practice. NZ Med J. 2010;123(1310):9–18.
43. Joshy G, Colonne CK, Dunn P, Simmons D, Lawrenson R. Ethnic disparities in causes of death among diabetes patients in the Waikato region of New Zealand. NZ Med J. 2010;123(1310):19–29.
44. Kenealy T, Elley CR, Robinson E, et al. An association between ethnicity and cardiovascular outcomes for people with type 2 diabetes in New Zealand. Diabetes Med. 2008;25(11):302–8.
45. Kenealy T, Elley CR, Collins JF, Moyes SA, Metcalf PA, Drury PL. Increased prevalence of albuminuria among non-European peoples with type 2 diabetes. Nephrol Dial Transplant. 2012;27(5):1840–6.
46. Kerr GD, Gamble GD, Doughty RN, Simmons D, Baker J. Mortality in individuals with type 2 diabetes and heart disease in a unique New Zealand population. Diabetes Med. 2006;23(12):1313–8.
47. Kerr AJ, McLachland A, Furness S, et al. The burden of modifiable cardiovascular risk factors in the coronary care unit by age, ethnicity, and socioeconomic status: PREDICT CVD-9. NZ Med J. 2008;121(1285):20–33.
48. Kolt GS, Schofield GM, Rush EC, Oliver M, Chadha NK. Body fatness, physical activity, and nutritional behaviours in Asian Indian immigrants to New Zealand. Asia Pac J Clin Nutr. 2007;16(4):663–70.
49. Lawrenson R, Gibbons V, Joshy G, Choi P. Are there disparities in care in people with diabetes? A review of care provided in general practice. J Prim Health Care. 2009;1(3):177–83.
50. Lim S, Chellumuthi C, Crook N, Rush E, Simmons D. Low prevalence of retinopathy, but high prevalence of nephropathy among Maori with newly diagnosed – Te Wai o Rona: diabetes prevention strategy. Diabetes Res Clin Pract. 2008;80(2):271–4.
51. New Zealand Ministry of Health. Annual Update of Key Results 2013/14: New Zealand Health Survey. 2014.
52. Robinson T, Simmons D, Scott D, et al. Ethnic differences in Type 2 diabetes care and outcomes in Auckland: a multiethnic community in New Zealand. NZ Med J. 2006;119(1235):U1997.
53. Robinson TE, Kenealy T, Garrett M, Bramley D, Drury PL, Elley CR. Ethnicity and risk of lower limb amputation in people with Type 2 diabetes: a prospective cohort study. Diabetes Med 2016;33:55–61.
54. Scott A, Toomath R, Bouchier D, et al. First national audit of the outcomes of care in young people with diabetes in New Zealand: high prevalence of nephropathy in Maori and Pacific Islanders. NZ Med J. 2006;119(1235):U2015.
55. Scott AR, Cheng A, Greenacre M, Devlin G. Implications of hyperglycaemia and ethnicity in patients with acute coronary syndromes in New Zealand. Diabetes Obes Metab. 2007;9(1):121–6.
56. Scott K, McGee MA, Schaaf D, Baxter J. Mental-physical comorbidity in an ethnically diverse population. Soc Sci Med. 2008;66(5):1165–73.
57. Simmons D, Rush E, Crook N. Prevalence of undiagnosed diabetes, impaired glucose tolerance, and impaired fasting glucose among Maori in Te Wai o Rona: diabetes prevention strategy. NZ Med J. 2009;122(1288):30–8.
58. Smith J, Jackson G, Orr-Walker B, et al. A population-based approach to the estimation of diabetes prevalence and health resource utilisation. NZ Med J. 2010;123(1310):62–73.
59. Tomlin AM, Tilyard MW, Dawson AG, Dovey SM. Health status of New Zealand European, Maori

and Pacific patients with diabetes in 242 New Zealand general practices. N Z Med J. 2006;119(1235):U2004.
60. Simmons, D. The epidemiology of diabetes and its complications in New Zealand. Diabetic Med. 1996;13:371–5.
61. Simmons D, Thompson C, et al. Polynesians: prone to obesity and Type 2 diabetes but not hyperinsulinemia. Diabet Med. 2001;18:193–8.
62. Ministry of Health and District Health Boards: Effectiveness of the "Get Checked" diabetes program. 2007. URL: http://www.oag.govt.nz/2009/performance-audits/get-checked.htm.
63. Joshy G, Lawrenson R, Simmons D. Retention of patients in the "Get Checked" free annual diabetes review program in New Zealand. NZ Med J. 2008;121(1270): U2945. URL: http://www.nzma.org.nz/__data/assets/pdf_file/0007/17818/Vol-121-No-1270-14-March-2008.pdf.
64. Review of the Diabetes "Get Checked" Programme. Report to ministry of health by Dr Brandon Orr-Walker, National Clinical Director for Diabetes. 2011. URL: https://www.beehive.govt.nz/release/diabetes-get-checked-programme-review.
65. Upfront: The new face of diabetes care in New Zealand. Best Pract J. 2012; Issue 44. URL: http://www.bpac.org.nz/BPJ/2012/may/upfront.aspx.
66. Ministry of Health Quality Standards for Diabetes Care Toolkit. 2014. URL: http://www.health.govt.nz/publication/quality-standards-diabetes-care-toolkit-2014.
67. United Nations Public Administration Network, New Zealand Health Improves Diabetes Policy with Big Data Analytics. 2013. URL: http://www.unpan.org/PublicAdministrationNews/tabid/115/mctl/ArticleView/ModuleID/1467/articleId/40103/Default.aspx.
68. Ministry of Health. Living well with diabetes: a plan for people at high risk of or living with diabetes 2015–2020. Wellington: Ministry of Health. 2015. URL: http://www.health.govt.nz/publication/living-well-diabetes.
69. New Zealand Parliament, Parliamentary support, Research Papers. Obesity and diabetes in New Zealand. 2014. URL: http://www.parliament.nz/en-nz/parl-support/research-papers/00PLLawRP2014041/obesity-and-diabetes-in-new-zealand.
70. Williams M, Rush ER, Crook N, Simmons D. Perceptions of a Te Rongoa kakariki: green prescription health service among Māori in the Waikato and Ngāti Tuwharetoa rohe. Mai J. 2015;4(2):118–33.
71. Williams, M. Te Rongoaa Kakariki: Kanohi-ki-te-kanohi, e pai ana? Auckland University of Technology. 2014. URL: https://aut.researchgateway.ac.nz/bitstream/handle/10292/8648/WilliamsM.pdf?sequence=6.
72. Pringle R. Health and physical activity promotion: a qualitative examination of the effect of receiving a Green Prescription (GRx). Hamilton: University of Waikato. Wif Malcolm Insititute of Educational Research; 2008.
73. Eating and Activity Guidelines for New Zealand Adults, Healthy Families NZ. 2015. URL: http://www.parliament.nz/en-nz/parl-support/research-papers/00PLLawRP2014041/obesity-and-diabetes-in-new-zealand.
74. Ministry of Health. Childhood obesity plan. 2015. URL: http://www.health.govt.nz/our-work/diseases-and-conditions/obesity/childhood-obesity-plan.
75. Swinburn B, Wood A. Progress on obesity prevention over 20 years in Australia and New Zealand. Obes Rev. 2013;14(Supp 2):60–8.
76. Rush E, McLennan S, Obolonkin V, Vandal AC, Hamlin M, Simmons D, Graham D. Project energize: whole-of region primary school nutrition and physical activity programme; evaluation of body size and fitness five years after the RCT. Br J Nutr. 2013;19:1–9.
77. Simmons D, Rush E, Crook N. Development and piloting of a community health worker based intervention for the prevention of diabetes among New Zealand Māori in Te Wai o Rona: diabetes prevention strategy. Public Health Nutr. 2008;11:1318–25.
78. Simmons D, Jelsma JG, Galjaard S, Devlieger R, van Assche A, Jans G, Corcoy R, Adelantado JM, Dunne F, Desoye G, Harreiter J, Kautzky-Willer A, Damm P, Mathiesen ER, Jensen DM, Andersen LL, Lapolla A, Dalfra M, Bertolotto A, Wender-Ozegowska E, Zawiejska A, Hill D, Rebollo P, Snoek FJ, van Poppel MN. Results from a European multicenter randomized trial of physical activity and/or healthy eating to reduce the risk of gestational diabetes mellitus: the DALI Lifestyle Pilot. Diabetes Care. 2015;38:1650–6.
79. Coppell KJ, Tipene-Leach DC, Pahau HL, Williams SM, Abel S, Iles M, Hindmarsh JH, Mann JI. Two-year results from a community-wide diabetes prevention intervention in a high risk indigenous community: the Ngati and Healthy project. Diabetes Res Clin Pract. 2009;85(2):220–7.

11 Diabetes in Eastern Europe

Mykolay Khalangot, Vitaliy Gurianov, Alexander Vaiserman, Ieva Strele, Vasile Fedash, and Victor Kravchenko

This review is dedicated to relevant diabetes mellitus-related aspects in several European countries that emerged after the breakup of the Soviet Union. After more than two decades of existence, these countries significantly differ according to their economic standing, demographic parameters, as well as presence, speed, and orientation of healthcare reforms (Table 11.1). The former "Soviet republics" that prior to 1991 had similar socioeconomic characteristics and identical healthcare system are now independent Eastern European and Baltic states that belong to different socioeconomic and political communities.

In this chapter we are trying to analyze some diabetes-related aspects in four lower middle (Armenia, Georgia, Moldova, Ukraine), two upper middle (Azerbaijan, Belarus), and two high (Latvia and Russia) income countries in accordance with the World Bank classification [1] in the former Soviet Union.

Lower middle-income countries are facing an epidemiological transition, with increases in the prevalence and mortality related to noncommunicable diseases such as diabetes [2, 3], but the differences in life expectancy at birth (Table 11.1) are not always directly related to economic characteristics. Genetic, ethnic, geographic, and cultural features may also influence health outcomes, e.g., the Caucasus region in the former Soviet Union was known for longevity of its population [4]. Furthermore, diabetes-related mortality data [5] and data on mortality with diabetes mellitus marked as the cause of death [6], obtained from different independent sources, also does not demonstrate any negative relationship with gross national income (GNI) per capita (Table 11.1). Even a positive association between GNI and mortality level can be revealed when using certain statistical methods ($p<0.001$, chi-square test for trend). These data raise doubts about methods of recording mortality, as well as about the possibility to efficiently influence this outcome in diabetes patients.

M. Khalangot, MD, ScD (✉)
Shupyk National Academy of Postgradual Medical Education, Kyiv, Ukraine
e-mail: nikhalangot@ukr.net

V. Gurianov, PhD
Bogomolets National Medical University, Kyiv, Ukraine

A. Vaiserman, ScD
Chebotariov Institute of Gerontology, National Academy of Medical Sciences, Kyiv, Ukraine

I. Strele, MD, PhD
Riga Stradins University, Riga, Latvia

V. Fedash, MD, PhD
Institute of Physiology and Sanocreatology of ASM, Chisinau, Moldova

V. Kravchenko, ScD
Komisarenko Institute of Endocrinology and Metabolism, National Academy of Medical Sciences, Kyiv, Ukraine

S. Dagogo-Jack (ed.), *Diabetes Mellitus in Developing Countries and Underserved Communities*, DOI 10.1007/978-3-319-41559-8_11

Table 11.1 Some total and diabetes-related characteristics of the Eastern European countries and Latvia

Country, income level [1]	GNI per capita, $ (2014) [1]	Total population, millions (2014) [1]	Life expectancy at birth, years (2013) [1]	Diabetes – related deaths (20–79), per 100,000 population 2013 [5]	No. of diabetes mellitus deaths cases, both sexes, all ages, per 100,000 population – 2012 [6, 7]
Armenia, LMIC	3,780	3,006	75	32.6	43.1^{2012}
Azerbaijan, UMIC	7,590	9,538	71	24.1	7.8^{2007}
Belarus, UMIC	7,340	9,470	72	79.6	3.6^{2009}
Georgia, LMIC	3,720	4,504	74	32.9	10.4^{2010}
Moldova, LMIC	2,550	3,556	69	37.1	10.7^{2010}
Russian Federation, HIC	13,210	143,8	71	137.2	6.3^{2010}
Ukraine, LMIC	3,560	45,36	71	45.5	4.9^{2012}
Latvia, HIC	15,660	1,990	74	57.9	23.6^{2012}

Comments:
GNI per capita (formerly GNP per capita) is the gross national income, converted to US dollars using the World Bank Atlas method, divided by the midyear population
LMIC lower middle-income countries ($1,046–4,125), *UMIC* upper middle-income countries ($4,126–12,735), *HIC* high income countries ($12,736 or more)
Life expectancy at birth indicates the number of years a newborn infant would live if prevailing patterns of mortality at the time of its birth were to stay the same throughout its life

It should be also noted that geographically most of Russia's territory lies within Asia, and this fact inevitably influences some epidemiologic features of diabetes mellitus.

Thus, the following analysis will be focused on revealing diabetes-related problems, common for Eastern Europe, taking into account particularities of separate countries. According to the World Bank classification, Latvia is related to Central, rather than to Eastern Europe, and together with Lithuania and Estonia makes up a subgroup of "Baltic states." Nevertheless, it is included into this review in order to facilitate possible comparisons, in the light of common Soviet historic background.

Classification and Unique Aspects of the Pathophysiology of Type 1 and Type 2 Diabetes in Region

Diabetes Epidemiology in Eastern Europe

Several epidemiologic diabetes-related features of seven Eastern European countries and Latvia were taken from the latest International Diabetes Federation (IDF) review [5] and presented in Table 11.2. The first glance at these data causes many questions and concerns.

- Diabetes prevalence among adults in all countries of Eastern Europe except Russia is given as a summary of epidemiologic studies conducted in other countries, e.g., diabetes prevalence in Ukraine and Azerbaijan is evaluated, based on studies, and performed among rural residents of Albania. The same assessments for Belarus are made according to research from Turkey, Poland, Russia, and Bulgaria [8]. It is surprising that the data from Turkey was not used for Azerbaijan, as the population of these countries is ethnically related, and extrapolations for Belarus are not limited by Polish data but are conducted according to Turkish and Bulgarian data among others [8].
- The biggest surprise is caused by diabetes prevalence data from Russia. The only paper, referenced by IDF experts [8], is a study about type 2 diabetes prevalence among several Siberian ethnic minorities [9]. To project these results onto all of Russia's territory, let alone to use it for epidemiologic descriptions of other counties, is wrong in our opinion. There are

Table 11.2 Some diabetes-related epidemiologic characteristics of the Eastern European countries extracted from the IDF diabetes atlas sixth edition [5]

Country	Adult population (20–79) in 1000s	Diabetes cases (20–79) in 1000s	Diabetes national prevalence (%)	Diabetes comparative prevalence (%)	Diabetes-related deaths (20–79)	Incidence type 1 diabetes (0–14) per 100,000	Mean diabetes-related expenditure per person with diabetes (USD)
Armenia	208,211	5,495	2,64[a]	2,46	979	n.a.	187
Azerbaijan	642,069	14,634	2,28[a]	2,45	2,300	n.a.	521
Belarus	711,219	44,525	6.26[a]	5.07	7,534	5.6	357
Georgia	315,113	9,342	2.96[a]	2.45	1,481	4.6	383
Moldova	260,604	7,209	2.77[a]	2.44	1,320	n.a.	287
Russian Federation	10,892,897	1,092,411	10.03	8.28	197,299	12.1	899
Ukraine	3,485,802	104,358	2.99[a]	2.45	20,654	8.1	314
Latvia	155,223	9,570	6.17	4.58	1,152	7.5	1,135

n.a. not applicable
[a]Estimate of diabetes prevalence based on extrapolation from other countries

recent epidemiologic studies of diabetes prevalence in Russia according to glucose tolerance test data that included 3,208 randomly selected persons from four Russian regions (Moscow, Rostov, Ekaterinburg, and Nizhniy Novgorod) aged 30–70 year. There were 1,757 (55 %) women and 1,454 (45 %) men included in the study. During the screening process, the general prevalence of diabetes in the above regions was 1.9 % [CI 95 % 1,48–2,47] ($n=62$ persons), impaired glucose tolerance 2.8 % [CI 95 % 2.29–3.47] ($n=91$ persons). Prevalence of previously undiagnosed type 2 diabetes in the above population is 1.9 %, which approximately corresponds to known T2D prevalence; thus, the actual diabetes prevalence in the studied population was 4.1 % [10]. An error during interpretation or presentation of data from Dogadin et al. [9] can be seen, as some of these same results were published in Russian [11] indicating a 1.1 % prevalence of previously undiagnosed diabetes among 18+ years old residents of Krasnoyarsk (Russia) [11]. Thus, the claim of IDF experts [5] that Russia is a European country with highest number of people with diabetes cannot be confirmed.

- The extrapolations regarding diabetes prevalence in Ukraine are not any less doubtful. Indeed, the assumption about the number of adults (20–79 years) living with diabetes (1,043,580 persons) does not significantly differ from the known number of diabetes patients in Ukraine, which allows to anticipate a significantly higher prevalence of diabetes. A recently started investigation of fasting glycemia and glucose tolerance in rural areas of Ukraine revealed that 12 % of persons over 44 years old have diabetes [12, 13] (Table 11.3).

Diabetes Mortality Trends in Ex-Soviet Eastern European Countries

Economic and political crisis of the last Soviet years and the first decade of independence led to a significant deterioration of the Soviet healthcare system, which in its turn should have led to increase of mortality in post-Soviet countries. It is notable that health systems play a key role in the control and management of diabetes [30], and lower middle-income countries (LMIC) are facing an epidemiological transition, with increases in the prevalence and mortality related to noncommunicable diseases, such as diabetes [2].

Deterioration of insulin access for T1D patients was of course the most anticipated reason for a rise in mortality among diabetics. The term “insulin supply crisis” was sometimes used to refer to problems with free insulin supply in

Table 11.3 Most recent diabetes-related epidemiologic characteristics of the Eastern European countries extracted from the national informational sources

Country, reference	Prevalence of the diagnosed diabetes cases, (%)	Prevalence[a] of the insulin-treated diabetes cases, (%)	Diabetes screening data, % (age group, population type)	Diabetes mellitus incidence in children and adolescents per 100,000 (age group available, years)	Diabetes mellitus prevalence in children and adolescents per 100,000 (age group available, years)
Armenia [14]	2.0	0.3	n.a.	7.9 (0–14)	38.9 (0–14)
Azerbaijan [15]	2.0	0.3	n.a.	n.a.	n.a.
Belarus [16–18]	2.9	0.7	n.a.	13.4 (0–14)	70.1 (0–14)
Georgia [19, 20]	1.7	n.a.	n.a.	10.4 (0–14)	42.7 (0–14)
Moldova [21]	2.4	0.4	n.a.	n.a.	47.0 (0–18)
Russian Federation [22–25]	2.6	0.6	1.9 (30–70, urban)	12.0 (0–14)	72.8 (0–14)
				15.3 (15–17)	186.4 (15–17)
Ukraine [13, 26, 27]	3.0	0.5	12.7 (45+, rural)	16.4 (0–14)	86.9 (0–14)
			13.7 (30–80, mixed)	13.1 (15–17)	210.1 (15–17)
Latvia [28, 29]	4.1	0.9	n.a.	16.2/22.1 (0–9) (mal/fem)	67.3/78.9 (0–9) (mal/fem)
				15.0/17.0 (10–19) (mal/fem)	247.6/232.2 (10–19) (mal/fem)

Comments:
n.a. not applicable
[a]Estimated by authors on the ground of the statistical data referenced

Ukraine [31]. In 2001, Maria Telishevska et al. demonstrated results of a regional (Lviv, West Ukraine) study. Its purpose was to reveal causes of a high death rate among young people with diabetes in Ukraine [32]. It seems that in other post-Soviet countries this issue was ignored until now.

Recently, chief Russian endocrinologists/diabetologists, Ivan Dedov and Marina Shestakova (2013), reported that adult T1D mortality in 2007 and 2012 was 4.81 and 3.26 cases per 100,000 persons, respectively, i.e., according to the authors, there was a “decrease of 28.4 %” [24]. Unfortunately in this case, there is no T1D patient mortality data for previous years, which prevents a more precise tendency assessment. We thought it would be reasonable to use an electronic WHO resource [6] to perform such mortality assessment for seven countries (Fig. 11.1).

The age of the deceased (15–24 years) allows us to relate them to T1D with high chances and that in its turn makes us assume that a multifold increase of mortality among young persons from 1985 to 2000 can reflect problems with insulin supply. Using the same source [6] and taking into account the number of people of the corresponding gender and age in Russia, Ukraine, and Belarus, we have calculated diabetes mortality indicators for males (Fig. 11.3a) and females (Fig. 11.3b) aged 15–34 years. The data are approximated by a parabolic relation (with high determination factor for Ukraine $R^2=0.897$ and Russia $R^2=0.879$ for males; $R^2=0.859$ and $R^2=0.889$ for females accordingly). For Belarus, the model was credible but less convincing, and, for four other counties, mortality during these years was not assessed or approximated due to a small number of cases.

It must be noted that WHO mortality database [6] only has data about mortality due to diabetes and not about all deceased persons with diabetes. During the Soviet period, all statistical indicators did not have any protection from manipulations at different levels. Sometimes a local health manager

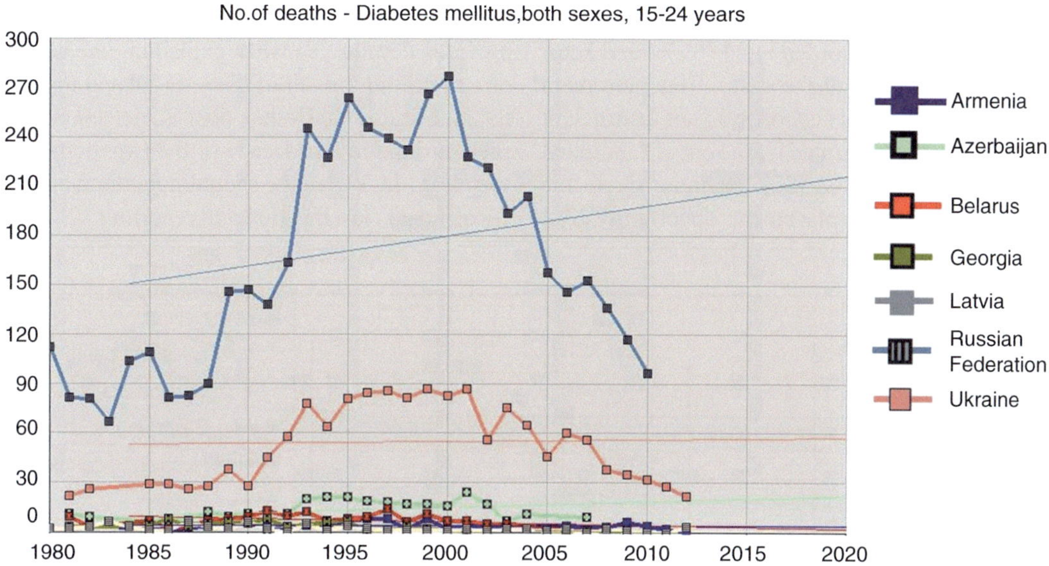

Fig. 11.1 Number of death cases due to diabetes mellitus, both sexes, 15–24 years (Extracted from WHO mortality database [6])

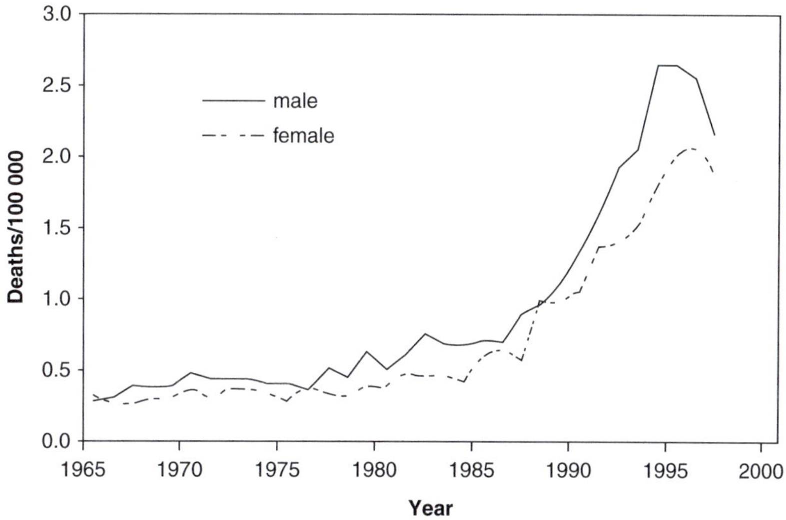

Fig. 11.2 Age standardized death rate from diabetes mellitus, ages 0±49, Ukraine 1965–1998. Source: INED/CHDE [32] (The figure is reproduced from Telishevska et al. [32] with permission of the publisher, John Wiley and Sons)

could demand for another cause of death to be recorded in a person with T1D, for example, pneumonia (that could have caused a fatal diabetic ketoacidosis) or chronic renal failure so that statistical indicators could be "improved" and diabetes remained unmentioned. Decrease of administrative pressure that started after 1986 in USSR could have led to a more honest classification of mortality causes; thus, an assessment of diabetes mortality growth marked in countries including Ukraine at the end of the twentieth century (Fig. 11.2) cannot be absolutely unambiguous.

In 60 out of 64 insulin-treated subjects who died in Lviv Oblast in 1998 and the first 8 months of 1999 and were under 50 years of age, as identified by Maria Telishevska, diabetes mellitus was listed as the underlying cause of death, and so they would have been recorded in official statistics as dying from diabetes [32]. Chronic renal failure was recorded in 44 (69 %) and keto-acidosis in 4 (6 %) of the cases. Thus, the main cause of death in this cohort was not insufficient insulin access (confirmed in one out of four lethal cases of ketoacidosis) [32] but more likely the absence of renal replacement opportunity. But such possibilities were extremely limited during previous decades, so when explaining the causes of a multifold growth of diabetes-related mortality in Ukraine and other post-Soviet countries, seen during the last decade of the twentieth century (Fig. 11.3a, b), we should note the factor of correct data classification and reporting.

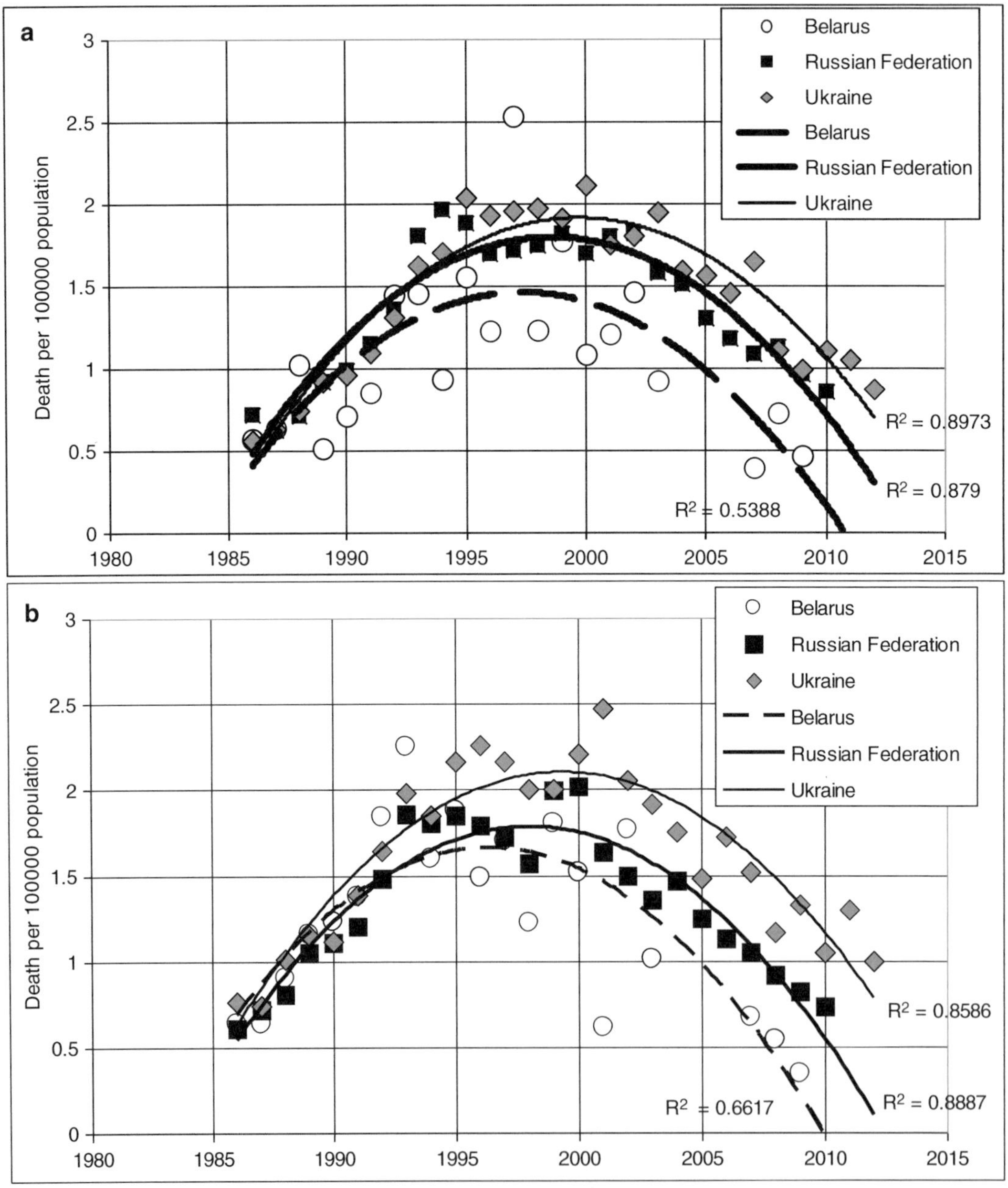

Fig. 11.3 (**a**) Changes of annual mortality due to diabetes (male, 15–34 years) for three countries. (**b**) Changes in diabetes mortality (females 15–34 years old) for three countries (Crude data extracted from WHO mortality database [6] with following annual mortality calculation and model approximation)

Diabetes related mortality indexes in Russian young adults (15–34 years old) that we calculated according to WHO mortality database [6] increased from 0.7 to 1.8 in men and from 0.6 to 2.0 in women per 100,000 population (1986 and 1999, respectively) with a gradual decrease to almost initial levels by 2010 (0.85 and 0.7). Taking into account recent recommendations about differentiation of diabetes mellitus clinical types, which use age at diagnosis <35 years as one of the two main hallmarks of the T1D [33, 34], most diabetes-related death cases in young adults (15–34 years old) can be considered T1D. These indicators are significantly lower than those, given by Russian authors for 2007 and 2012 (4.81 and 3.26 death cases per 100,000 adult population, respectively) as portrayal of T1D mortality [24]; however, in the latter case the data involves mortality of T1D adults of any age from all causes. The data about mortality dynamics, recently reported by Russian authors, are based on information from a diabetes patient register, updated annually since 2007 [24]; therefore, it would be logical to expect an evaluation of mortality cases in relation to the number of registered patients, i.e., with due account for the number of person-years (PY) of observation, and not relative to adult population. Such exact mortality evaluations can be seen in an assessment of data from a Latvian diabetes register: Mortality in a population with diabetes decreased statistically significantly from 57.76 per 1,000 PY in 2000 to 45.33 per 1,000 PY in 2012. The age-standardized mortality ratio of the population with diabetes to the population of Latvia decreased from 1.71 (95 % CI 1.62–1.81) in 2000 to 1.23 (95 % CI 1.19–1.27) in 2012 [35]. Mortality tendency for men and women with diabetes in Latvia are shown in Fig. 11.4. Unfortunately, there is no analysis of mortality tendencies of two main types of diabetes (T1D and T2D) according to this register's data.

Ivan Dedov [36] points out that the average life expectancy among men with T2D in Russia somewhat exceeds the one for the general Russian population (according to Russian official healthcare data in 2009 average life expectancy was 62.9 years for men and 75 years for women). According to the author, this is associated with a thorough health monitoring of T2D patients, who

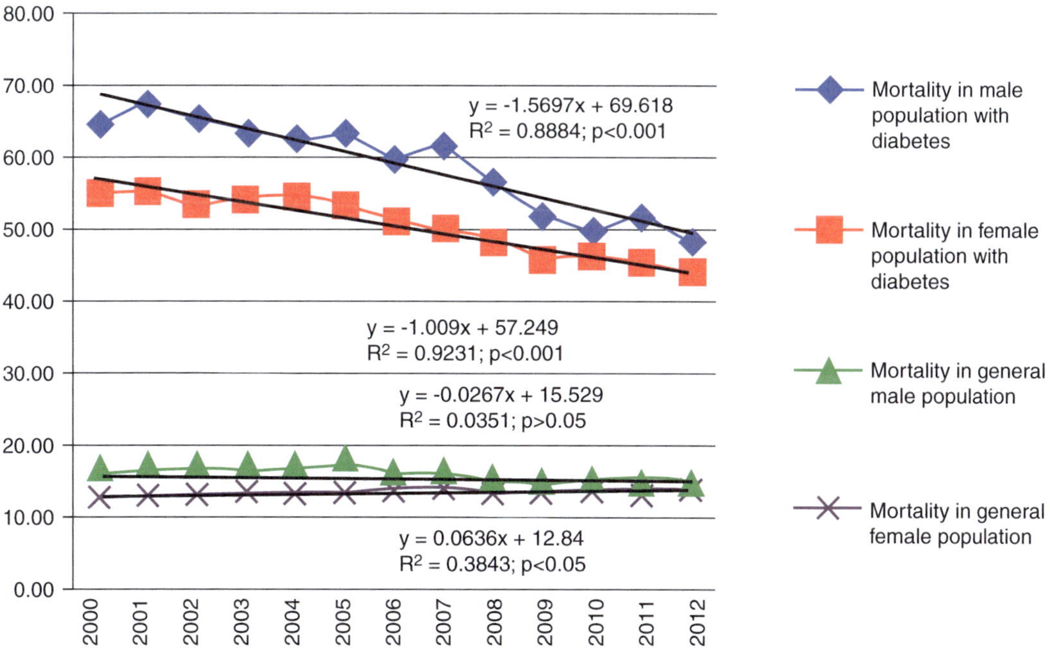

Fig. 11.4 Mortality rate differences by gender in a population with diabetes and general population of Latvia 2000–2012, per 1,000 PY (The figure is reproduced from Pildava et al. [35] with permission of the publisher, Elsevier)

frequent the doctor to correct glucose-lowering treatment and other risk factors of cardiovascular mortality: arterial blood pressure, lipid metabolism, and blood clotting [36]. These reasons can be accepted only as explanation for the increasing of average age at death of diabetic patients, recently recorded by various population registers (in Ukraine [37, 38], Belarus [17], and Russia [24]). Comparing average life expectancy (according to age at the time of death) of T2D patients in this case is inappropriate, as the frequency of T2D grows with age, i.e., it is wrong to compare average life expectancy in general population at birth with a T2D population, the average age at the time of diagnosis in Ukraine was 57.3 years [38]. That is why, for example, patients with Alzheimer's disease die later, comparing to the general population not because of a more intensive treatment but due to this illness being diagnosed later in life.

Our cross-sectional analysis of nationwide Ukrainian diabetes mellitus patients register discovered an increase of age at the time of death among T2D patients in 2007, comparing to 2002. This increase was much greater for those being treated with oral antidiabetic drugs (OAD) comparing to insulin-treated patients [37, 38]. Age at death of insulin-treated T2D patients, from 2002 to 2007, increased by 1.54 (95 % CI 0.81–2.26) years, and those who used OAD – by 6.27 (95 % CI 3.67–8.87) years. Life expectancy for the general population of Ukraine, which survived until they were 55 years old in 1989, was about 22 years (Fig. 11.**5**). According to WHO life tables, life expectancy for Ukrainians in 55–59 age group was 20.4 years in 2006. Life expectancy at age 60 years for Ukrainians was 17 in 2000 and 18 years in 2012 [39]. In other words, life expectancy for type 2 diabetes patients achieved in 2007 (age at the time of death = 68.68 years for insulin treated and 72.72 years for OAD treated) remains lower than in the general Ukrainian population. These data correspond to an analysis based on the data from the Framingham Heart Study, according to which diabetic men and women 50 years and over lived on average 7.5 and 8.2 years less than their non-diabetic equivalents [40].

Gender and Age-Related Aspects of Diabetes Patient Mortality: Issues of Recording and Classifying Death Cases

Using a constantly functioning patient register[1] allows to study the epidemiology of T1D diagnosed in adults and to consider gender differences. The aim of this study is to analyze mortality among T1D patients in Ukraine within the gender aspect. We have used a database with 384,080 DM patients with the first entry made on 12 February 1998 and the last entry on 28 December 2007. We have grouped patients according to probable DM type (T1D – age at the time of diagnosis <30 years in case of receiving insulin treatment), as well as grouping according to gender and age. General assessment of observation duration in age groups of this cohort was performed using the calculation of person-years. We have analyzed the vital status in groups from 15 to 64 years during the whole observation period, as well as for 2003, 2004, and 2005 (for each year separately). Standardization according to age group and gender was conducted according to official Ukrainian mortality data in 2003. Odds ratios (ORs) and 95 % confidence intervals (CIs) were calculated. In the same way, the relation of mortality risk, associated with the male gender, was evaluated using ORs in T1D patients. Data about general mortality in Ukraine was taken from the official WHO website 11 December 2006.

We have created a large cohort of T1D patients (29,791 persons, Table 11.4). In general, mortality among men exceeds such among women: mortality ORs for men and women = 1.37 (95 % CI 1.24–1.5) $p<0.0001$. Women with T1D from this cohort also have higher average age and

1 Such register was functional in Ukraine for some time (2000–2009), and several studies in the field of T1D [41, 42] as well as T2D [43–47] were based on its data. Some investigations, based on the Ukrainian Diabetes Mellitus Register, were published in local journals in Ukrainian [48–51]; therefore, here we are giving a more detailed presentation of some of that published data about gender aspects of mortality among diabetes patients.

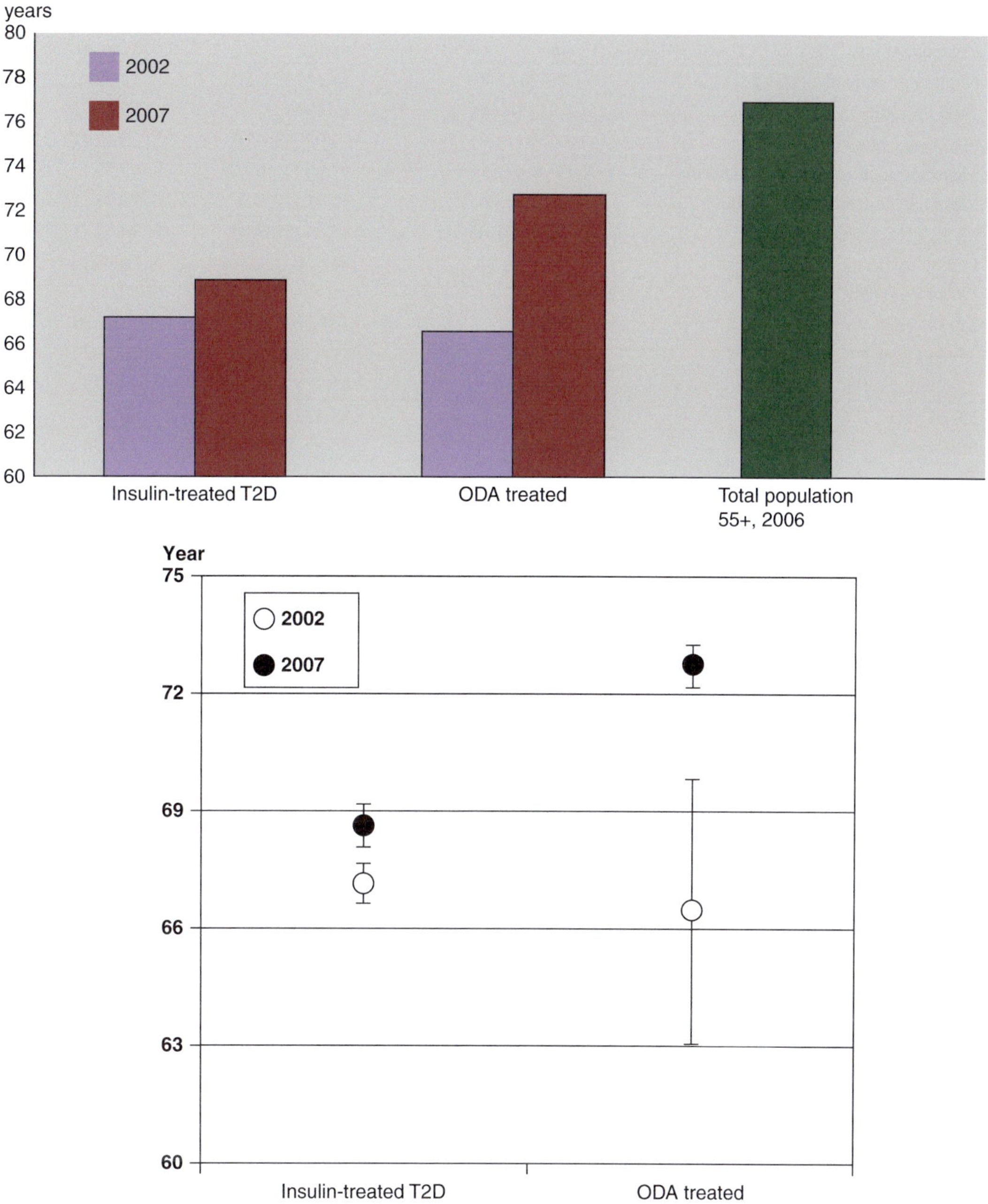

Fig. 11.5 Changes in life expectancy of type 2 diabetes patients in Ukraine, estimated by analyzing the average age at the time of death of those who died in 2002 ($N=1228$) and 2007 ($N=2050$) according to the analysis of diabetes register. *Lower panel* presents mean age and 95 % CI of the insulin-treated and OAD-treated T2D groups [37]

disease duration ($p<0.0001$) comparing to men. At the same time, average life expectancy, calculated according to average age at the time of death, did not significantly differ depending on gender ($p=0.47$). We should note a very low (40.23 years) average life expectancy of T1D patients in Ukraine.

Stratification of observation period duration according to age groups is given in Table 11.4. The highest number of person-years of observation

Table 11.4 Same characteristics of T1D patient cohorts [48]

Characteristics	All	Men	Women
Number of patients, *n* (%)	29,721 (100)	15,187 (51.1)	14,515
Total mortality cases, *n* (%)	1,917 (6.45)	1,119*	798
Mean age, years (SD)	32.54 (11.91)	31.98 (11.45)*	33.12 (12.34)
Mean age at diagnosis, years (SD)	17.74 (7.5)	17.96 (7.46)	17.52 (7.52)
Mean age at death, years (SD)	40.23 (13.04)	40.41 (12.50)	39.98 (13.76)
Mean T1D duration, years	13.91 (11.05)	13.34 (10.83)*	14.52 (11.25)
Follow-up period in age groups:	151,018	76,566	74,452
15–24 years, PY			
25–34 years, PY	246,252	134,602	111,650
35–44 years, PY	222,302	114,382	107,920
45–54 years, PY	175,750	81,125	94,625
55–64 years, PY	62,639	29,122	33,517
65–74 years, PY	21,456	9,966	11,490
75 + years, PY	3,126	1,396	1,730

Modified from Khalangot [48]
*$P<0.001$ versus women
PY person-years

Table 11.5 Relative mortality rate of T1D patients who are in the Ukrainian register of diabetes in comparison to general population of Ukraine by age groups (15–64 years old)

	2003		2004		2005	
Age	OR	95 % CI	OR	95 % CI	OR	95 % CI
A – women						
15–24	9.44	6.21–14.3	9.6	6.25–14.7	8.6	5.34–13.8
25–34	10.6	8.08–13.9	6.64	4.72–11.34	8.37	6.21–11.3
35–44	6.67	5.0–8.89	5.71	4.18–7.8	4.14	2.86–5.99
45–54	3.18	2.28–4.44	4.08	3.06–5.43	2.5	1.75–3.56
55–64	2.38	1.51–2.36	2.15	1.38–3.36		
B – men						
15–24	3.21	2.14–4.83				
25–34	3.09	2.43–3.95	3.28	2.59–4.14	2.41	1.83–3.16
35–44	2.77	2.21–3.46	2.69	2.15–3.37	1.95	1.49–2.54
45–54	1.49	1.12–1.99	1.54	1.17–2.02		
55–64						

Modified from Khalangot [48]
ORs are shown only in cases when they are significantly different from one

coincides with the age period between 15 and 64 years, which justifies further analysis of mortality in these age groups. We should mention that only a small preponderance of person-years of observation for women starts only at 45 years old which differs significantly from the gender-age distribution of the general population of Ukraine.

Relation of mortality risks for persons with T1D in relation to the general population of Ukraine somewhat decrease with age and is significantly higher for women than for men (Table 11.5a, b). For women with T1D aged 15–34 years, there is no mortality gender difference, usually for the general population of Ukraine (Table 11.6).

Thus, according to a short observation period of nearly all Ukraine T1D population, the absolute mortality of young women and men of the

Table 11.6 Risks of all-cause mortality for men relative to women among T1D patients and the general population Ukraine stratified by age

	T1D		Total population (Ukraine, 2002)	
Age group, years	OR (95 % CI)	*P*	OR (95 % CI)	*P*
15–24		0.197	2.95 (2.81–3.09)	<0.001
25–34		0.110	3.49 (3.37–3.61)	<0.001
35–44	1.79 (1.50–2.13)	<0.001	3.64 (3.56–3.73)	<0.001
45–54	1.60 (1.32–1.93)	<0.001	3.22 (3.17–3.28)	<0.001
55–64	1.39 (1.06–1.82)	0.021	2.61 (2.58–2.65)	<0.001

ORs are shown only in cases when they are significantly different from one [48]

Table 11.7 The relative mortality rate of diabetic patients who are in the register of diabetes in comparison to general population of Latvia by age groups

	Male		Female	
Age group	RR	95 CI	RR	95 CI
<20	2.37	1.13–4.97	2.47	0.93–6.59
20–29	4.47	3.31–6.02	11.34	7.34–17.45
30–39	4.33	3.37–5.03	6.67	5.21–8.78
40–49	2.47	2.23–2.69	3.42	2.99–3.89
50–59	1.62	1.54–1.70	2.25	2.12–2.39
60–69	1.34	1.29–1.38	1.99	1.93–2.06
70–79	1.30	1.27–1.34	1.65	1.62–1.69
80+	1.04	0.99–1.08	1.12	1.09–1.15

Data extracted from Pildava et al. [35]

corresponding age turned out to be the same, unlike in the general population. And relative mortality of young women was several times higher, comparing to relative mortality among males.

The comparison of mortality rate indicators of diabetic patients with the mortality of the general population of Latvia showed that women with diabetes had higher relative mortality rate than men (Table 11.7). For example, in the 20- to 29-year-old women group with diabetes, the mortality rate was 11 times higher than that of women in the population of Latvia in the same age group, but in the 30–39 age group – nearly seven times bigger. The mortality rate of men with diabetes compared to that of men in the population of Latvia was increased most in the 20–29 age group – by more than four times [35].

This way, analysis of diabetic registers in Ukraine and Latvia shows a significantly higher risk of all-cause mortality in young women with diabetes comparing to women without diabetes, than in men with diabetes comparing to women without diabetes.

Investigation of a T1D patient cohort from the UK, which like the Ukrainian diabetic register was created based on data from primary care doctors (7,713 patients, last observation 1999), concluded that the risk of death in relation to persons without diabetes is the highest for young T1D patients, and it is greater among young women, than men [52]. A study from Ukraine [48] confirms this conclusion, complementing the fact that the gender difference of mortality among T1D patients 15–34 years old can disappear. This increase of mortality risk among young women with T1D has not been sufficiently explained. One possible explanation can be the following: Ischemic heart disease (IHD) in T1D patients is observed at a younger age [53], and women get it at the same frequency as men [54]. Premenopausal women, due to higher levels of nitrogen oxide that men, have a more intensive endothelium-dependent vasodilation. Diabetes leads to endothelial disfunction which neutralizes this difference between men and women [55]. Data about the increase of general mortality relative

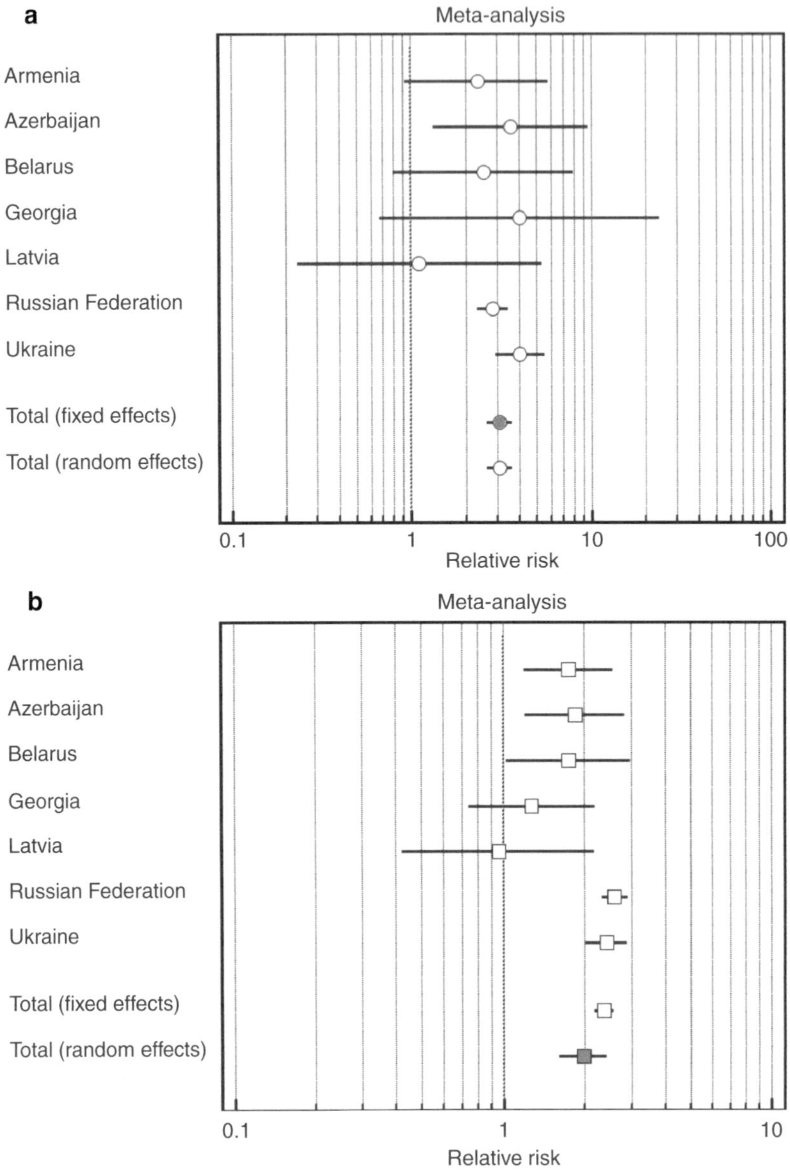

Fig. 11.6 Diabetes-related mortality risks (in relation to general mortality for a specific age group in men and women) for women comparing to men in 15–34 (**a**) and 35–54 (**b**) year age group

risk for women with T1D that were obtained as a result of analyzing population registers of some Eastern European and Baltic states can be seen as an epidemiologic confirmation of the need to continue fundamental research into the reasons of gender differences of the clinical progression and consequences of T1D.

While trying to reveal causes of the described phenomenon, we performed a meta-analysis (Fig. 11.6a, b) of diabetes-related mortality data comparing to the general mortality in seven countries. The data were extracted from WHO mortality database [6].

Increase of diabetes-related mortality risk (in relation to general mortality for a specific age group in men and women) for women comparing to men in Russia, Ukraine, and Azerbaijan in 15–34-year age group (Fig. 11.6a) and in Russia,

Ukraine, Azerbaijan, Armenia, and Belarus (Fig. 11.6b) in 35–54 age group was demonstrated. A generalization of relative risks for this age group was performed for all seven countries in order to confirm the assessment in 15–34 age group (Fig. 11.6a). During heterogeneity testing ($p=0.45$), the homogeneity hypothesis was not rejected; therefore, the Mantel-Haenszel model was chosen (generalized RR = 3.1 (95 % CI 2.6–3.6). In 35–54 age group, the homogeneity hypothesis was rejected ($p=0.008$); therefore, the random effects model was chosen (generalized RR = 2.0 (95 % CI 1.6–2.4).

Thus, the fraction of death cases "from diabetes" within the general mortality for females aged 15–54 turned out to be greater, than the corresponding number for males. This pattern is more prominent in young women.

Thus, it seems that the female gender lowers the chances of survival of diabetic women not only as a result of activating cardiovascular pathology and not only in the youngest women.

EURODIAB has reported an SMR of 2.0 in 12 European countries that followed 28,887 children with T1D (141 deaths during 219,061 person-years) with a range of SMR from 0 to 4.7 among the countries included in the study [52]. Life expectancy of T1D patients in Ukraine in 2007, assessed according to age at the time of death, did not exceed 40.2 years [48]. In the UK, according to similar cohort study, this value is 55 years [52]; however, the British cohort also included children, which could influence the assessment of average T1D duration and age at the time of death. Renal failure is the leading cause of death (28.4 %) in Ukrainian T1D patient cohort [50], whereas according to a British study of diabetes mellitus patient register containing primary care data, the leading cause of death among T1D patients was CVD [56]. Similar results were obtained by a European study, EURODIAB [57]. Comparison of main causes of death according to EURODIAB data and Ukrainian Diabetes Register (UDR) data is shown in Fig. 11.7. Apparently, death from renal failure among T1D patients in Ukraine prevails several times over other causes, while in other parts of Europe the main cause of death is CVD. It was previously noted by epidemiologists that the main cause of death for T1D patients is renal failure [58]; however, these data were relevant in 1960s–1970s. Today's experts believe that the shift in mortality structure toward CVD happened due to intensification of hypotensive therapy and insulin treatment [59]; therefore, the mortality structure of T1D patients that we have revealed when analyzing UDR can be assumed to conform to earlier time period of clinical practice. An earlier investigation that we have previously cited [32] also indicates that renal failure is the main cause of death among young diabetic patients in Ukraine [32].

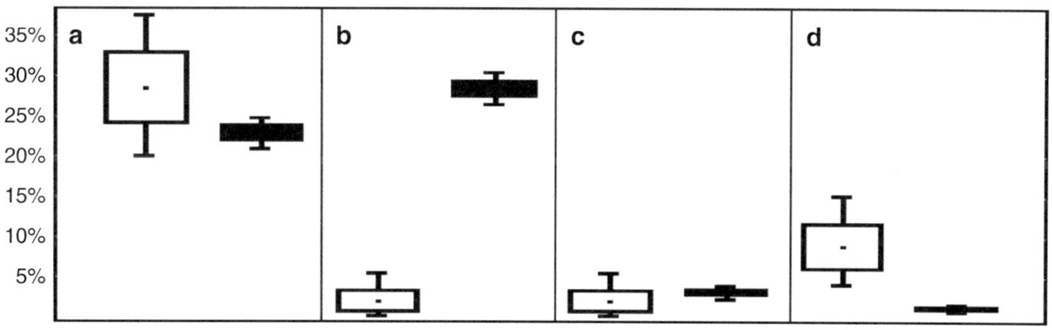

Fig. 11.7 Interval estimation of structure (%) of the main death causes among T1D patients, diagnosed before 30 years of age according to EURODIAB data (*white boxes*) and the Ukrainian Diabetes Register (*black boxes*). Death causes: CVD (**a**); renal failure (**b**); DKA or coma (**c**); cancer (**d**). *Note*: given means (%) ± SE (the *dot* within the *box* and height of boxes, respectively), 95 % CI (*lines* that emerge above and below the boxes) (Data from Ukrainian Diabetes Register given according to Khalangot et al. [50]; EURODIAB given according to Soedamah-Muthu et al. [57])

In summary, the performed analysis of diabetes mortality trends in ex-Soviet Eastern European countries allows to make the following conclusions:

- For 15 years after 1985, the WHO mortality databases recorded a multifold diabetes-related mortality growth in several East European countries, including Russia, Ukraine, and Belarus.
- After the year 2000, there is a gradual reduction of diabetes-related mortality in these countries.
- The analysis conducted in Ukraine indicates that the main cause of death for T1D patients is renal failure. As renal dialysis therapy in USSR was scarce, one may assume that post 1985 diabetes-related mortality growth can reflect not just issues with insulin supply, but also a decrease of administrative pressure, when recording the cause of death in corresponding documents.
- Reduction of general mortality, demonstrated by some diabetes population registers (Latvia), and an increase of average age at the time of death (Ukraine, Russia, Belarus) allows to assume that the decrease of diabetes-related death cases, recorded by WHO mortality databases, is a real phenomenon, rather than a reflection of change of policy toward recording the cause of death in corresponding certificates.
- According to data from diabetic registers in Latvia and Ukraine, the phenomenon of female gender-related increase of general mortality in young women was confirmed. We saw this for the first time when comparing the fraction of those who died due to diabetes within general male and female mortality in East European countries according to WHO mortality databases.

Some Aspects of the Pathophysiology of Type 1 and Type 2 Diabetes in Ukraine

Association Between Early-Life Events and Risk for Diabetes Mellitus in Ukraine Population

The "thrifty phenotype" hypothesis proposed by Hales and Barker [60] suggests that inadequate nutrition during in utero development can result in long-term adaptive changes in glucose-insulin metabolism (including reduced capacity for insulin secretion and insulin resistance) that, due to an enhanced ability to store fat, improve survival under postnatal conditions of nutritional deprivation. However, windows of plasticity close early in life, and postnatal environmental exposures may lead to the selected trajectory of becoming inappropriate, resulting in adverse effects on adult health. If mismatch exists between the environment predicted in utero and the actual environment experienced in subsequent life (e.g., excess food consumption), diabetes and other features of the metabolic syndrome will result. To study this prediction, associations between early-life conditions and the risk of developing diabetes mellitus in adulthood have been studied in Ukraine population. The main findings of these studies are presented in subchapters below.

Association Between Prenatal Exposure to the Ukraine Famine of 1932–1933 and Type 2 Diabetes

Nutrition during pregnancy has been proposed as an explanation for the occurrence of type 2 diabetes later in life, but direct measures are hard to obtain. To better identify any effects of early nutrition, studies of man-made famines can offer distinct opportunities for the unbiased comparison of individuals born under such conditions with unexposed controls [61]. These approaches can provide information about specific pregnancy exposures, especially if the population at risk, the timing and degree of exposure and relevant health outcomes can be accurately defined. For type 2 diabetes in later life, studies of the Dutch famine of 1944–1945 Lumey et al. [62], the Chinese famine of 1959–1962 Li et al. [63], and three famines in twentieth century Austria Thurner et al. [64] all suggest a relation with early-life nutrition. All these studies have a particular strength: The timing of the famine in relation to the stage of gestation was particularly well defined in the Dutch study, as was the risk of adult hyperglycemia in the Chinese study, and a large number of patients receiving antidiabetic drugs over a long time period was included in the nationwide Austrian study. However, no study combines all these strengths. To overcome the limitations of previous approaches, the setting of the Ukraine famine of 1932–1933 was used to study the association between early-life nutrition and late-life type 2 diabetes in a large population, in cohorts well defined with respect to the timing of the famine in relation the stage of pregnancy and the severity of the famine around the time of birth [65].

This study included all patients with type 2 diabetes diagnosed at age 40 years or older in the Ukraine national diabetes register 2000–2008 and used all individuals born between 1930 and 1938 from the 2001 Ukraine national census as the reference population. The studied population included individuals born before and after the famine period as controls and those from regions that experienced extreme, severe, or no famine. The prevalence odds ratios (ORs) were used as the measure of association between type 2 diabetes and early famine exposure, with stratification by region, date of birth, and sex for comparisons of diabetes prevalence in specific subgroups.

The odds of type 2 diabetes by date and region of birth in 43,150 patients with diabetes and 1,421,024 individuals born between 1930 and 1938 were compared (Fig. 11.8). With adjustment for season of birth, the OR for developing type 2 diabetes was 1·47 (95 % CI 1.37–1.58) in individuals born in the first half of 1934 in regions with extreme famine, 1·26 (1·14–1·39) in individuals born in regions with severe famine, and there was no increase (OR 1·00, 0·91–1·09) in individuals born in regions with no famine, compared with births in other time periods (Fig. 11.9).

The associations between type 2 diabetes and famine around the time of birth were similar in men and women. These findings show a dose-response relation between famine severity during prenatal development and odds of type 2 diabetes in later life and suggest that early gestation is a critical time window of development.

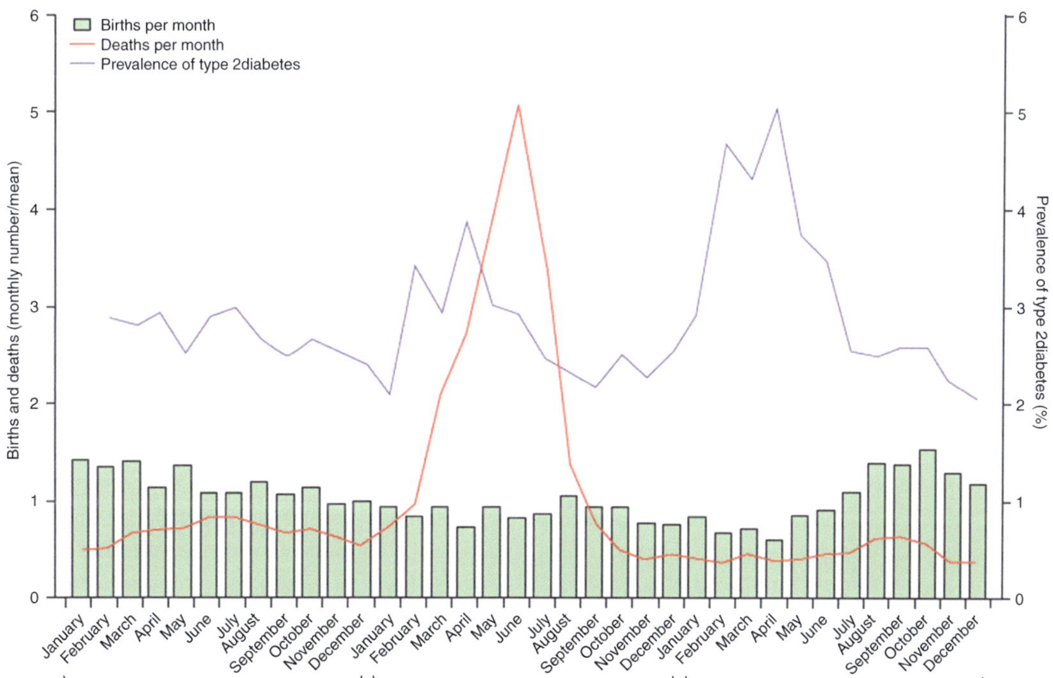

Fig. 11.8 Monthly births and deaths in eastern Ukraine in 1932–1934 and prevalence of type 2 diabetes between 2000 and 2008, by year and month of birth. Ratio of monthly values to overall mean. Deaths rates are per 1,000 population, birth counts are from the Ukraine 2001 census, and prevalence of type 2 diabetes is from the Ukraine national diabetes register (The figure is reproduced from Lumey et al. [65] with permission of the publisher, Elsevier Science Ltd.)

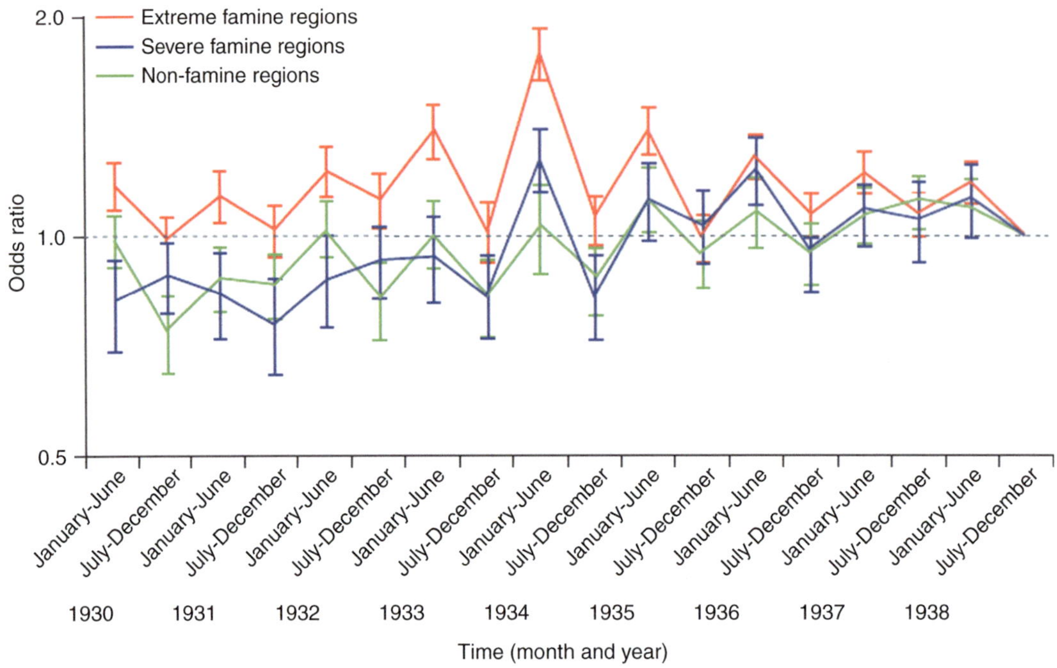

Fig. 11.9 Odds for registered cases of type 2 diabetes (2000–2008) by month and year of birth and famine severity in the region of birth (1932–1933). Odds ratios comparing the odds of type 2 diabetes among births by half year to the odds for births from July to December, 1938 (reference group). *Error bars* show 95 % CIs (The figure is reproduced from Lumey et al. [65] with permission of the publisher, Elsevier Science Ltd.)

Seasonality of Birth in Diabetic Patients in Ukraine

Season of birth provides another type of "natural experiment" to examine the association between early-life conditions and later health outcomes. Month of birth is a good instrument that can help assess the effects of early growth on adult health independent of life-course factors. This is true because in decades past, there were important seasonal differences in nutrition, especially in developing countries. The food supply (variety, quantity, and freshness of fruits, vegetables, cereals, and animal protein) was varied according to season. These differences in access to high quality food supply can potentially influence intrauterine growth depending on the month of gestation. Other possible triggering factors for disease progression such as infections, sunlight/photoperiod, productions of vitamin D and melatonin, and outdoor temperature also tend to change seasonally. Seasonal patterns of birth for both type 1 and type 2 diabetic patients were determined in Ukraine population.

Type 1 Diabetes

Seasonal pattern of birth in type 1 diabetic patients has been repeatedly described around the world (see, e.g., [66]). Significant seasonality of birth in persons with type 1 diabetes was revealed in Ukraine population [67]. The data consisted of prevalent cases of type 1 diabetes in Ukraine by the end of 2003. Cases were restricted to individuals born after 1 January 1960 and diagnosed with type 1 diabetes before age 30 ($n=20{,}117$). People who were born during the same time in general population ($n=29{,}105{,}560$) served as a reference standard. A significant seasonal pattern of type 1 diabetes incidence rates was found ($p<0.001$), with the lowest rates in December and the highest in April (Fig. 11.10). The rate ratio between the extremes was 1.32 (95 % CI 1.27–1.39). Tests for seasonal pattern in subgroups defined by sex and age or by sex and date of birth were all significant with p-values less than 0.02. No interactions with sex or age at diagnosis were revealed, while a strong interaction with period of birth ($p<0.0001$) was demonstrated.

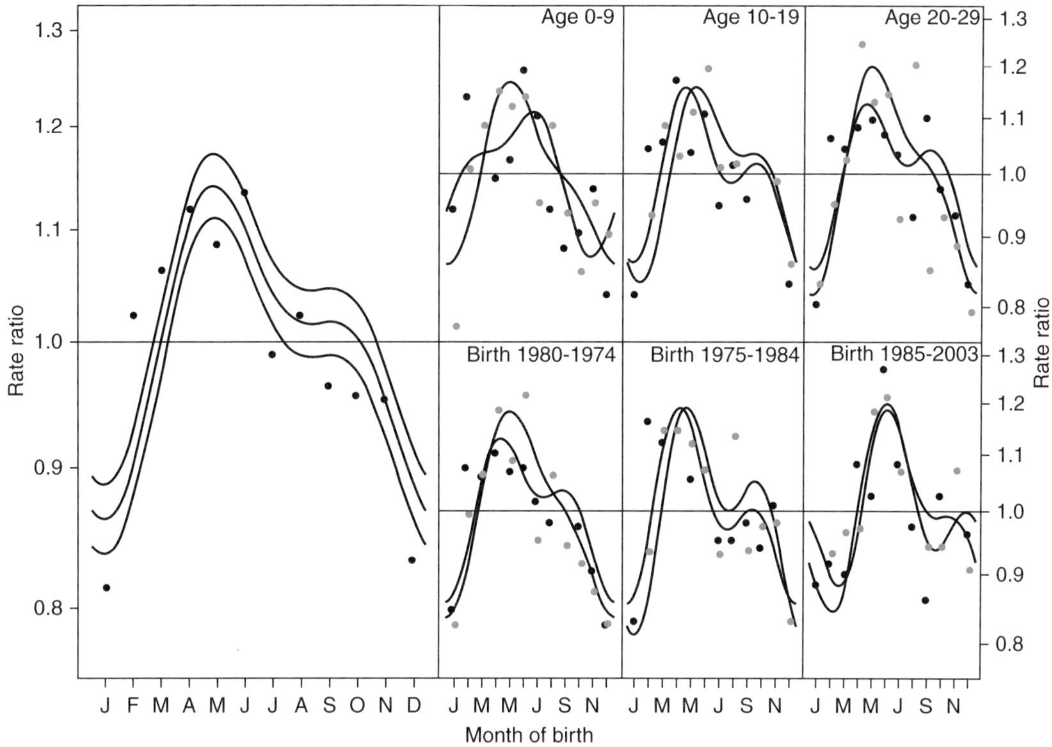

Fig. 11.10 Effect of month of birth on the risk of developing type 1 diabetes. *Left-hand panel*, the overall effect with the 95 % CI, controlled for sex, age at diagnosis and period of birth. The points are observed rate ratios for single months. *Right-hand panel*, analyses subdivided by sex and broad categories of date of birth. Men: *dark*; women: *light* (The figure is reproduced from Vaiserman et al. [67] with permission of the publisher, Elsevier Science Ltd.)

Type 2 Diabetes

In contrast to the well-described birth seasonality in childhood diabetes persons, the seasonality of birth in adult type 2 diabetes patients has been reported only in few papers. In Ukraine, seasonality of birth was strongly evident in type 2 diabetes patients [68]. In this study, cases were restricted to type 2 diabetes patients from three large Ukrainian regions (Chernigiv: $n=18{,}594$; Kherson: $n=19{,}738$; Rivne: $n=13{,}882$) born before 31 December 1959 and diagnosed with diabetes after age 39. Reference populations were based on the Ukraine census 2001 depersonalized data ($n=1{,}567{,}917$). Seasonality of birth was evident in type 2 diabetes patients (male: peak in 12 April, nadir in 22 November, amplitude 28.9 %, $p<0.001$; female: peak in 22 April, nadir in 15 December, amplitude 36.4 %, $p<0.001$). Similar pattern with peaks between mid-March and mid-May and nadirs between mid-October and mid-December was obtained in all regions studied (Fig. 11.11). This pattern was substantially uniform for all birth cohorts over the study period.

Similar Birth Seasonality in Type 1 and Type 2 Diabetics and Underlying Mechanisms Proposed

The results obtained indicate that early-life factors linked to seasons are implicated in the subsequent development of both type 1 diabetes and type 2 diabetes in Ukraine. In the study population, individuals born in April experienced fetal life largely in the nutritionally marginal months from late autumn to early spring and passed the first postnatal months in a season of relative plenty. These individuals were found to have increased risk of diabetes. In contrast, a decreased risk was found for those born in November–December. In this

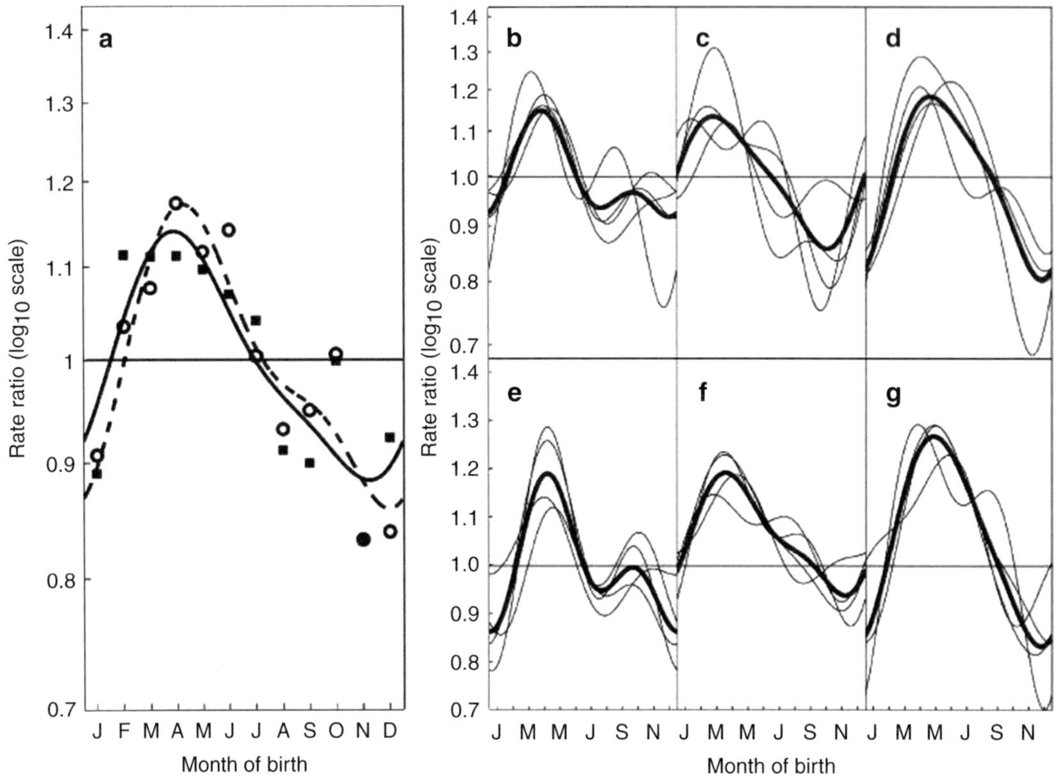

Fig. 11.11 Effect of month of birth on the risk of developing type 2 diabetes. (**a**) The overall effect for men (*solid line* and *black squares*) and women (*dashed line* and *white circles*). (**b**–**g**) Analyses subdivided by sex and regions. Chernigiv men (n=6,411) (**b**); Kherson men (n=6,145) (**c**); Rivne men (n=4,954) (**d**); Chernigiv women (n=12,183) (**e**), Kherson women (n=13,593) (**f**), Rivne women (n=8,928) (**g**). In each of the panels, the estimated patterns subdivided by birth cohort are drawn as *thin lines*; the overall effects are drawn as the *thick lines* (The figure is reproduced from Vaiserman et al. [68] with permission of the publisher, Elsevier Science Ltd)

group, fetal development in a nutritionally favorable season would have been followed by early infancy in a season of relative shortage (winter-spring). Obviously, the first scenario is more high-risk for diabetes development than the second one. These results are highly consistent with the "thrifty phenotype" hypothesis by Hales and Barker [60].

Interestingly, in the very recent research by Jensen et al. [69], no evidence of seasonality of birth in adult type 2 diabetes in Denmark was obtained. The authors have suggested that differences in the effects observed in Denmark and Ukraine can be explained by the differences in latitude or the standard of living between these countries. Indeed, since seasonal variation in both nutrition and weather was much more extreme in Ukraine than in Denmark during the study periods, and, since Ukraine is a lower middle-income country, the people might have experienced the extremes more pronounced here than in a more affluent country like Denmark.

Surprisingly, the month-of-birth patterns obtained for children and young adults (0–29 years) with type 1 diabetes and for middle-to-old aged type 2 diabetes patients in Ukraine were quite similar. The finding that type 1 and type 2 diabetes share similar seasonality of birth led to hypothesis that early-life triggers can be common to both phenotypes in Ukraine population [70]. These findings are consistent with the "accelerator hypothesis" [71] which argue that type 1 and type 2 diabetes, despite the marked differences in pathogenesis, are merely poles of a single pathological spectrum.

Correlation Between the Prevalence of Type 1 Diabetes with the Daily Insulin Dose and the Autoimmune Process Against Glutamic Acid Decarboxylase in Adults

The purpose of this diabetes register-based study in Ukraine [41] was to determine whether the insulin requirement can change systematically in T1D patients and whether this requirement depends on the same factors that determine its prevalence. The rate of insulin requirement among adults with type 1 diabetes (T1D) in 24 Ukrainian regions was compared. The data included the prevalent cases of T1D in Ukraine at the end of 2006. Only persons aged over 14 years at the time of inclusion into the Ukrainian register and diagnosed with diabetes before 30 years of age were included in this study ($n = 26{,}796$). As the average duration of the disease was found to be 14.86 years, the average daily insulin doses were calculated for each year of the duration, from 0 (<1) to 15 years.

For patients with a disease duration (DD) of up to 15 years ($n = 13{,}677$), the daily insulin dose (DID) was observed to increase linearly with DD ($R = 0.899$, $p < 0.001$), see Fig. 11.12. A further increase in the disease duration in the range of 16–31 years was not accompanied by regular changes in the insulin dose. The regular rise of insulin dose, observed with the increase in the duration of T1D in adults diagnosed before the age of 30 years, is still an unknown phenomenon.

Furthermore, the differences in the T1D prevalence among the 24 Ukrainian regions were obtained ($p < 0.001$). In the "minimal" regional cluster (MIC), the prevalence rate was 6 (5–6), and, in the "maximal" (MAC) regional cluster, it was 9 (8–9) per 10,000 adults.

Insulin doses standardized according to the disease duration within the range of 0–15 years in the minimal prevalence cluster of T1D prevalence were significantly lower, when compared with the intermediate and maximal prevalence clusters. The values in the intermediate prevalence cluster

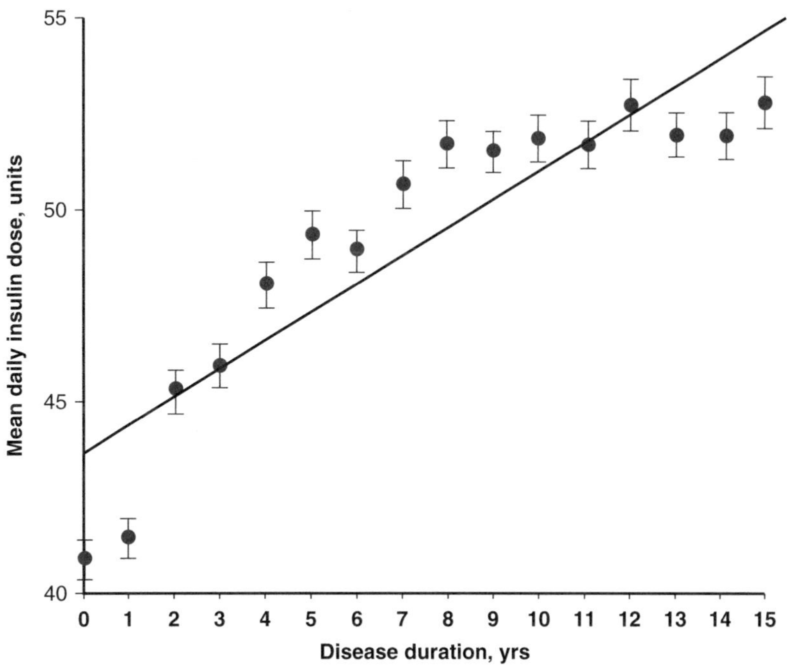

Fig. 11.12 Average (Mean ± SE) daily insulin doses of type 1 diabetes mellitus patients depending on the disease duration in the range of 0–15 years (The figure is reproduced from Khalangot et al. [41] with permission of the publisher, Elsevier Ltd.)

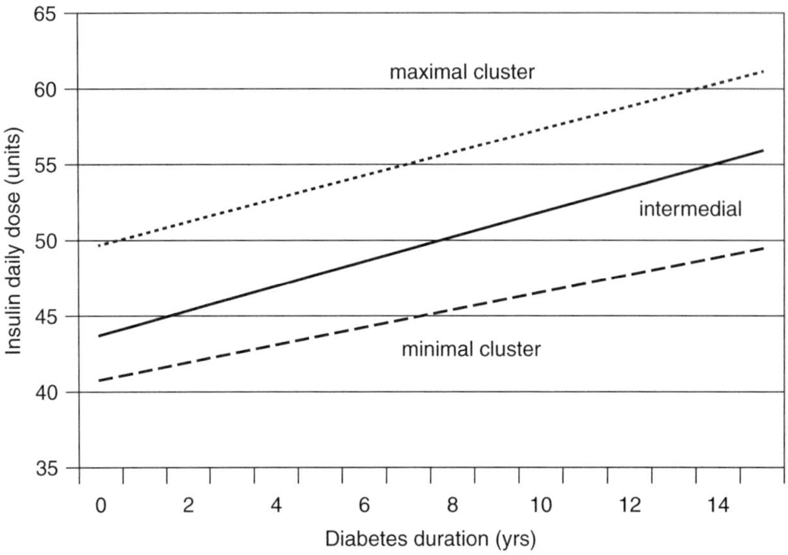

Fig. 11.13 Average daily insulin doses of diabetes mellitus type 1 patients depending on the disease duration (in the range of 0–15 years) as well as on the territorial cluster, selected according to disease prevalence (The figure is reproduced from Khalangot et al. [41] with permission of the publisher, Elsevier Ltd)

were lower than those in the maximal prevalence cluster (Fig. 11.13).

The median insulin doses were standardized according to DD, and the values were lowest in the MIC and highest in the MAC populations: 45.89 (45.28–47.19) and 56.59 (53.33–57.88) U/24 h, respectively ($p<0.01$). Furthermore, the level of HbA1c in the MAC of T1D patients was observed to be higher than that in the MIC (9.52 ± 2.24 %, $n=240$, and 8.57 ± 3.29 %, $n=111$, respectively; $p<0.01$).

The glutamic acid decarboxylase 65 antibody (GADA) comparisons: A total of 86 T1D patients with a mean age of 27.5 years (0.86) and a mean diabetes duration of 10.3 (0.72) years (SE) were randomly selected from four regional diabetes registers. The GADA and the plasma c-peptide levels were also determined. The logistic regression model was used, and the odds ratio (OR) and 95 % confidence interval (CI) were calculated. The GADA levels and persistence in the MAC patients ($n=38$) were higher than that of the MIC patients ($n=48$): 14.1 ± 4.6 and 3.2 ± 1.2 U/ml, respectively, mean ± SE; $p=0.028$; OR = 9.66 (3.31–28.17), $p<0.001$. Adjusting for age, gender, and duration of the diabetes affected the results only slightly: OR = 7.91 (2.44–25.57), $p<0.001$.

Thus, adult type 1 diabetics living on territories with high prevalence of this disease may require higher daily insulin doses. This phenomenon may be explained by more intense autoimmunity in patients residing on these territories. Similar comparisons of GADA levels and persistence in populations that differ significantly according to T1D prevalence (e.g., in countries of Northern Europe and Japan or Korea) seem very desirable to us, but, as far as we know, they have not been performed yet.

Genomic Landscape of Diabetes in Region

For the last two decades, diabetes-related genetic studies in Eastern Europe were conducted mostly in Russia and concerned in assessing T1D risks and complications, as well as T2D and some genes associated with genetic polymorphism. In particular, Dimitry Chistiakov et al. demonstrated that human cytotoxic T lymphocyte-associated antigen-4 gene is strongly associated with and linked to T1D in a Russian population [72] and suggest a protective role of the 262 T allele of the catalase gene against the rapid development of diabetic neuropathy in T1D [73]. But association studies of these polymorphisms in KCNJ11 and ABCC8 (E23K and ABCC8 exon 31 variants) were only conducted in the regions of Russia near Europe [74], but not Siberia. Most recent study assessed whether SNPs rs5219 and rs757110 are associated with a predisposition to T2DM in Siberians (1,384 T2D patients; 414 healthy individuals, all belong to a Russian ethnic group) and found that neither SNP was associated with the disease [75]. Thus, "genomic landscape" of T2D differs significantly between European and Asian parts of Russia.

Ukraine as well has some studies, looking at genetic aspects of diabetes. In particular, it has been shown that 49A/G polymorphism of CTLA4 gene – as in type 1 diabetes mellitus – plays an important role in genetic predisposition to latent autoimmune diabetes of adults (LADA) in Ukrainian population. 49G/G genotype CTLA4 is associated with the risk of developing T1D, T2D, and LADA [5]. It is interesting that there were no 49A/G polymorphism of CTLA4 differences between T1D and T2d found in the study. Just recently, Ukraine saw its first assessment of neonatal diabetes in patients with onset of diabetes during the first 9 months of life [76]: the incidence of neonatal diabetes in Ukraine over a 36-month period (2012–2014) was calculated to be 1 in 126,397 live births. Genetic testing was undertaken for 42 patients with permanent or transient diabetes diagnosed within the first 6 months of life ($n=22$) or permanent diabetes diagnosed between 6 and 9 months ($n=20$). KCNJ11 and ABCC8 mutations was the most common cause (52 %) of neonatal diabetes. Ukraine has a similar incidence of neonatal diabetes as other European countries [77, 78] and K_{ATP} channel gene mutations are the most common cause. All 11 patients with KCNJ11 and ABCC8 mutations were successfully switched from insulin injections to oral sulfonylurea therapy with an improvement in their glycemic control [76].

Diagnosis of Diabetes and Prediabetes in Region

For the last 15 years in Eastern Europe, diabetes was diagnosed according to WHO recommendations (1999) [79]. The corresponding diagnostic criteria in Russia and Ukraine are mentioned in documents approved by government healthcare organizations [80, 81]. Categories of prediabetes, Impaired fasting glucose (IFG) or impaired glucose tolerance (IGT), are known only as given by WHO (1999) [79]. Stretching of IFG from 6.1–6.9 to 5.6–6.9 mmol/l, as was done by the experts from the American Diabetes Association (ADA) [82, 83] in the process of preventing diabetes development, is not used. We know of only one example of comparative assessments of hyperglycemia criteria between WHO and ADA: the screening study involving 2,368 adult residents of the Moscow region [84]. The prevalence of early disorders of carbohydrate metabolism and T2D are 17.1 and 7.2, respectively, using WHO criteria and 40.0 and 5.9 % by ADA criteria. Alexander Dreval et al. [84] believe that "refusal to undergo oral glucose tolerance test (OGTT) during screening decreases detectability of early metabolic disorders by 28.8 and 6.1 % using WHO and ADA criteria, respectively. When screening is aimed to diagnose T2D alone, OGTT can be omitted in subjects with fasting plasma glucose level below 4.7 mmol/l. If it is aimed to diagnose both T2D and impaired glucose tolerance, OGTT is not needed in subjects with fasting plasma glucose level below 4.2 mmol/l" [84]. Screening for T2D and prediabetes in other Russian cities based on OGTT only in those who had IFG levels of plasma glucose revealed the following structure prevalence (%) of blood glucose categories according to WHO 1999: isolated IFG – 7.4 (95 % CI 6.7–8.1); IFG + IGT – 1.6 (95 % CI 1.2–1.9); unknown T2D – 5.2 (95 % CI 4.6–5.8). Previously known T2D prevalence in this study population of Chelyabinsk city (Ural region) aged 20–74 years old was 1.8 (95 % CI 1.4–2.1) % [85]. When using similar design in another study, carried out in Abakan city (Khakassia region), prevalence of screen-detected

T2D, IGT, and IFG were only 1.25 (95 % CI 0.94–1.56); 0.34 (95 % CI 0.18–0.56); and 0.04 %, respectively. Prevalence of known T2D in Khakassia was 2.13 % [86]. Thus, in Russia known T2D prevalence in different regions does not differ significantly and is equal to 1.8–2.13 %, whereas screen-detected T2D prevalence has more substantial regional differences – from 7.2 to 1.25 %. A small OGTT-based study in Ukraine (rural population, age 45+) revealed new T2D prevalence of 12.7 % and normal fasting glucose and tolerance only in 36.6 % of the studied persons [13].

Complications of Diabetes in Region

Complication prevalence assessments in a population of T1D patients based on diabetic register data from Ukraine and Russia are compared with results of multinational, multi-center, observational, cross-sectional survey assessing diabetes secondary care in Central and Eastern Europe (DEPAC Survey) – (Table 11.8). A total of seven countries, including two Baltic states (Latvia and Lithuania), took part in the DEPAC Survey [87].

A cohort consisting of 29,721 adult T1D patients can be viewed as full population data on this illness in Ukraine. Inclusion criterion for this cohort was diabetes diagnosis before the age of 30. This hallmark was not used in two other cases, which could theoretically increase the possibility of false allocation of T2D or other diabetic type patients to T1D insulin-treated. Nevertheless, comparing average age and gender distribution of Ukrainian and DEPAC Survey patients rather indicates their similarities. Average HbA1c and BMI levels in Ukraine and DEPAC Survey did not differ significantly, and fractions of patients whose HbA1c reached <7 % in Russia, Ukraine and DEPAC Survey were

Table 11.8 Same characteristics of T1D patients according to cross-sectional data analysis

Characteristics	Ukraine [37, 50]	Russia [22, 24]	DEPAC Survey [87]
Number of patients, *n*	29,721	294,257	2,497
Gender: females (%)	47.02	n.a.	48.4 (43.0–50.9)
Mean age, years	34.47 (12.91)	n.a.	36.9 (25.2–42.2)
Mean T1D duration, years	17.32 (11.02)	n.a.	13.7 (9.4–16.6)
BMI, kg/m^2	23.16 (4.10)	n.a.	24.0 (21.7–25.7)
Systolic BP, mmHg	125.91 (19.75)	n.a.	124 (116–133)
Diastolic BP, mmHg	78.15 (10.94)	n.a.	76 (68–82)
Mean HbA1c, %	8.75 (2.57)	n.a.	8.2 (7.7–9.8)
HbA1c <7 %	18.78 %	26.1 %	23.9 %
Nephropathy (any stage), %	32.14	23.0	27.8 (12.0–55.4)
Renal failure, %	4.96	9.0	n.a.
End-stage renal failure, %	2.78	n.a.	0.44 (0.0–2.3)
Amputation (any level), %	2.71	1.2	1.2 (0.0–4.6)
Foot ulcer, %	4.19	5.6	2.1 (0.7–7.7)
Retinopathy (any stage), %	55.1	34.7	40.9 (19.0–87.6)
Blindness, %	3.47	1.54	0.48 (0.0–3.4)
Insulin analogues, %	9.84	20–80	49 (38–95)

Data are means or %. (SD or country lowest mean value – country highest mean value)
HbA1c data were registered in 8.6 and 13 % T1D cases in Ukrainian and Russian diabetes registers, respectively. BMI was measured in 25 % of T1D cases (Russian register). Percentage of patients with measurements of protein excretion according to Russian register data is as follows: microalbuminuria – 6.37 %, proteinuria – 5.77 % of T1D cases. In case of the Russian register the "diabetic foot" category is used and can include foot ulcers and/or amputation cases. Data are means or %., (SD or country lowest mean value-country highest mean value). Insulin analogues fraction presented as regional lowest – highest value
n.a. not applicable

close. There is no gender, age, or diabetes duration data in the Russian register, and most quantitative data are given as category distribution, which makes a lot of comparisons difficult. It is quite unusual that 11.6 % of T1D patients in Russia have insufficient body mass (<18.5 kg/m^2) and that can indicate a lack of effect from insulin treatment. It should be noted that the corresponding BMI category among T2D patients is only 0.2 % [22] according to Russian register data.

The data on high prevalence of end-stage renal failure, amputation, foot ulcers, and blindness in Ukraine seems disturbing. But all this indicators seem comparable with highest country mean value of DEPAC Survey (Table 11.8).

Less than 10 % of T1D patients in Ukraine and 49 % according to DEPAC Survey data receive insulin analogs. In Russia the use of insulin analogues depends on the level of economic prosperity of the region [24]. It seems that frequent use of these drugs is becoming an issue of image or status of the patient and the healthcare system. Some experts are currently criticizing the policy toward government procurement in some post-Soviet states, e.g., Kyrgyzstan [3], where an insulin analog, which is not included on the WHO EML, has significantly higher costs and has been shown to have little added clinical value [88] is also purchased.

Results of a similar cross-sectional review are also presented for T2D patients (Table 11.9). Among the most significant differences is the higher percentage of women among T2D patients in Ukraine, comparing to DEPAC Survey. It cannot go unnoticed that myocardial infarction is four times less frequent in Ukrainian and Russian

Table 11.9 Same characteristics of T2D patients according to cross-sectional data analysis

Characteristics	Ukraine [37, 51]	Russia [22, 24]	DEPAC Survey [87]
Number of patients, *n*	105,480	3,705,102	8,231
Gender: females (%)	67.17	n.a.	52.7 (48.1–71.8)
Mean age, years	66.6 (10.9)	n.a.	62.2 (60.5–64.4)
Mean T2D duration, years	8.98 (7.4)	n.a.	10.2 (8.4–11.1)
BMI, kg/m^2	28.64 (4.7)	n.a.	30.6 (30.1–32.6)
Systolic BP, mmHg	144.16 (18.7)	n.a.	141 (138–149)
Diastolic BP, mmHg	85.97 (10.4)	n.a.	83 (80–88)
Mean HbA1c, %	8.88 (4.9)	n.a.	7.7 (7.5–8.3)
Total cholesterol (mmol/l)	5.41 (1.2)	5.43	5.39 (5.13–5.89)
Triglycerides (mmol/l)	2.23	1.8	2.12 (1.93–2.43)
Nephropathy (any stage), %	n.a.	4.9	25.3 (17.6–39.8)
End-stage renal failure, %	0.26	n.a.	0.44 (0.0–2.3)
Amputation (any level), %	n.a.	1.2	1.2 (0.0–4.6)
Foot ulcer, %	2.97	2.4	2.1 (0.7–7.7)
Retinopathy (any stage), %	n.a.	15.3	40.9 (19.0–87.6)
Blindness, %	n.a.	0.62	0.34 (0.1–0.7)
Myocardial infarction, %	3.24	3.7	12.4 (9.1–16.6)
Stroke or TIA, %	4.46	4.4	7.2 (4.0–13.3)
Any antihypertensive agents, %	35.99	n.a.	82.5 (75.8–91.4)
ACE inhibitors, %	25.27	n.a.	66.5 (57.0–84.1)
Statins, %	3.18	n.a.	48.3 (13.7–55.5)
OAD + Insulin, %	3.6	n.a.	16 (4–34)
Insulin only, %	22.5	n.a.	n.a.

Data are means or % (SD or country lowest mean value – country highest mean value); HbA1c levels registered in 7.4 and 8.4 % T2D cases of Ukrainian and Russian diabetes registers, respectively; BMI measured in 22 % of T2D cases from Russian registers; percentage of patients with measurements of protein excretion are as follows: microalbuminuria 8 %, proteinuria 13.8 % of T2D cases

T2D patients, then in DEPAC Survey. There are no such significant differences in stroke prevalence. That said, the use of statins, any antihypertensive agents, or ACE inhibitors in Ukraine is several times less, then in the DEPAC Survey. It is likely that in this case we are dealing with a long known paradox – Russia and Ukraine have highest CVD mortality levels and lowest myocardial infarction mortality levels in Europe: mortality from ischemic heart disease (ICD-9: 410–414) in 1999 in Ukraine was 399.86 and 229.53, whereas acute myocardial infarction (ICD-9: 410) mortality levels were 18.89 and 6.58 per 100,000 males and females, respectively [89]. This is most likely explained by an insufficient lifetime diagnostics of myocardial infarction. It is remarkable that ECG was performed for 81 (50–90) % of DEPAC Survey T2D patients [87].

Recently, two more possibilities for evaluating diabetes treatment in Ukraine in the framework of an international assessment had been used: EUCCLID – a European cross-sectional primary care diabetes survey in conjunction with the EASD study group. In this study, patients will be randomly selected from a list of all patients known to the participating GPs with T2D for whom the GP is the main diabetes care provider [90]. In another investigation, only glycemic control (HbA1c) of type 1 diabetes in clinical practice [91] was compared.

Due to a small number of patients from each country, data are not identified by individual country names in the final report [90]. However, data from individual countries have been seen and discussed at the local level. Ukrainian T2D EUCCLID data was generally close to data from Table 11.9, occupying lower positions in the assessment of treatment quality, comparing to other European countries. When assessing HbA1c levels in T1D patients in another international study [91], Ukrainian data were one of the better ones. One possible explanation for this could be the fact that Ukraine was represented by one of its Western regions – Volyn, which belongs to a group of regions with minimal adult T1D prevalence. Earlier we have revealed a positive correlation between intensity of insulin treatment, HbA1c and GADA levels, and T1D prevalence in adults [41, 42]. According to earlier healthcare reports, western Ukraine had lower T2D prevalence, compared to Ukraine's average [92].

Coordination and Delivery of Diabetes Care Services

Assessments of diabetes patient treatment quality, based on interviewing, recently performed in several post-Soviet countries by independent researchers revealed many specific issues related to accessibility of specialized aid and medications and also a great degree of treatment dissatisfaction. In particular, British investigators conducted 15 semi-structured interviews with patients with diabetes and physicians in Russian rural and urban settings, in public and private sectors. Patients worried about high and rising costs of care, while physicians noted concerns about lack of time to treat patients adequately. Although all specifically diabetes-related services are free of charge, patients requiring urgent surgery often face high user fees, either to bypass waiting lists in state facilities or to be treated immediately in a private institution. These "hidden," out-of-pocket payments impact adversely on equity and act as a barrier to timely care [93]. The same or close problems are revealed in Georgia [19], and the reforms of health insurance in Moldova [94–96] give us some hope.

The problem of organizing and financing renal replacement treatment cannot go unmentioned. According to a recent statement from the head of the Belarus endocrinology service, 126 persons died in 2012 due to diabetes-related causes (177 persons in 2011). Of these, 82 died as a result of chronic renal failure (115 in 2011), 39 from gangrene (56 in 2011), and 5 from coma (6 in 2011) [18]. Thus, renal failure is considered the main cause of death, which is considered diabetes-related in Belarus. Coverage indicators of renal replacement therapy in this country (hemodialysis, peritoneal dialysis, and kidney transplant) in 2012 were 432 patients per million population (189.3) in 2007) [18]. We attempted to clarify the meaning of "coverage" regarding the source of financing of this therapy and to what extent the need in such treatment could be satisfied in each of the mentioned post-Soviet countries. According to a 2006 review [97] dedicated to epidemiology of renal replacement in Central and Eastern Europe, the availability and outcome of renal replacement therapy in most of these countries have become comparable with what is seen in Western Europe. However, there are still large differences between individual countries. In particular, there is an urgent need for improvement in Belarus and Russia. The best correlation of transplantation/dialysis was noted in the Baltic states and the worst in Russia. According to the authors, there is no data on Ukraine and Moldova, despite numerous efforts to collect this data. We can confirm that during that period diabetes patients were discriminated against, when being selected for hemodialysis, and peritoneal dialysis was virtually unavailable. Since then, there were positive changes in Moldova and Ukraine. This type of treatment became available and covered by insurance (Moldova) or by direct government funding (Ukraine). Recently, a first assessment of renal replacement therapy (RRT) in Ukraine was published [98]. According to nephrologic register data, there were 5,985 prevalent RRT patients on 31 December 2012 (131.2 persons per million population). Mean age was 46.5 ± 13.8 years, 56 % men and 74 % received hemodialysis, while peritoneal dialysis and kidney transplantation both represented 13 %. Twelve percent of patients with end-stage renal disease had diabetes. In 2012, 1,129 patients started dialysis (incidence 24.8 per million population), with 80 % on hemodialysis. Mean age was 48 ± 14 years, 58 % men and 20 % had diabetes. Two years diabetes mellitus patient's survival on dialysis was 64.5 % (Fig. 11.14). The transplant rate in 2012 was 2.1 per million population. The incidence and prevalence of RRT and the transplantation rate in Ukraine are among the lowest in Europe, suggesting that the need for RRT is not being met. Strategies to reduce the RRT deficit include the development and improvement of transplantation and home-based dialysis programs. Further evaluation of the quality of Ukrainian RRT care is needed.

Peritoneal dialysis recently became widely accessible in Ukraine, and diabetes patients even prevailed among those, who received this treatment [98]. At the time of this chapter's preparation, 553

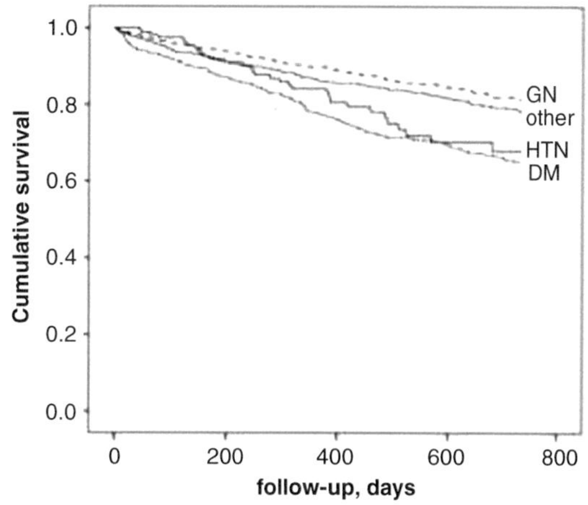

	90 days	1 year	2 years
N at risk			
GN, n=1.179	1.005	649	282
Other, n=1.143	967	644	281
HTN, n=167	141	74	20
DM, n=605	490	304	115
Events			
GN	42	101	147
Other	54	133	177
HTN	5	22	33
DM	45	111	149
Survival, %			
GN	96.3	89.7	81.3
Other	95.1	86.1	77.7
HTN	96.8	83.0	65.0
DM	92.3	77.7	64.5

Fig. 11.14 Kaplan-Meier curves for patient survival from day 1, by primary renal disease. *GN* glomerulonephritis, *HTN* hypertension, *DM* diabetes mellitus, *y* years (Modified from Kolesnyk et al. [98])

patients are receiving RRT in Moldova, including 80 diabetes mellitus patients (Adrian Tanase; personal communications data, 2016).

In summary, after this review of diabetes clinical aspects, we can state the following:

- Effect of economic prosperity of the country upon T1D treatment is best seen in the usage of insulin analogs.
- T2D treatment in Ukraine is characterized by significantly lower use of statins, any antihypertensive agents, ACE inhibitors, comparing to Central European and Baltic countries.
- Prevalence of myocardial infarction in T2D patients in Ukraine and Russia is significantly

lower comparing to Central European and Baltic countries.
- Financial welfare itself does not always affect the efficacy of diabetes treatment in expected fashion or to a sufficient level.
- Issue of renal replacement therapy of patients with diabetic nephropathy is far from being solved in Eastern Europe. Recently, there is some progress in providing RRT in Ukraine; however, its volume and quality is still in need of improvement.

Non-pharmacological Management

Current treatment strategies aim at achieving the best possible control include a non-pharmacological approach consisting of lifestyle interventions using physical exercise and modification of nutrition intakes in the early stage of type 2 diabetes [99]. Physical activity, independent of weight loss, has a beneficial effect on diabetic mortality [100]. Mentions and some descriptions of such lifestyle interventions can be found in patient education literature, as well as in guidelines for doctors that exist in Eastern Europe. For example, the guidelines of T2D primary and secondary care in Ukraine contain short recommendations on lifestyle modifications with dietary advice (calculation of carbohydrate units and food glycemic index, saturated fats and fiber intake) [81]; however, practical use of these and other recommendations is difficult due to a lack such health workers, as dietologists. The Soviet health system had such medical specialization, and it remains in some post-Soviet countries till this day; however, the number of such specialists is clearly inadequate, comparing to the number of patients with diabetes.

A similar situation exists in the field of physiotherapy: Rehabilitation and physical training experts are not currently a mass category of professionals in Ukrainian, as well as other post-Soviet healthcare systems. On the other hand, there are physiotherapy doctors, who work in large hospitals, walk-in clinics, and health resorts, where they administer treatment, using various electromagnetic devices, mineral water therapy, massage, etc.

One of the typical reviews of these methods that are recommended for treating diabetes and its complications [101] does not mention any verification of its clinical efficacy. Clearly, it will be very difficult to perform such verification using evidence-based medicine.

Rational Selection of Anti-diabetes Medications

We have previously mentioned several evaluations and comparisons of anti-diabetes medications use, including the frequency of insulin use (and its analogs) for diabetes treatment (see section "Complications of Diabetes in Region"). Diabetes patient registry-based Ukrainian study revealed that glibenclamide treatment of T2D is associated with greater risk of all-cause mortality versus gliclazide or glimepiride treatment and cardiovascular disease (CVD) mortality versus gliclazide treatment [38]. Danish registry-based observational study showed an increase of all-cause and cardiovascular mortality risks in T2D patients with and without previous myocardial infarction, receiving such common insulin secretagogues as glibenclamide, glimepiride, and glipizide versus metformin, whereas gliclazide versus metformin had no such risks [102]. Recently, using four different methodological approaches, when analyzing retrospective cohorts of T2D patients, we discovered an elevated total mortality risk for glibenclamide-treated versus gliclazide and metformin-treated patients, in case of using three of this approaches (models). Direct comparison of gliclazide versus metformin, when using one of these models discovered a lower mortality risk for gliclazide-treated [47]. The advantage of most oral anti-diabetes medications in comparison to glibenclamide were known, whereas the results of comparison of gliclazide and metformin seems new.

Unlike insulin, other anti-diabetes medications are not free for patients in most post-Soviet countries of Eastern Europe [31, 51, 103, 104]. This establishes a negative relationship between the frequency of using cheap drugs and populations' economic situation. Glibenclamide belongs to such type of medications, with the greatest hypoglycemic effect. This makes its chances of leaving Eastern European market quite low. For example, 5 years ago in one region of Central Ukraine, most oral-treated T2D patients received glibenclamide [51].

Thus, treatment algorithms used for glycemic control of diabetes patients in Europe are also practiced in its Eastern European part; however, their wide implementation is often limited by economic factors.

Translating Primary Prevention of Type 2 Diabetes

The lifestyle intervention using physical exercise and modification of nutrition is efficient in preventing type 2 diabetes in patients with impaired glucose tolerance [99]. Clinical trials confirm that lifestyle interventions (dietary modification and increased physical activity) reduce the risk of progressing from impaired glucose tolerance to type 2 diabetes [105]. Assessing T2D risk according to FINDRISK scale [106] is quite common in Eastern Europe [107]. We should acknowledge that today's strategies of primary prevention of type 2 diabetes [106] are still not considering the fact that "Prior to the development of type 2 diabetes, glucose levels increase into the pre-diabetic states of isolated impaired fasting glycaemia (i-IFG), isolated impaired glucose tolerance (i-IGT), or combined IFG/IGT" [108]. Physical activity was associated with a lower progression to diabetes in individuals with i-IGT category, a condition characterized by muscle insulin resistance. Physical activity did not predict progression to diabetes in individuals with i-IFG category, a condition characterized by hepatic insulin resistance [109]. These findings suggest distinct pathophysiological mechanisms of i-IFG and i-IGT although the T2D prevention relevance of these observations requires further clarification. Detecting new phenotypical differences of i-IFG and i-IGT that was recently performed in Ukraine [110] may possibly facilitate this.

Several alternative approaches to diabetes prevention are starting to be investigated in Ukraine. Several studies have indicated that the amount of oxygen to which tissues are exposed may substantially impact cardio-metabolic health [111–114]. Interestingly, living at high altitude (hypobaric hypoxia) seems to be associated with improved glucose homeostasis and a decreased prevalence of T2D [111] and doing interval normobaric hypoxic training is an effective method of improving resistance to hypoxia and correcting prediabetic carbohydrate metabolism disorders [114].

Organizing and Conduction Diabetes Research in Region

Diabetes research in the former Soviet Union was always carried out in the framework of experimental and clinical endocrinology, with three research and clinical facilities, as centers of this research.

- Kharkov Institute of Endocrinology – founded in 1919 by physiologist Vasyl Danilevsky, in 1927 insulin production began (mass production of insulin continued for over 50 years). In 1923, Victor Kohan-Yasniy was the first in the country to extract insulin from pancreatic tissue and to administer it to a diabetic coma patient. Back in the 1930s, Semen Henes determined that the main objective of treating diabetes patients is giving them the opportunity to take up normal amounts of carbohydrates. Together with O. Reznytska they designed a diet therapy plan for diabetes patients http://www.ipep.com.ua/.
- Kyiv Institute of Endocrinology and Metabolism was founded in 1965 by endocrinologist Vasyl Komisarenko. Andriy Yefimov headed clinical research in the field of diabetes for many years. Prof. Yefimov is considered to be the founder of Ukrainian diabetology. http://www.iem.net.ua/
- Endocrinology Research Center (Moscow) – founded in 1922 by Prof. Vasyl Shervinskiy, who is considered the founding father of Russian endocrinology. Human insulin was synthesized in 1972 under the leadership of N. Yudaev. http://www.endocrincentr.ru/about/diabed/

Future Directions: Unmet Needs, Unanswered Questions, and Unquestioned Answers

One of the unanswered questions that no one seems to ask is the reason why according to Russian diabetes registers the prevalence of T2D among women is 2.5 times higher than in men [115]. The same was noticed in Ukraine [116, 117] but has not been seen in other parts of Europe [118]. Epidemiological studies based on hyperglycemia screening conducted in Russia [11, 85] and more recently in Ukraine [13] did not confirm the fact of gender differences of the real T2D prevalence, whereas a British study of the trends in diabetes awareness (a self-reported doctor diagnosis) showed that diabetes awareness was three time more frequent in women (6 %) than men (2 %) [119]. Awareness was lower in rural and less-educated respondents. High body mass index predicted diabetes awareness in women but did not explain gender or socioeconomic differences. More than half of those reporting a diabetic diagnosis reported receiving no conventional medical treatment, and insulin use was less frequent than in Western populations [119].

Thus, in the future we still need to find the reason for better diagnostic efficacy of T2D in women compared to men in post-Soviet countries.

Effects of childhood starvation on the risk of developing T2D later in life is another topic that should be discussed. The effect of famine on increasing the risk of being diagnosed with diabetes in Ukraine and some other countries was assessed only based on analysis of large administrative patient databases [65, 120], whereas current prevalence of screen-detected type 2 diabetes (SDDM) among those who survived the famine during childhood and are still alive today remains unknown. The developmental origins hypothesis proposes that "undernutrition during early development is associated with an increased type 2 diabetes risk in adulthood" [121]. If we were to assume that this phenomenon is a consequence of a more rapid T2D development in persons with "diabetic genotype," then the population that is studied today, surviving for more than 70 years, not diagnosed with diabetes, may have had a decreased SDDM prevalence several decades after the famine episodes. It is assumed that this unexpected effect can be explained by a situation, where the carriers of a corresponding genes were already diagnosed with diabetes.

Possibly some recent assessments of SDDM prevalence in those Ukrainians who reported famine exposure [13] could be an indirect confirmation of this situation. A recent genotyping of those who survived the Leningrad siege [122] also led to unexpected results: In case of UCP3 gene, "normal" allele C and C/C genotype prevailed in women, whereas "mutated" allele T, associated with atherosclerosis, T2D, and obesity were significantly less common. When explaining these results we cannot overlook the possibility, that carriers of atherogenic and diabetogenic genotype could have greater chances of surviving during famine but could not live till being genotyped in the twenty-first century due to early development of atherosclerosis. It is clear that conducting epidemiologic studies in Eastern Europe using individual famine exposure data can clarify causa relation between undernutrition during postnatal development and type 2 diabetes risk in adulthood.

This review did not attempt to cover all significant diabetes research conducted during the last few years in Eastern Europe or even Ukraine, Latvia, and Moldova. In particular, some substantial clinical and immunological investigations in Ukraine [123, 124] remained beyond its reach. Nevertheless, we tried to concentrate on the most familiar to us: issues of diabetes epidemiology, aspects of diagnostic, and treatment practice of East European countries that could be compared, as well as some pathophysiologic aspects, the study of which was based on the analysis of population registers. We can point to the absence of credible epidemiologic data on diabetes in Eastern Europe or their insufficiently adequate interpretation as one of the main conclusion. We can also note a generally significant range of treatment quality in European countries regarding diabetes. The only thing that we can count on now is that collaboration with the EU will lead to gradual improvements of diabetes care in Eastern Europe and will facilitate new fundamental research in the field of diabetes. The experience of Baltic states gives certain ground for such hopes.

References

1. The World Bank Data. Countries and economies. http://data.worldbank.org/country. Retrieved 11 Jan 2015.
2. Narayan KM, Ali MK, Koplan JP. Global noncommunicable diseases—where worlds meet. N Engl J Med. 2010;363(13):1196–8. doi:10.1056/NEJMp1002024.
3. Beran D. The impact of health systems on diabetes care in low and lower middle income countries. Curr Biabetes Rep. 2015;15(4):1–13.
4. Wilmoth JR, Lundström H. Extreme longevity in five countries. Eur J Popul/Rev Eur Démogr. 1996;12(1):63–93.
5. International Diabetes Federation, Diabetes Atlas. 6th ed. Brussels. 2013. http://www.idf.org/diabetesatlas.
6. http://apps.who.int/healthinfo/statistics/mortality/whodpms/.
7. Turcanu G, Domente S, Buga M, Richardson E. Republic of Moldova: health system review. Health Syst Transit. 2012;14(7):1–151.
8. Whiting DR, Guariguata L, Weil C, Shaw J. IDF diabetes atlas: global estimates of the prevalence of diabetes for 2011 and 2030. Diabetes Res Clin Pract. 2011;94(3):311–21.
9. Dogadin SA, Mashtakov BP, Taranushenko TE. Prevalence of type 2 diabetes in northern populations of Siberia. Int J Circumpolar Health. 2001;60:205–10.
10. Шишкина НС, Сунцов ЮИ, Болотская ЛЛ, Максимова ВП, Смирнов СВ, Дедов ИИ. Распространенность сахарного диабета 2 типа (по данным скрининга). Сахарный диабет. 2005;2:7–8. http://cyberleninka.ru/article/n/rasprostranennost-saharnogo-diabeta-2-tipa-po-dannym-skrininga.
11. Догадин СА, Крижановская ЕВ, Виноградова СВ. Результаты скрининга жителей Красноярска на сахарный диабет. Сахарный диабет № 1, 2004, с. 8–10. http://cyberleninka.ru/article/n/rezultaty-skrininga-zhiteley-krasnoyarska-na-saharnyy-diabet.
12. Khalangot MD, Kravchenko VI, Pisarenko Yu M, Okhrimenko NV, Lerman NG, KovtunVA. Prevalence of diabetes mellitus, impaired glucose regulation, and their anthropometric risk factors in elderly residents of rural. Ukraine Endocrynologia. 2014;19(2):119–25. http://nbuv.gov.ua/j-pdf/enkrl_2014_19_2_7.pdf. [Article in Ukrainian]. n.d.
13. Khalangot M, Gurianov V, Okhrimenko N, Luzanchuk I, Kravchenko V. Neck circumference as a risk factor of screen-detected diabetes mellitus: community-based study. Diabetol Metabol Syndr. 2016;8:12.
14. Martirosyan H, Petrosyan V, Crape B, Melkomian DM, Koshkakaryan M, Sahakyan Y, Truzyan N. Rapid appraisal of diabetes care in Armenia: a qualitative research. Yerevan: Center for Health Services Research and Development, American University of Armenia; 2012.
15. State Statistical Committee of the Republic of Azerbaijan, Baku 2015. www.stat.gov.az.
16. Kharchanka A, Roubuts T. Morbidity dynamics of diabetes in children living in the West region of Belarus. Endocr Abstr. 2014;35:P805. doi:10.1530/endoabs.35.P805.
17. Shepelkevich AP. Int J Endocrinol. 2015;4(68):119–21. (In Russian) www.mif-ua.com/archive/article/40847.
18. Особенности оказания диабетологической помощи в Республике Беларусь на современном этапе / Шепелькевич А.П. [и др.]. (2012) Ars. Medica 15(70):6–11. http://natbookcat.org.by/isgbi/marcview.do?id=1067461&position=2.
19. Balabanova D, McKee M, Koroleva N, Chikovani I, Goguadze K, Kobaladze T, … Robles S. Navigating the health system: diabetes care in Georgia. Health Pol Plan. 2009;24(1):46–54.
20. Georgia Statistical yearbook_2013_eng www.ncdc.ge.
21. Ministerul Sănătății al Republicii Moldova Centrul Național de Management în Sănătate. ANUARUL STATISTIC AL SISTEMULUI DE SĂNĂTATE DIN MOLDOVA ANUL 2013. Chișinău, 2014.
22. Dedov II, Shestakova MV, Vikulova OK. National register of diabetes mellitus in Russian Federation: status on 2014 (Article in Russian) Сахарный диабет. 2015;18(3):5–23. http://endojournals.ru/index.php/dia/article/view/7235.
23. Shiryaeva TYu, Andrianova EA, Suntsov YuI. Type 1 diabetes mellitus in children and adolescents of Russian Federation: key epidemiology trends (article in Russian) Сахарныйдиабет. 2013;(3):21–29. http://dx.doi.org/10.14341/2072-0351-813.
24. Дедов ИИ, Шестакова МВ (2013). Результаты реализации подпрограммы «Сахарный диабет» федеральной целевой программы «Предупреждение и борьба с социально значимыми заболеваниями 2007–2012 годы». Сахарныйдиабет, (2S).Спецвыпуск [Federal targeted programme "Prevention and Management of Socially Significant Diseases (2007–2012)": results of the "Diabetes mellitus" sub-programme] (article in Russian). http://cyberleninka.ru/article/n/rezultaty-realizatsii-podprogrammy-saharnyy-diabet--federalnoy-tselevoy-programmy-preduprezhdenie-i-borba-s-sotsialno-znachimymi#ixzz3r1FgzdzE.
25. Suntsov YuI. Modern antihyperglycemic agents prescribed in Russia for type 2 diabetes mellitus. (arti-

cle in Russian) Сахарный диабет. 2012;(1):6–9. http://cyberleninka.ru/article/n/sovremennye-saharosnizhayuschie-preparaty-ispolzuemye-v-rossii-pri-lechenii-saharnogo-diabeta-2-tipa.
26. Chernobrov AD, editors. Main indicators of endocrinological care of Ukraine for 2015: review. Kyiv: V.P. Komisarenko Institute of Endocrinology and Metabolism of the Acad Med Sci, Ukraine Ministry of Health. Endocrynologia. 2014;19(1) Supplement 1 (data set in Ukrainian).
27. Mankovsky B. The prevalence of undiagnosed type 2 diabetes mellitus in Ukraine. Diabetologia. 2007;50 Suppl 1:0376.
28. The Center for Disease Prevention and Control of Latvia. http://www.spkc.gov.lv/about-SPKC/. Accessed 11 June 2015.
29. The Central Statistics Bureau of Latvia. http://www.csb.gov.lv/en. Accessed 11 June 2015.
30. Atun R, Jaffar S, Nishtar S, Knaul FM, Barreto ML, Nyirenda M, et al. Improving responsiveness of health systems to noncommunicable diseases. Lancet. 2013;381(9867):690–7.
31. Khalangot M, Tronko M. Primary care diabetes in Ukraine. Prim Care Diabetes. 2007;1(4):203–5.
32. Telishevska M, Chenet L, McKee M. Towards an understanding of the high death rate among young people with diabetes in Ukraine. Diabet Med. 2001;18(1):3–9.
33. Shields BM, Peters JL, Cooper C, Lowe J, Knight BA, Powell RJ, Hattersley AT. Can clinical features be used to differentiate type 1 from type 2 diabetes? A systematic review of the literature. BMJ Open. 2015;5(11):e009088.
34. Royal College of General Practitioners and NHS Diabetes. Coding, classification and diagnosis of diabetes. Secondary coding, classification and diagnosis of diabetes. 2011. http://www.sdrn.org.uk/sites/sdrn.org.uk/files/nhs%20diagnosis%20classification% 20report.pdf.
35. Pildava S, Strēle I, Briģis Ģ. The mortality of patients with diabetes mellitus in Latvia 2000–2012. Medicina. 2014;50(2):130–6.
36. Dedov II. Diabetes mellitus – a dangerous treat to the mankind. [Article in Russian]. Vestn Ross Akad Med Nauk. 2012;(1):7–13. http://europepmc.org/abstract/med/22550704.
37. Khalangot MD. Epedemiologic characteristics of diabetes mellitus type1 and 2 according to data from national population-based patient register. [Manuscript in Ukrainian]. Thesis for the Degree of Doctor of Medical Sciences. V.P. Komisarenko Institute of Endocrinology and Metabolism AMS of Ukraine, Kiev; 2009.
38. Khalangot M, Tronko M, Kravchenko V, Kovtun V. Glibenclamide-related excess in total and cardiovascular mortality risks: data from large Ukrainian observational cohort study. Diabetes Res Clin Pract. 2009;86(3):247–53.
39. http://apps.who.int/gho/data/view.main.680.
40. Franco OH, Steyerberg EW, Hu FB, Mackenbach J, Nusselder W. Associations of diabetes mellitus with total life expectancy and life expectancy with and without cardiovascular disease. Arch Intern Med. 2007;167(11):1145–51.
41. Khalangot M, Kravchenko V, Tronko M, Gur'ianov V. Correlation between the prevalence of type 1 diabetes with the daily insulin dose and the autoimmune process against glutamic acid decarboxylase in adults. Eur J Intern Med. 2009;20(6):611–5.
42. Khalangot M, Tronko M, Okhrimenko N, Kravchenko V, Gurianov V, Tronko M. Prevalence of type 1 diabetes correlates with daily insulin dose, adverse outcomes and with autoimmune process against glutamic acid decarboxylase in adults. Rijeka, Croatia: INTECH Open Access Publisher; 2011.
43. Khalangot M. Current practice of insulin and oral hypoglycaemic agents treatment of diabetes mellitus type 2 patients according to diabetes mellitus register data analysis in the city of Donetsk, Ukraine. Prim Care Diabetes. 2007;1(4):224.
44. Khalangot M, Hu G, Tronko M, Kravchenko V, Guryanov V. Gender risk of nonfatal stroke in type 2 diabetic patients differs depending on the type of treatment. J Womens Health (Larchmt). 2009;18(1): 97–103.
45. Khalangot M, Tronko M, Kravchenko V, Kulchinska J, Hu G. Body mass index and the risk of total and cardiovascular mortality among patients with type 2 diabetes: a large prospective study in Ukraine. Heart. 2009;95(6):454–560.
46. Khalangot M, Tronko M, Kravchenko V, Kulchinska J, Hu G. The joint effects of different types of glucose-lowering treatment and duration of diabetes on total and cardiovascular mortality among subjects with type 2 diabetes. Diabetes Res Clin Pract. 2008;82(1):139–47.
47. Khalangot M, Kovtun V. Evaluation approach can significantly influence oral glucose-lowering drugs total mortality risks in retrospective cohorts of type 2 diabetes mellitus patients. Curr Diabetes Rev. 2014;10(5):336–42.
48. Khalangot ND. Age related and sex peculiarities of mortality from diabetes mellitus type 1 (based on analysis of data of Ukraine's diabetes mellitus Register) [Article in Ukrainian]. Problemy starenia I dolgoletia. 2008;17(1):75–82. http://www.geront.kiev.ua/psid-2010/2008_1.pdf#page=75.
49. Khalangot MD, Kravchenko VI, Okhrimenko NV, Kovtun VA, Tronko EM. Analysis of mortality, proliferative retinopathy prevalence, and arterial hypertension among type 1 diabetic patients residing in areas that differ in prevalence of this disease. Endocrinologia. 2009;14(1):77–85. Article in Ukrainian.
50. Khalangot MD, Tronko MD, Kravchenko VI, Kovtun VA, Okhrimenko NV, Bolgarska SV. Some mortality risk factors for type 1 diabetes mellitus patients in Ukraine evaluated according to data from National Register. Endocrinologia. 2010;15(1):62–70. Article in Ukrainian.

51. Khalangot MD, Kovtun VA, Okhrimenko NV, Sokolova LK, Bolgarska SV. Approaches to an assessment of probable funds required for treatment of patients with diabetes mellitus in Ukraine УКР. МЕД. ЧАСОПИС, 3 (89) – V/VI 2012|[Article in Ukrainian]. http://www.umj.com.ua/article/12340/.
52. Soedamah-Muthu SS, Fuller JH, Mulnier HE, Raleigh VS, Lawrenson RA, Colhoun HM. All-cause mortality rates in patients with type 1 diabetes mellitus compared with a non-diabetic population from the UK general practice research database, 1992–1999. Diabetologia. 2006;49:660–6.
53. Krolewski AS, Kosinski EJ, Warram JH, Leland OS, Busick EJ, Asmal AC, Rand LI, Christlieb AR, Bradley RF, Kahn CR. Magnitude and determinants of coronary artery disease in juvenile-onset insulin-dependent diabetes mellitus. Am J Cardiol. 1987;59:750–5.
54. Lloyd CE, Kuller LH, Ellis D, Becker DJ, Wing RR, Orchard TJ. Coronary artery disease in IDDM: gender differences in risk factors but not risk. Arterioscler Thromb Vasc Biol. 1996;16:720–6.
55. Steinberg HO, Paradisi G, Cronin J, Crowde K, Hempfling A, Hook G, Baron AD. Type II diabetes abrogates sex differences in endothelial function in premenopausal women. Circulation. 2000;101: 2040–6.
56. Laing SP, Swerdlow AJ, Slater SD, Botha JL, Burden AC, Waugh NR, Smith AW, Hill RD, Bingley PJ, Patterson CC, Qiao Z, Keen H. The British Diabetic Association Cohort Study, II: cause-specific mortality in patients with insulin-treated diabetes mellitus. Diabet Med. 1999;16(6):466–71.
57. Soedamah-Muthu SS, Chaturvedi N, Witte DR, Stevens LK, Porta M, Fuller JH, EURODIAB Prospective Complications Study Group. Relationship between risk factors and mortality in type 1 diabetic patients in Europe: the EURODIAB Prospective Complications Study (PCS). Diabetes Care. 2008;31(7):1360–6.
58. Dorman JS, Laporte RE, Kuller LH, Cruickshanks KJ, Orchard TJ, Wagener DK, Becker DJ, Cavender DE, Drash AL. The Pittsburgh insulin-dependent diabetes mellitus (IDDM) morbidity and mortality study. Mortality results. Diabetes. 1984;33(3): 271–6.
59. Maahs DM, Rewers M, editors. Mortality and renal disease in type 1 diabetes mellitus—progress made, more to be done. J Clin Endocrinol Metab. 2006;91(10):3757–59.
60. Hales CN, Barker DJ. The thrifty phenotype hypothesis. Br Med Bull. 2001;60:5–20.
61. Lumey LH, Stein AD, Susser E. Prenatal famine and adult health. Annu Rev Public Health. 2011;32:237–62.
62. Lumey LH, Stein AD, Kahn HS. Food restriction during gestation and impaired fasting glucose or glucose tolerance and type 2 diabetes mellitus in adulthood: evidence from the Dutch Hunger Winter Families Study. J Dev Orig Health Dis. 2009;1:S164.
63. Li Y, He Y, Qi L, et al. Exposure to the Chinese famine in early life and the risk of hyperglycemia and type 2 diabetes in adulthood. Diabetes. 2010;59: 2400–6.
64. Thurner S, Klimek P, Szell M, et al. Quantification of excess risk for diabetes for those born in times of hunger, in an entire population of a nation, across a century. Proc Natl Acad Sci U S A. 2013;110: 4703–7.
65. Lumey LH, Khalangot MD, Vaiserman AM. Association between type 2 diabetes and prenatal exposure to the Ukraine famine of 1932–33: a retrospective cohort study. Lancet Diabetes Endocrinol. 2015;3:787–94.
66. Laron Z, Lewy H, Wilderman I, et al. Seasonality of month of birth of children and adolescents with type 1 diabetes mellitus in homogenous and heterogeneous populations. Isr Med Assoc J. 2005;7:381–4.
67. Vaiserman AM, Carstensen B, Voitenko VP, et al. Seasonality of birth in children and young adults (0–29 years) with type 1 diabetes in Ukraine. Diabetologia. 2007;50:32–5.
68. Vaiserman AM, Khalangot MD, Carstensen B, et al. Seasonality of birth in adult type 2 diabetic patients in three Ukrainian regions. Diabetologia. 2009;52: 2665–7.
69. Jensen CB, Zimmermann E, Gamborg M, et al. No evidence of seasonality of birth in adult type 2 diabetes in Denmark. Diabetologia. 2015;58:2045–50.
70. Vaiserman A, Khalangot M. Similar seasonality of birth in type 1 and type 2 diabetes patients: a sign for common etiology? Med Hypotheses. 2008;71: 604–5.
71. Wilkin TJ. Changing perspectives in diabetes: their impact on its classification. Diabetologia. 2007;50:1587–92.
72. Chistiakov DA, Savost'anov KV, Nosikov VV. CTLA4 gene polymorphisms are associated with, and linked to, insulin-dependent diabetes mellitus in a Russian population. BMC Genet. 2001;2(1):6.
73. Chistiakov DA, Zotova EV, Savost'anov KV, Bursa TR, Galeev IV, Strokov IA, Nosikov VV. The 262T> C promoter polymorphism of the catalase gene is associated with diabetic neuropathy in type 1 diabetic Russian patients. Diabetes Metabol. 2006;32(1):63–8.
74. Chistiakov DA, Potapov VA, Khodirev DC, Shamkhalova MS, Shestakova MV, Nosikov VV. Genetic variations in the pancreatic ATP-sensitive potassium channel, beta-cell dysfunction, and susceptibility to type 2 diabetes. Acta Diabetol. 2009;46:43–9.
75. Sokolova EA, Bondar IA, Shabelnikova OY, Pyankova OV, Filipenko ML. Replication of *KCNJ11* (p.E23K) and *ABCC8* (p.S1369A) association in Russian Diabetes Mellitus 2 type cohort and meta-analysis. PLoS ONE. 2015;10(5): e0124662.
76. Globa E, Zelinska N, Mackay DJ, Temple KI, Houghton JA, Hattersley AT, Flanagan SE, Ellard

S. Neonatal diabetes in Ukraine: incidence, genetics, clinical phenotype and treatment. J Pediatr Endocrinol Metab. 2015;28(11–12):1279–86.

77. Grulich-Henn J, Wagner V, Thon A, Schober E, Marg W, et al. Entities and frequency of neonatal diabetes: data from the diabetes documentation and quality management system (DPV). Diabet Med. 2010;27:709–12.
78. Iafusco D, Massa O, Pasquino B, Colombo C, Iughetti L, Early Diabetes Study Group of ISPED, et al. Minimal incidence of neonatal/infancy onset diabetes in Italy is 1:90,000 live births. Acta Diabetol. 2012;49:405–8.
79. World Health Organization. Definition, diagnosis, and classification of diabetes mellitus and its complications: report of a WHO consultation. Part 1: diagnosis and classification of diabetes mellitus. Geneva: World Health Org; 1999. WHO/NCD/NCS/99.2.
80. Дедов И.И., Шестакова М.В., Максимова М.А. Федеральная целевая программа «Сахарный диабет» (Методические рекомендации).- М., 2003.- С.42–46. http://www.voed.ru/fcp_sd.htm.
81. УНІФІКОВАНИЙ КЛІНІЧНИЙ ПРОТОКОЛ ПЕРВИННОЇ ТА ВТОРИННОЇ (СПЕЦІАЛІЗО ВАНОЇ) МЕДИЧНОЇ ДОПОМОГИ ЦУКРОВИЙ ДІАБЕТ 2 ТИПУ Approved by Health Ministry of Ukraine, 21.12.2012 №1118. http://www.moz.gov.ua/docfiles/dod1118_2_2012.pdf.
82. The Expert Committee on the Diagnosis and Classification of Diabetes Mellitus. Follow-up report on the diagnosis of diabetes mellitus. Diabetes Care. 2003;26:3160–7.
83. American Diabetes Association. Diagnosis and classification of diabetes mellitus. Diabetes Care. 2014;37(Supplement 1):S81–90.
84. Dreval' AV, Misnikova IV, Barsukov IA, Ponchakova GV, Kuznetsov AV. Prevalence of type 2 diabetes mellitus and other abnormalities of carbohydrate metabolism depending on diagnostic criteria Сахарный диабет, 2010 (1) 116–120. http://cyberleninka.ru/article/n/rasprostranennost-saharnogo-diabeta-2-tipa-i-drugih-narusheniy-uglevodnogo-obmena-v-zavisimosti-ot-kriteriev-diagnostiki.
85. Vaychulis IA, Shaposhnik II, Vaychulis TN. Результаты скрининга сахарного диабета2 типа и других нарушений углеводного обмена среди работающего населения Челябинска. Сахарный диабет. 2006;9(4):51–5. http://cyberleninka.ru/article/n/rezultaty-skrininga-saharnogo-diabeta-2-tipa-i-drugih-narusheniy-uglevodnogo-obmena-sredi-rabotayuschego-naseleniya-chelyabinska.
86. Dogadin SA, Artemenko GP, Tsyplyakova NB, Subrakova NI, Dazidenko LN, Boyko SA, … & Veselkin DA. Результаты скрининга сахарного диабетау жителей г. Абакана (Республика Хакасия). Сахарный диабет. 2008;11(2):55–58. http://endojournals.ru/index.php/dia/article/viewFile/5761/3539.
87. Andel M, Grzeszczak W, Michalek J, Medvescek M, Norkus A, Rasa I, Niewada M, Kamiński B, Kraml P, Madacsy L, DEPAC Group. A multinational, multi centre, observational, cross sectional survey assessing diabetes secondary care in Central and Eastern Europe (DEPAC Survey). Diabetic Medicine. 2008;25(10):1195–203.
88. Gill GV, Yudkin JS, Keen H, Beran D. The insulin dilemma in resource-limited countries. A way forward? Diabetologia. 2010. doi:10.1007/s00125-010-1897-3.
89. WHO, World Health Statistics. Annual electronic File, July, 2001 version. Geneve. Retrieved 30 Jan 2004.
90. Gorter KJ, Wens J, Khunti K, Claramunt XC, Topsever P, Drivsholm T, … Rurik I. The European EUCCLID pilot study on care and complications in an unselected sample of people with type 2 diabetes in primary care. Prim Care Diabetes. 2010;4(1):17–23.
91. McKnight JA, Wild SH, Lamb MJE, Cooper MN, Jones TW, Davis EA, Hofer S, Fritsch M, Schober E, Svensson J, Almdal T, Young R, Warner JT, Delemer B, Souchon PF, Holl RW, Karges W, Kieninger DM, Tigas S, Bargiota A, Sampanis C, Cherubini V, Gesuita R, Strele I, Pildava S, Coppell KJ, Magee G, Cooper JG, Dinneen SF, Eeg-Olofsson K, Svensson AM, Gudbjornsdottir S, Veeze H, Aanstoot HJ, Khalangot M, Tamborlane WV, Miller KM. Glycaemic control of type 1 diabetes in clinical practice early in the 21st century: an international comparison. Diabet Med. 2015;32(8):1036–50.
92. Kravchenko VI, Tronko ND, Pankiv VI, Venzilovich YM, Prudius FG. Prevalence of diabetes mellitus and its complications in the Ukraine. Diabetes Res Clin Pract. 1996;34:S73–8.
93. Kühlbrandt C, Basu S, Mckee M, Stuckler D. Looking at the Russian health care system: through the eyes of patients with diabetes and their physicians. Br J Diabetes Vasc Dis. 2012;12(4):181–4.
94. Richardson E, Roberts B, Sava V, Menon R, McKee M. Health insurance coverage and health care access in Moldova. Health Policy Plan. 2012;27(3):204–12.
95. Shishkin S, Jowett M. A review of health financing reforms in the Republic of Moldova, Health financing policy paper no. 1. Copenhagen: WHO Regional Office for Europe; 2012.
96. Domente S, Turcanu G, Habicht J, Richardson E. Developments in primary health care in the Republic of Moldova: essential steps to improving access to services. Eurohealth. 2013;19(2):28–31.
97. Rutkowski B. Highlights of the epidemiology of renal replacement therapy in Central and Eastern Europe. Nephrol Dial Transplant. 2006;21(1):4–10.
98. Kolesnyk I, Noordzij M, Kolesnyk M, Kulyzky M, Jager KJ. Renal replacement therapy in Ukraine: epidemiology and international comparisons. Clin Kidney J. 2014;7(3):330–5.

99. Buysschaert M, Hermans MP. Non-pharmacological management of type 2 diabetes. Acta Clin Belg. 2004;59(1):14–9.
100. Diamond J. The double puzzle of diabetes. Nature. 2003;423:599–602.
101. Kyrylyuk M. Balneotherapy, pelotherapy and physiotherapy of diabetes mellitus. Клінічна ендокринологія та ендокринна хірургія. 2010;(1):68–76. https://scholar.google.com/scholar?q=+Kyrylyuk+M.+%282010%29+Balneotherapy%2C+pelotherapy+and+physiotherapy+of+diabetes+mellitus.
102. Schramm TK, Gislason GH, Vaag A, et al. Mortality and cardiovascular risk associated with different insulin secretagogues compared with metformin in type 2 diabetes, with or without a previous myocardial infarction: a nationwide study. Eur Heart J. 2011;32:1900–8.
103. Perlman F, Balabanova D. Prescription for change: accessing medication in transitional Russia. Health Policy Plan. 2011;26(6):453–63.
104. Khalangot M. Current practice of insulin and oral hypoglycaemic agents treatment of diabetes mellitus type 2 patients according to diabetes mellitus register data analysis in the city of Donetsk, Ukraine. Prim Care Diab. 2007;1(4):224.
105. Yung LM, Yung M, Yao X, Chen ZY, Huang Y, Leung FP. Exercise, vascular wall and cardiovascular diseases. Sports Med. 2009;39(1):45–63.
106. Lindström J, Neumann A, Sheppard KE, Gilis-Januszewska A, Greaves CJ, Handke U, … Roden M. Take action to prevent diabetes – the IMAGE toolkit for the prevention of type 2 diabetes in Europe. Horm Metabol Res. 2010;42:S37–55.
107. Schepelkevich AP, Kholodova EA, Salko OB, et al. Assessment of risk of type 2 diabetes mellitus development in the republic of Belarus (in Russian). Zdravookhranenie. 2012;11:4–8. http://rsml.med.by/diab/p19.pdf.
108. Færch K, Borch-Johnsen K, Holst JJ, Vaag A. Pathophysiology and aetiology of impaired fasting glycaemia and impaired glucose tolerance: does it matter for prevention and treatment of type 2 diabetes? Diabetologia. 2009;52(9):1714–23.
109. Engberg S, Glümer C, Witte DR, Jørgensen T, Borch-Johnsen K. Differential relationship between physical activity and progression to diabetes by glucose tolerance status: the Inter99 Study. Diabetologia. 2010;53(1):70–8.
110. Khalangot ND, Kravchenko VI, Okhrimenko NV, Pysarenko YuM, Koliasa OS, Kovtun VA, Gurianov VG, Tronko MD. Anthropometric differences of persons with various types of screen-detected hyperglycemia in rural Ukraine. Zurnal NAMN Ukrainy. 2015;21(3–4):342–50.
111. Vogel M, Blaak E, Goossens G. Moderate hypoxia exposure: a novel strategy to improve glucose metabolism in humans? EMJ Diabetes. 2015; 3(1):73–9.
112. Serebrovska TV, Shatilo VB. Remote ischemic preconditioning versus intermittent hypoxia training: a comparative analysis for cardioprotection. Fiziolohichnyi zhurnal. 2014;61(3):99–117.
113. Korkushko OV, Shatilo VB, Chyzhova VP, Naskalova SS, Osmak YeD, Gremiakov AV, Antoniuk-Scheglova IA, Gavalko GV, Naumchuk NS. Organism reaction to dosed hypoxic hypoxia in the healthy subjects and individuals with prediabetic metabolism disturbances Fiziolohichnyi zhurnal. 2016 (in press).
114. Shatilo VB, Korkushko OV, Chizhova VP, Naskalova SS, Gavalko AV, Antoniuk-Shcheglova IA, Gremiakov AV, Osmak D, Zhuravleva D, Yu B. Efficacy of using interval normobaric hypoxic exercise training in elderly patients with prediabetic derangements of carbohydrate metabolism. Problemy stareniia I dolgoletia. 2015;24:3–4 (in press).
115. Suntsov YuI, Bolotskaya LL, Maslova OV, Kazakov IV. Epidemiology of diabetes mellitus and prognosis of its prevalence in the Russian Federation. Сахарный диабет, (1). http://cyberleninka.ru/article/n/epidemiologiya-saharnogo-diabeta-i-prognoz-ego-rasprostranennosti-v-rossiyskoy-federatsii.
116. Tronko M, Khalangot M, Kravcenko V, et al. Gender distribution in Ukrainian adult insulin-treated diabetics depending of age at diagnosis. Endocr Abstr. 2006;11:298. http://www.endocrine-abstracts.org/ea/0011/ea0011P298.htm.
117. Khalangot MD, Gurianov VG, Vaiserman AM. Gender differences in prevalence of diagnosed type 2 diabetes and patient's body mass index in five Ukraine regions with diverse historical backgrounds. BIO. 2012;2:1–10.
118. Gale EA, Gillespie KM. Diabetes and gender. Diabetologia. 2001;44:3–15.
119. Perlman F, McKee M. Diabetes during the Russian transition. Diabetes Res Clin Pract. 2008;80(2):305–13.
120. Thurner S, Klimek P, Szell M, Duftschmid G, Endel G, Kautzky-Willer A, Kasper DC. Quantification of excess risk for diabetes for those born in times of hunger, in an entire population of a nation, across a century. Proc Natl Acad Sci. 2013;110(12):4703–7.
121. van Abeelen AF, Elias SG, Bossuyt PM, Grobbee DE, van der Schouw YT, Roseboom TJ, Uiterwaal CS. Famine exposure in the young and the risk of type 2 diabetes in adulthood. Diabetes. 2012;61(9):2255–60.
122. Polyakova IV, Glotov OS, Khoroshinina LP, Turjeva LV, Ivashchenko TE, Baranov VS. Genotype and allele frequencies of UCP and PPAR gene families in residents of besieged Leningrad and in the control group. Adv Gerontol. 2014;27(3):418–24.
123. Mankovsky BN, Metzger BE, Molitch ME, Biller J. Cerebrovascular disorders in patients with diabetes mellitus. J Diabetes Complicat. 1996;10(4):228–42.
124. Popova V, Zak K, Gruzov M, Afanasyeva V, Simeonova T, Mankovsky B. The prognostic value of the immunological phenotype of lymphocytes in subjects positive for diabetes-associated autoantibodies. Diabetologia. 2006;49:280–1. 233.

Diabetes in Ethnic Minorities and Immigrant Populations in Western Europe

12

Oliver Razum and Helmut Steinberg

The issue of diabetes in immigrant, ethnic minorities, and underserved communities in Europe is complex; it is complex due to diverse geographical and ethnic background of immigrant populations and differences in health-care systems across European countries. In addition, the availability and quality of data differ between countries and, therefore, are not possible to perform systematic comparisons between countries. The overarching results demonstrate that immigrant and underserved populations tend to have a higher prevalence of diabetes when compared to the "native population" while not necessarily different from populations where they originate from. Risk factors for diabetes appear to be similar between populations, mostly insulin resistance, obesity, and sedentary lifestyle with possible genetic differences contributing to the increased susceptibility. Some data suggest a greater prevalence of microvascular complications, especially diabetic retinopathy, and lower rates of macrovascular disease in some immigrant populations. While health-care coverage is almost universal in Europe albeit delivered by country-specific systems, immigrant populations face different and often additional barriers; often they tend to be less educated and have difficulty with the native language and different cultural and/or religious values that may interfere with effective diabetes prevention and treatment. Immigrants who receive medical care appear to be provided with the same medications as the natives although there appear to be differences in the utilization of insulin. While there is research conducted in specific populations, this is often done locally or regionally which hampers the generalization of results. Countries that have National Health Services (e.g., UK, the Netherlands, and Scandinavian countries) tend to have more and possibly more representative data compared to countries that have statutory health insurance systems such as Germany. Some data originate from small local or regional studies where the results are often being published as progress reports in the native language that are difficult to obtain. Researchers agree that standardized large-scale and representative studies that allow comparison of different populations throughout specific countries or even Europe are wanting.

O. Razum
Fakultät fürGesundheitswissenschaften, School of Public Health, Universität Bielefeld,
Postfach 10 01 31, 33501 Bielefeld, Germany
e-mail: oliver.razum@uni-bielefeld.de

H. Steinberg, MD (✉)
Division of Endocrinology, Diabetes and Metabolism, Department of Medicine, University of Tennessee Health Science Center Memphis, 920 Madison Avenue, Suite #300, Memphis, TN 38163, USA
e-mail: hsteinb1@uthsc.edu

S. Dagogo-Jack (ed.), *Diabetes Mellitus in Developing Countries and Underserved Communities*,
DOI 10.1007/978-3-319-41559-8_12

Heterogeneity of Immigrant Populations

Immigration in Europe, especially Western Europe, has in principle three origins: resettling from colonial territories, need for additional labor, and asylum policies for political refugees. This explains a large part of the differences in the ethnic backgrounds of immigrants between European countries (Table 12.1). For example, the main immigrant groups in England are from South Asian, Black Caribbean, and East African background, while the main immigrant groups in Germany are from Turkey and Southern Europe, and North African immigrants are found mostly in France, Belgium, and the Netherlands which in addition also has a large group of Surinamese Indians. Newer established immigrant populations in Western Europe come from former communist countries such as Poland, Romania, or Russia. In some of these countries, Roma people are an underserved minority who, when migrating to Western Europe, remain at risk of low access to care and discrimination [9, 32].

Recording of ethnicity has not been uniform through time and between countries. Early on, ethnicity was assessed based on the country of birth or original citizenship or place of birth of the parents. However, this has changed in some European countries over the last two to three decades due to more modern concepts of ethnicity and also the fact that there are now third and even fourth generations of immigrant populations who were born in Europe. While an updated and modern concept of ethnicity is appropriate to better inform about specifics of health-care disparities, it makes it difficult to compare old and new findings in the literature, as well as between countries with differing concepts, unless one has access to the original definitions and raw data.

Table 12.1 Estimated proportion of ethnic/immigrant minorities in the population of some Western European countries

Country	Proportion (%)	Major ethnic groups
France	6.4	North African, South East Asian
Germany	8.5	Turkish, Italian, Greek, Polish
Italy	3.2	African, Asian, Eastern European
The Netherlands	4.7	Turkish, North African, Surinamese
United Kingdom	7.9	African (Caribbean, East African), Indian, Pakistani

Diagnosis and Pathophysiology

The methods of ascertaining the diagnosis of diabetes in reports have been varied; the diagnosis of diabetes or prediabetes has been based on self-report or on glucose/HbA1c screening, often in high-risk groups, according to the recommendations by the EASD/ADA, or it has been based on reports to registries from participating physicians. The majority of subjects suffer from type 2 diabetes which has been consistently reported to occur earlier (by up to two decades) in minority populations. The pathogenesis of type 2 diabetes appears to be related to increased caloric intake, to (central) obesity, and to insulin resistance and beta cell failure, and these do not appear to be different between populations. The excess incidence of diabetes in South Asian women correlates with more prevalent central obesity but this is not the case for men [51, 52]. One study estimates that up to 90 % of Asian immigrant women may be at risk for diabetes [21]. The most and the earliest data supporting this statement come from studies in subjects of South Asian ethnicity; more recent studies from Turkey do confirm and extend these results to other ethnic minorities [44]. However, when waist circumference is used to assess central obesity, the risk for diabetes in South Asians significantly increases at lower values compared to African or Caucasian populations. In addition, it has been proposed that differences in suppression of nonesterified fatty acids may act as mediators of glucose intolerance in Indian Asian populations [40]. In minority subjects of African descent as compared to subjects in the country of origin, increased caloric intake from protein and fat has been shown to be associated with higher rates of diabetes [2]. Similar findings have been reported in migrants from South Asia (Pakistan and Sri Lanka) who settled in Norway [54]. This pattern of increasing food consumption is similar to populations in developing countries who move from rural to urban settings with an increase in calorie consumption and more sedentary lifestyle [45].

Few studies have compared genetic determinants of type 2 diabetes between immigrant and native populations. Some studies in South Asian (Indian) populations suggest that genetic differences may exist [17, 30], but larger studies are needed to get better insight into this issue.

Prevalence Estimates

The prevalence of diabetes in minorities is affected by ethnicity and country of residence. In one study in the UK [59], standardized prevalence rates for diabetes were 1.7, 5.3, and 8.9 % in white, African Caribbean, and Pakistani/Bangladeshi groups. In a more recent study [51], incidences of diabetes over an up to 20-year time period were 14 % for European, 33 % for Indian Asian, and 30 % for African Caribbean subjects. Based on these findings, it is estimated that by age 80, approximately 50 % of Indian Asian and African Caribbean subjects versus approximately 20 % of Europeans will have developed diabetes. A study from Oslo, Norway [25], compared the prevalence of diabetes between South Asian and Western subjects in a low-income population; diabetes prevalence rates were 27.5 % and 2.9 % for South Asian and Western women and 14.3 % and 5.9 % for South Asian and Western men, respectively. The age-adjusted odds ratios for South Asians versus Westerners were 11.0 for women and 3.0 for men; adjustment for waist-hip ratio reduced these ratios to 7.7 and 2.6 in the South Asian women and men, respectively.

A study from Amsterdam [47], Netherlands, compared the prevalence of diabetes between Dutch, Turkish, and Moroccan subjects. Unadjusted diabetes prevalence rates were 5.1 %, 11.0 %, and 18.8 % in Dutch, Turkish, and Moroccan men, respectively; unadjusted diabetes prevalence rates were 2.9 %, 8.4 %, and 16.1 % in Dutch, Turkish, and Moroccan women, respectively. A different study from Amsterdam [7], Netherlands, that was conducted around the same time compared the prevalence of diabetes between Dutch, Hindustani Surinamese, and African Surinamese groups. Age-adjusted prevalence was 5.5 %, 14.2 %, and 26.7 % for the Dutch, African Surinamese, and Hindustani Surinamese groups, respectively. In a univariate analysis, a history of CVD and waist circumference demonstrated the strongest association with diabetes. In a multivariate analysis, a history of CVD, a first-degree relative with diabetes, and Hindustani Surinamese were the strongest determinants of diabetes. While increased rates of diabetes have been found in groups of Indian and African descent in England and the Netherlands, it appears that these minorities living in the Netherlands have almost twice the prevalence than that observed in England [1]; it is unclear whether these differences between countries are due to differences in the studied populations (e.g., genetic or social/ethnic variability) or due to differences in the environment.

Germany has the second highest number of diabetic subjects in Europe (IDF-Atlas 7th edition 2015) after the Russian Federation and with Austria and Spain the highest population prevalence in Western Europe. There are few studies assessing the prevalence and incidence in ethnic minorities in Germany which is due to privacy laws as well as the way these data are collected. Most of these studies are small and likely affected by sampling bias. The estimate for diabetes prevalence in Turkish subjects has been reported in a range from 3 %, which is lower than the prevalence in native Germans, to 14 % which is 50–100 % higher compared to native Germans (Icks et al. Deutscher Gesundheitsbericht Diabetes 2011, pp 148–154; www.diabetesde.org). Most experts agree that the prevalence of type 2 diabetes is likely to be higher than in the native population [43], where it is assumed to be 7.2 % [18].

Roma, in earlier literature referred to as gypsies and travelers, do most likely represent one of the oldest of all migrant minorities in Europe; it is well documented that they do have poorer health and decreased life expectancy. One study from England [39] demonstrated a 4.0 % self-reported prevalence of diabetes in the gypsy/traveler group which was not different from the native group. In contrast, a study from Hungary [20, 31] reported an 18.4 % prevalence of undiagnosed diabetes, nearly one-and-a-half-fold higher than the 7.5 % observed in the native Hungarian population.

Gestational diabetes seems to be more common among ethnic minorities, e.g., among Turkish women in Germany (183 per 1,000 pregnancies compared to 138 per 1,000 pregnancies in German women) [42]. Rates of gestational diabetes have been reported to be elevated also in groups of South Asian and African descent whether they lived in Norway [26] or in other countries [27]. This may explain some of the increased perinatal complications seen in minority groups [29].

Children of migrants are often more obese and more sedentary suggesting an increased future risk of type 2 diabetes. For type 1 diabetes, however, it appears that children born to immigrants have a lower risk [13, 22, 23]. However, minority children with type 1 diabetes have worse glycemic control, more severe hypoglycemic episodes, and a higher rate of hospitalization [46].

Complications of Diabetes

Few data are available regarding diabetic complications in different ethnic groups. The available data indicate that Asian Indians suffer more from retinopathy and nephropathy compared to the native populations. In subjects in the UK with early onset of type 2 diabetes (age <40 years), South Asians exhibited more retinopathy (17.5 % vs. 7.9 %) and more nephropathy (18.1 % vs. 7.8 %). In the same study [8], macrovascular disease was also more prevalent in the South Asian group (15.7 % vs 9.4 %). These results were confirmed in a larger and more recent study [49] that observed a 52 %, 42 %, and 38 % prevalence of any diabetic retinopathy in African/Afro-Caribbeans, South Asians, and white Europeans, respectively. In the same study, sight-threatening diabetic retinopathy was also nearly twice as common in both African/Afro-Caribbeans and South Asians compared to white Europeans. Diabetic nephropathy was reported in several studies to progress more rapidly in Asian Indians [11, 12] with the latter study observing a 40-fold increased risk of end-stage diabetic nephropathy compared to the native Dutch population. However, more recent studies were not able to confirm higher rates of complications [19, 56] or faster progression of renal disease in minority groups [38]. While ethnic differences may be explained, at least in part, by the higher prevalence, earlier onset of diabetes, and higher glucose levels, those variables do not appear to completely account for the differences.

Diabetic neuropathy was less common in Asian Indians when compared to African or Caucasian groups [56]. Macrovascular disease appears less common with African ethnicities [56] which is mostly explained by lower rates of smoking in this group [33].

Coordination and Delivery of Diabetes Care Services

Health care is almost universally available in all European countries and includes diabetes care and education, and the patients' expenses for their care including medications are often negligible. All health-care services do have guidelines for diabetes care that are modeled after ADA/EASD recommendations. Nevertheless, for a number of reasons that are not all well understood, minorities do not obtain the same benefits from the health-care system as their native counterparts as often evidenced by higher average glucose levels and lower attainment of treatment goals for other cardiovascular risk factors such as hypertension [19].

Data on health-care delivery and utilization in minorities are scarce, mostly due to lack of recording ethnicity in the primary care setting

[5]. One study [15] revealed that Indian patients with diabetes were less likely to be seen by a primary care physician, but a later study [36] showed no differences in access to health care for diabetes between white and South Asian Indian groups. However, the latter study showed a tendency toward lower control rates of diabetes in the minority groups. A study from Italy [4] supports these findings in minorities; while minorities with diabetes were cared for in similar proportions as the native population, they were less likely to be tested for HbA1cA and had worse glucose control.

A number of barriers to health-care delivery have been identified [35, 55] (Miriam McHardy – Master Thesis Necessity, Concepts and Feasibility of Culturally Tailored Diabetes Education for Migrants in the Netherlands and the United Kingdom: A Qualitative Study on Experts' Views); they include language barriers and lack of transportation (driver's license and car), especially in first-generation immigrants and subjects with low educational status, low health literacy, and cultural and religious norms [58], as well as differences in illness perception between patients and providers [57] (Table 12.2). Even if advice is provided in a culturally appropriate context and understanding, implementation of changes can be a struggle within the routines of already established food habits [14].

Efforts to overcome those barriers come from both the provider (health-care delivery) and the consumer side. For example, case workers and "community links" have been shown to improve diabetes care and outcomes. The use of translators [48] can improve communication of certain issues and concepts but also has the potential to change the tone of the conversation by removing humor and adding the interpreter's own opinions. Self-help groups and social clubs are used by minority patients to improve self-management of their diabetes [16], but not all minority groups find them acceptable.

Table 12.2 Potential barriers to health-care delivery

Language
Different perception of illness
Low health literacy
Low educational status
Cultural norms
Religious norms
Lack of acceptable healthy food choices
Lack of transportation

Non-pharmacological Management

Diet and exercise are the cornerstone of any diabetes treatment regimen; it is also the cornerstone of diabetes prevention. Diet and exercise have been shown to improve glycemia and lipids in ethnic minorities and prevent progression to the metabolic syndrome [50]. There are no studies comparing the efficacy of these modalities between native and minority populations. As pointed out above, minority groups face additional barriers when attempting to change eating and exercise habits; healthy food items have to be available, affordable, and useable for established food patterns. Increasing physical activity can be difficult for some minority groups, especially women who are not permitted to show body parts or exercise in the company of men. Because of these additional barriers, it is important to develop and deliver culturally competent diabetes care interventions [58].

Rational Selection of Antidiabetic Medications

Drugs for the treatment of diabetes are available to all subjects diagnosed with this disease and cost is covered completely in most countries. Most common older and newer diabetes drugs are available in Europe where the European Medicinal Agency is in control of approving the applications for marketing by the drug companies; however, coverage and reimbursement rates of drugs are decided separately by the unique regulatory agencies in each country which affects utilization by the patients. There are no studies comparing efficacy and safety of different antidiabetic drugs between immigrant and native populations, and, therefore, no recommendations in regard to the first- and second-line choices can be made. In the absence of studies that could provide guidance for drug selection and in the absence of significant differences in the pathophysiology of diabetes development between immigrant and native populations, drug prescription should follow the guidance by ADA/EASD. A study from the Netherlands [10] showed underutilization of diabetes drugs in Turkish and Moroccan immigrants but not in Surinamese and Antillean immigrants. A study from England [6] provided a more granular listing of the use of antidiabetic drugs; the utilization of oral drugs, predominantly metformin and sulfonylurea, was similar between groups. However, minorities were less likely to utilize insulin alone or insulin plus oral drugs. The utilization of lipid-lowering and antihypertensive drugs was similar between groups. Lower utilization of insulin and lipid-lowering agents in migrants was also reported in a study from Italy [34]. The reasons for these differences, especially the lower rate of insulin use, are not clear; this may be due to the younger age of immigrants, lower prescription rates by the providers, or lower acceptance by the patient. Additionally, based on the results from a large Austrian/German registry study, there is a difference in the utilization of continuous insulin infusion therapy between Turkish and German/Austrian children [24]. The fact that this "underutilization" occurs in the face of universal healthcare coverage points to social and cultural issues in the ethnic minority groups that are not well understood. Whether this underutilization of insulin pump therapy contributes to worse glycemic control, more severe hypoglycemic episodes, and a higher rate of hospitalization [46], as pointed out above, is not clear.

Translating Primary Prevention of Type 2 Diabetes

Ethnic minorities are at high risk of developing diabetes; it is estimated that half of Indian Asian subjects may be diabetic by age 80. Therefore, prevention of type 2 diabetes is of utmost importance in these groups. Progress has been slow in part due to barriers that are present in those groups; in addition, different barriers exist in minorities from different origin. Johnson et al. [28] describe a number of these barriers such as lack of access to exercise facilities, family and work commitments, cost, language, religious differences, and cultural norms; in addition, differences in illness perception contribute [57]. Taking these considerations into account [53], one prevention study that adapted the design of the Finnish Diabetes Prevention Study in a culturally sensitive way was conducted in Scotland. The study was unable to recruit sufficient numbers of participants to assess the effect of the intervention on progression to diabetes; the (revised) primary question was whether clinically meaningful weight loss can be achieved. The results of this 3-year study, the PODOSA (Prevention Of Diabetes and Obesity in South Asians), demonstrated more weight loss associated with a decrease in central obesity and a trend toward lower fasting and 2-h post OGTT values; importantly, there was less progression to diabetes, and this has to be taken with a grain of salt since the study was not powered to view this result with sufficient confidence. A similar diabetes prevention study, the DH!AAN study, in Surinamese Asians is currently underway in the Netherlands [37] (Health Promotion International, Vol. 29 No. 4). The results of the PODOSA and the DH!AAN study will be compared with those of a similar, currently ongoing study in India, the D-CLIP study [3]. Together, the results will guide development of more targeted diet and exercise programs to prevent diabetes in these populations.

Organizing and Conducting Diabetes Research and Future Directions

Diabetes research of ethnic minorities has been conducted mostly at a local or regional level and was more qualitative than quantitative. Results of this research point to the increased risk of developing type 2 diabetes in a higher proportion of minorities and possibly higher rates of complications. Results of this research have also identified a number of barriers to achieving lifestyle changes that are associated with a decreased risk of obesity, the metabolic syndrome, and diabetes. More recent outcome studies demonstrate the feasibility of implementing intensive lifestyle changes that are culturally adapted and lead to promising outcomes. Results from these ongoing intervention studies will be available in a few years.

Future research should use the locally/regionally acquired information and knowledge to design studies that are more representative of national or even Europe-wide ethnic populations. This can be accomplished by large registries that include data from multiple countries obtained in standardized fashion and/or by sufficiently large random samples throughout the different countries or, ideally, throughout Europe. This will help define the current state of diabetes and its complications in minorities in Europe while accounting for secular changes in the native population and environment. In addition, larger intervention studies that include several distinct minority groups (e.g., groups of Turkish, Asian Indian, and African descent) should be designed; results from such a study might identify intervention elements that are generally applicable to achieve improved outcomes as well as elements that require more group specific, ethnic, or local adaptation [41]. The final goal of these efforts is to support the development of culturally competent health-care systems, health-care systems that provide culturally and linguistically appropriate services which will reduce racial and ethnic health disparities and improve outcomes.

References

1. Agyemang C, Kunst AE, Bhopal R, Anujuo K, Zaninotto P, Nazroo J, Nicolaou M, Unwin N, van Valkengoed I, Redekop WK, Stronks K. Diabetes prevalence in populations of South Asian Indian and African origins: a comparison of England and the Netherlands. Epidemiology. 2011;22:563–7.
2. Anderson SG, Younger N, Heald AH, Tulloch-Reid MK, Simukonda WP, Mbanya JC, Jackson MD, Balkau B, Sharma S, Tanya A, Forrester T, Wilks R, Cruickshank JK. Nutrient intakes and dysglycaemia in populations of West African origin. Br J Nutr. 2011;105:297–306.
3. Anjana RM, Ranjani H, Unnikrishnan R, Weber MB, Mohan V, Narayan KM. Exercise patterns and behaviour in Asian Indians: data from the baseline survey of the Diabetes Community Lifestyle Improvement Program (D-CLIP). Diabetes Res Clin Pract. 2015;107:77–84.
4. Ballotari P, Caroli S, Ferrari F, Romani G, Marina G, Chiarenza A, Manicardi V, Giorgi Rossi P. Differences in diabetes prevalence and inequalities in disease management and glycaemic control by immigrant status: a population-based study (Italy). BMC Public Health. 2015;15:87.
5. Baradaran HR, Jamieson J, Gardee R, Knill-Jones RP. Scottish survey of diabetes services for minority ethnic groups. BMC Health Serv Res. 2006;6:130.
6. Benhalima K, Song SH, Wilmot EG, Khunti K, Gray LJ, Lawrence I, Davies M. Characteristics, complications and management of a large multiethnic cohort of younger adults with type 2 diabetes. Prim Care Diabetes. 2011;5:245–50.
7. Bindraban NR, van Valkengoed IG, Mairuhu G, Holleman F, Hoekstra JB, Michels BP, Koopmans RP, Stronks K. Prevalence of diabetes mellitus and the performance of a risk score among Hindustani Surinamese, African Surinamese and ethnic Dutch: a cross-sectional population-based study. BMC Public Health. 2008;8:271.
8. Chowdhury TA, Lasker SS. Complications and cardiovascular risk factors in South Asians and Europeans with early-onset type 2 diabetes. QJM. 2002;95:241–6.
9. Correspondent EUR. Commission calls to break circle of Roma health exclusion across Europe. Eureporter. 2014.
10. Denktaş S, Koopmans G, Birnie E, Foets M, Bonsel G. Underutilization of prescribed drugs use among first generation elderly immigrants in the Netherlands. BMC Health Serv Res. 2010;10:176.
11. Dreyer G, Hull S, Mathur R, Chesser A, Yaqoob MM. Progression of chronic kidney disease in a multi-ethnic community cohort of patients with diabetes mellitus. Diabet Med. 2013;30:956–63.
12. Earle KK, Porter KA, Ostberg J, Yudkin JS. Variation in the progression of diabetic nephropathy according to racial origin. Nephrol Dial Transplant. 2001;16:286–90.
13. Ehehalt S, Popovic P, Muntoni S, Willasch A, Hub R, Ranke MB, Neu A, Baden-Wuerttemberg DG. Incidence of diabetes mellitus among children of Italian migrants substantiates the role of genetic factors in the pathogenesis of type 1 diabetes. Eur J Pediatr. 2009;168:613–7.
14. Fagerli RA, Lien ME, Wandel M. Experience of dietary advice among Pakistani-born persons with type 2 diabetes in Oslo. Appetite. 2005;45:295–304.
15. Goyder EC, McNally PG, Botha JL. Inequalities in access to diabetes care: evidence from a historical cohort study. Qual Health Care. 2000;9:85–9.
16. Guell C. Tactics of diabetes control Turkish immigrant experiences with chronic illness in Berlin. Germany: The University of Edinburgh; 2009. 265 p.

17. Gujral UP, Pradeepa R, Weber MB, Narayan KM, Mohan V. Type 2 diabetes in South Asians: similarities and differences with white Caucasian and other populations. Ann N Y Acad Sci. 2013;1281:51–63.
18. Heidemann C, Du Y, Schubert I, Rathmann W, Scheidt-Nave C. Prevalence and temporal trend of known diabetes mellitus: results of the German Health Interview and Examination Survey for Adults (DEGS1). Bundesgesundheitsblatt Gesundheitsforschung Gesundheitsschutz. 2013;56:668–77.
19. Hewitt J. Ethnicity and prevalence of diabetic complications in elderly patients. In: Gallen I, editor. Pract Diabetes Int. 2004;139–42.
20. Hidvegi T, Hetyesi K, Biro L, Nadas J, Jermendy G. Screening for metabolic syndrome within a minority ethnic group (adult gypsy people) in Hungary. Bratisl Lek Listy. 2012;113:721–4.
21. Hjellset VT, Bjørge B, Eriksen HR, Høstmark AT. Risk factors for type 2 diabetes among female Pakistani immigrants: the InvaDiab-DEPLAN study on Pakistani immigrant women living in Oslo. Norway: J Immigr Minor Health. 2011;13:101–10.
22. Hjern A, Söderström U. Parental country of birth is a major determinant of childhood type 1 diabetes in Sweden. Pediatr Diabetes. 2008;9:35–9.
23. Hussen HI, Yang D, Cnattingius S, Moradi T. Type I diabetes among children and young adults: the role of country of birth, socioeconomic position and sex. Pediatr Diabetes. 2013;14:138–48.
24. Icks A, Razum O, Rosenbauer J, Bachle C, Hungele A, Monkemoller K, Muller-Godeffroy E, Heidtmann B, Kapellen T, Scheuing N, Holl RW, D. P. V. I. for the, E, The German Federal Ministry For, M. Research Competence Network Diabetes. Lower frequency of insulin pump treatment in children and adolescents of Turkish background with type 1 diabetes: analysis of 21,497 patients in Germany. Diabetes Technol Ther. 2012;14:1105–9.
25. Jenum AK, Holme I, Graff-Iversen S, Birkeland KI. Ethnicity and sex are strong determinants of diabetes in an urban western society: implications for prevention. Diabetologia. 2005;48:435–9.
26. Jenum AK, Mørkrid K, Sletner L, Vangen S, Vange S, Torper JL, Nakstad B, Voldner N, Rognerud-Jensen OH, Berntsen S, Mosdøl A, Skrivarhaug T, Vårdal MH, Holme I, Yajnik CS, Birkeland KI. Impact of ethnicity on gestational diabetes identified with the WHO and the modified International Association of Diabetes and Pregnancy Study Groups criteria: a population-based cohort study. Eur J Endocrinol. 2012;166:317–24.
27. Jenum AK, Sommer C, Sletner L, Mørkrid K, Bærug A, Mosdøl A. Adiposity and hyperglycaemia in pregnancy and related health outcomes in European ethnic minorities of Asian and African origin: a review. Food Nutr Res. 2013;57. doi:10.3402/fnr.v57i0.18889.
28. Johnson M, Everson-Hock E, Jones R, Woods HB, Payne N, Goyder E. What are the barriers to primary prevention of type 2 diabetes in black and minority ethnic groups in the UK? Qual Evid Synth Diabetes Res Clin Pract. 2011;93:150–8.
29. Khalil A, Rezende J, Akolekar R, Syngelaki A, Nicolaides KH. Maternal racial origin and adverse pregnancy outcome: a cohort study. Ultrasound Obstet Gynecol. 2013;41:278–85.
30. Kodama K, Tojjar D, Yamada S, Toda K, Patel CJ, Butte AJ. Ethnic differences in the relationship between insulin sensitivity and insulin response: a systematic review and meta-analysis. Diabetes Care. 2013;36:1789–96.
31. Kósa Z, Moravcsik-Kornyicki Á, Diószegi J, Roberts B, Szabó Z, Sándor J, Ádány R. Prevalence of metabolic syndrome among Roma: a comparative health examination survey in Hungary. Eur J Public Health. 2015;25:299–304.
32. Kühlbrandt C, Footman K, Rechel B, McKee M. An examination of Roma health insurance status in Central and Eastern Europe. Eur J Public Health. 2014;24:701–2.
33. Leggetter S, Chaturvedi N, Fuller JH, Edmonds ME. Ethnicity and risk of diabetes-related lower extremity amputation: a population-based, case-control study of African Caribbeans and Europeans in the United Kingdom. Arch Intern Med. 2002;162:73–8.
34. Marchesini G, Bernardi D, Miccoli R, Rossi E, Vaccaro O, De Rosa M, Bonora E, Bruno G. Undertreatment of migrants with diabetes in a universalistic health care system: the ARNO observatory. Nutr Metab Cardiovasc Dis. 2014;24:393–9.
35. McHardy M. Necessity, concepts and feasibility of culturally tailored diabetes education for migrants in the Netherlands and the United Kingdom: a qualitative study on experts' views. Hamburg: Hamburg University of Applied Sciences; 2014. 134 p.
36. Nazroo JY, Falaschetti E, Pierce M, Primatesta P. Ethnic inequalities in access to and outcomes of healthcare: analysis of the Health Survey for England. J Epidemiol Community Health. 2009;63:1022–7.
37. Nicolaou M, Vlaar E, van Valkengoed I, Middelkoop B, Stronks K, Nierkens V. Development of a diabetes prevention program for Surinamese South Asians in the Netherlands. Health Promot Int. 2014;29:680–91.
38. Pallayova M, Rayner H, Taheri S, Dasgupta I. Is there a difference in progression of renal disease between South Asian and white European diabetic adults with moderately reduced kidney function? J Diabetes Complications. 2015;29:761–5.
39. Parry G, Van Cleemput P, Peters J, Walters S, Thomas K, Cooper C. Health status of Gypsies and Travellers in England. J Epidemiol Community Health. 2007;61:198–204.
40. Patel JV, Vyas A, Prabhakaran D, Bhatnagar D, Durrington PN, Heald A, Hughes EA, Mackness MI, Reddy KS, Cruickshank JK. Nonesterified fatty acids as mediators of glucose intolerance in Indian Asian populations. Diabetes Care. 2005;28:1505–7.
41. Razum O, Spallek J. Addressing health-related interventions to immigrants: migrant-specific or diversity-sensitive? Int J Public Health. 2014;59:893–5.
42. Reeske A, Zeeb H, Razum O, Spallek J. Differences in the incidence of gestational diabetes between

women of Turkish and German Origin: an analysis of Health Insurance Data from a Statutory Health Insurance in Berlin, Germany (AOK), 2005–2007. Geburtshilfe Frauenheilkd. 2012;72:305–10.
43. RKI. Gesundheit in Deutschland. In: Koch-Institut R, editor, Gesundheitsberichterstattung des Bundes. Gemeinsam getragen von RKI und Destatis. Berlin: Robert Koch-Institut; 2015. p. 516.
44. Satman I, Omer B, Tutuncu Y, Kalaca S, Gedik S, Dinccag N, Karsidag K, Genc S, Telci A, Canbaz B, Turker F, Yilmaz T, Cakir B, Tuomilehto J, Group T-IS. Twelve-year trends in the prevalence and risk factors of diabetes and prediabetes in Turkish adults. Eur J Epidemiol. 2013;28:169–80.
45. Satman I, Yilmaz T, Sengül A, Salman S, Salman F, Uygur S, Bastar I, Tütüncü Y, Sargin M, Dinççag N, Karsidag K, Kalaça S, Ozcan C, King H. Population-based study of diabetes and risk characteristics in Turkey: results of the Turkish diabetes epidemiology study (TURDEP). Diabetes Care. 2002;25:1551–6.
46. Scheuing N, Wiegand S, Bächle C, Fröhlich-Reiterer E, Hahn E, Icks A, Ludwig KH, Mönkemöller K, Razum O, Rosenbauer J, Holl RW, Initiative D. Impact of maternal country of birth on type-1-diabetes therapy and outcome in 27,643 children and adolescents from the DPV Registry. PLoS One. 2015;10:e0135178.
47. Schrier AC, Ujcic-Voortman JK, de Wit MA, Verhoeff AP, Kupka R, Dekker J, Beekman AT. Ethnic differences in the association between cardiovascular risk factors and psychological distress in a population study in the Netherlands. BMC Public Health. 2012;12:1090.
48. Seale C, Rivas C, Kelly M. The challenge of communication in interpreted consultations in diabetes care: a mixed methods study. Br J Gen Pract. 2013;63: e125–33.
49. Sivaprasad S, Gupta B, Gulliford MC, Dodhia H, Mohamed M, Nagi D, Evans JR. Ethnic variations in the prevalence of diabetic retinopathy in people with diabetes attending screening in the United Kingdom (DRIVE UK). PLoS One. 2012;7:e32182.
50. Telle-Hjellset V, Råberg Kjøllesdal MK, Bjørge B, Holmboe-Ottesen G, Wandel M, Birkeland KI, Eriksen HR, Høstmark AT. The InnvaDiab-DE-PLAN study: a randomised controlled trial with a culturally adapted education programme improved the risk profile for type 2 diabetes in Pakistani immigrant women. Br J Nutr. 2013;109:529–38.
51. Tillin T, Hughes AD, Godsland IF, Whincup P, Forouhi NG, Welsh P, Sattar N, McKeigue PM, Chaturvedi N. Insulin resistance and truncal obesity as important determinants of the greater incidence of diabetes in Indian Asians and African Caribbeans compared with Europeans: the Southall and Brent REvisited (SABRE) cohort. Diabetes Care. 2013;36:383–93.
52. Tillin T, Hughes AD, Mayet J, Whincup P, Sattar N, Forouhi NG, McKeigue PM, Chaturvedi N. The relationship between metabolic risk factors and incident cardiovascular disease in Europeans, south Asians, and African Caribbeans: SABRE (Southall and Brent revisited) – a prospective population-based study. J Am Coll Cardiol. 2013;61:1777–86.
53. Wallia S, Bhopal RS, Douglas A, Bhopal R, Sharma A, Hutchison A, Murray G, Gill J, Sattar N, Lawton J, Tuomilehto J, Mcknight J, Forbes J, Lean M, Sheikh A. Culturally adapting the prevention of diabetes and obesity in South Asians (PODOSA) trial. Health Promot Int. 2014;29:768–79.
54. Wandel M, Råberg M, Kumar B, Holmboe-Ottesen G. Changes in food habits after migration among South Asians settled in Oslo: the effect of demographic, socio-economic and integration factors. Appetite. 2008;50:376–85.
55. Wilson C, Alam R, Latif S, Knighting K, Williamson S, Beaver K. Patient access to healthcare services and optimisation of self-management for ethnic minority populations living with diabetes: a systematic review. Health Soc Care Community. 2012;20: 1–19.
56. Winkley K, Thomas SM, Sivaprasad S, Chamley M, Stahl D, Ismail K, Amiel SA. The clinical characteristics at diagnosis of type 2 diabetes in a multi-ethnic population: the South London Diabetes cohort (SOUL-D). Diabetologia. 2013;56:1272–81.
57. Yilmaz-Aslan Y, Brzoska P, Bluhm M, Aslan A, Razum O. Illness perceptions in Turkish migrants with diabetes. Qual Study Chron Illn. 2014;10: 107–21.
58. Zeh P, et al. Cultural barriers impeding ethnic minority groups from accessing effective diabetes care services: a systematic review of observational studies. Divers Equal Health Care. 2014;11:9–33.
59. Nazroo JY. The health of Britian's ethnic minorities: findings from a national survey. London: Policy Studies Institute, 1997.

Diabetes Among Indigenous Canadians

13

Sudaba Mansuri and Anthony J. Hanley

Background

Indigenous Peoples of Canada

According to the Canadian Constitution Act of 1982, three distinct groups of Indigenous Canadians are recognized: First Nations, Métis, and Inuit, with each group having their own set of unique languages, traditions, art, and culture [1]. First Nations people are currently the largest Indigenous group in Canada [2, 3]. The Métis are the second largest group, and their history dates back to the mid-seventeenth century when European (predominantly French and Scottish) fur traders married Indigenous (Cree, Ojibway, Algonquin, and other First Nations) women [3, 4]. The third largest Indigenous group is the Inuit, who traveled from Western Alaska around 1000 CE to the Arctic [3, 5].

Over 1.4 million Canadians are self-identified with Indigenous identity, accounting for 4.3 % of the total Canadian population, according to the 2011 National Household Survey [3]. Of those who identified with Indigenous identity, 60.8 % identified as First Nations, 32.3 % identified as Métis, and 4.2 % identified as Inuit [3].

Indigenous communities are found in all areas of Canada, including urban, rural, and isolated areas. While many Indigenous communities are in close proximity to non-Indigenous cities or towns, or are otherwise accessible by permanent road, a substantial proportion of Indigenous communities are remote or isolated, accessible only by air or water. The largest population of Indigenous Canadians is found in Ontario and the Western provinces, with eight in ten Indigenous Canadians living in these provinces [3]. Métis communities are concentrated in Alberta, British Columbia, Ontario, Manitoba, and Saskatchewan. The traditional territory of the Inuit is in the Arctic regions of Canada (Nunavut, Northwest Territories, and Northern Quebec). Roughly 40 % of First Nations communities are located on federally recognized lands called reserves [3]. However, according to national survey data, off-reserve Indigenous Canadians are one of the fastest growing groups in Canada, with 56 % of Indigenous people living in urban areas in 2011, up from 49 % in 1996 [3].

Indigenous peoples in Canada speak over 60 distinct languages which are grouped into 12 language families [6]. According to the 2011 Census, over 200,000 people reported speaking their Indigenous mother tongue, and of these people,

S. Mansuri, MSc
Department of Nutritional Sciences, Faculty of Medicine, University of Toronto, Toronto, ON, Canada

A.J. Hanley (✉)
Departments of Nutritional Sciences and Public Health Sciences, Faculty of Medicine, University of Toronto, Toronto, ON, Canada
e-mail: anthony.hanley@utoronto.ca

S. Dagogo-Jack (ed.), *Diabetes Mellitus in Developing Countries and Underserved Communities*, DOI 10.1007/978-3-319-41559-8_13

almost all of them reported speaking their mother tongue regularly [6]. The most common language family is the Algonquin family, with over 144,000 people reporting that their mother tongue belonged to this family. The languages that fall under this family include Cree languages, Ojibway, Innu/Montagnais, and Oji-Cree. The Inuit and Athapaskan language families are the second and third largest language families, with Inuktitut being the mother tongue among the Inuit family and Dene being the mother tongue of the Athapaskan family. Despite the vast diversity in languages among Indigenous Canadians, those who speak Cree, Inuktitut, and Ojibway account for almost two-thirds of the languages spoken [6].

The age structure of the Canadian Indigenous population is vastly different from the general Canadian population. As a result of higher fertility rates and shorter life expectancy, the Indigenous population is younger than the non-Indigenous population, with the median age of the Indigenous population being 28 years, notably lower than the median age of the non-Indigenous population at 41 years [7]. According to the 2011 National Household Survey, Indigenous children aged 14 and under represented 28 % of the total Indigenous population compared to 7 % of the population of children in the general population in Canada [8]. Indigenous youth aged 15–24 represented 18.2 % of the total Indigenous population and 5.9 % of the youth in the general population of Canada [8]. Whereas Indigenous seniors aged 65 and older made up only 5.9 % of the total Indigenous population, non-Indigenous seniors represent 14.2 % of the non-Indigenous population. Among the three Indigenous groups, Inuit were the youngest, with a median age of 23 years, First Nations people had a median age of 26, and the Métis had a median age of 31.

Since initial contact with Europeans approximately 400 years ago, seismic sociocultural changes in the lives of Indigenous Canadians have significantly impacted their health and well-being. The imposition of colonial institutions, including the fur trade, the system of reserves, and the residential school system, has led to loss of land, language, and sociocultural knowledge and resources. These effects are still present in Indigenous communities where there are poor living conditions, high rates of unemployment, low literacy and educational attainment, income inadequacy, and inadequate community resources [9].

Prevalence and Incidence of Type 2 Diabetes

The burden of type 2 diabetes mellitus (DM) is disproportionately higher in Indigenous Canadians compared to non-Indigenous Canadians [10, 11]. Although the prevalence of diabetes was extremely rare in this population prior to the 1950s [12], chart reviews a few decades later revealed notably high rates of this condition in the Mohawk community of Kahnawake, the First Nations community of Sandy Lake, and the James Bay Cree of Northern Quebec [13–16]. Data from surveillance studies documented a doubling of type 2 DM prevalence among Indigenous people in Saskatchewan between 1980 and 1990 [17] and an increase in prevalence of 45 % between 1985 and 1994 among the First Nations population of the Sioux Lookout Zone in Northwestern Ontario [18].

The prevalence rates of diabetes among Indigenous Canadians have been established using a variety of approaches, including self-reported diagnoses in national surveys, administrative data, and more detailed surveys using oral glucose tolerance tests (OGTTs). Prevalence rates vary considerably according to the methodology that was used. National data from the 2008–2010 First Nations Regional Longitudinal Health Survey and the 2009–2010 Canadian Community Health Survey found that age-standardized rates of self-reported diabetes among the First Nations population were 17.2 % for individuals 18 years and older living on-reserve and 10.3 % among First Nations living off-reserve compared to the prevalence in the

	Source	Age	Age-standardized Prevalence (%) (95 % confidence interval)
Non-aboriginal	2009–2010 CCHS	12+	5.0 (4.3–5.7)
First-Nations (on-reserve)	2008–2010 RHS	18+	17.2 (16.5–19.0)
First-Nations (off-reserve)	2009–2010 CCHS	12+	10.3 (3.4–17.2)
Inuit	2006 APS	15+	NA
Métis	2009–2010 CCHS	12+	7.3 (2.2–12.5)

Fig. 13.1 Prevalence of self-reported diabetes among Indigenous peoples aged 12 years and older, Canada, 2006, 2008–2010, 2009–2010 (Source: Public Health Agency of Canada (2011), using data from 2009 to 2010 Canadian Community Health Survey (Statistics Canada); First Nations Information Governance Centre (2011), using data from the 2008–2010 First Nations Regional Longitudinal Health Survey (Phase 2) (First Nations Information Governance Centre); Social and Aboriginal Statistics Division, *Aboriginal Peoples Survey, 2006: Inuit Health and Social Conditions*: Ottawa, ON: Statistics Canada; 2008. Statistics Canada. Public Health Agency of Canada. 2011)

general population which was 6 % (12 years and older) (Fig. 13.1) [19–21].

Administrative data from Manitoba reported a prevalence rate of type 2 DM that was 4.5 times higher than that in the non-First Nation population of Manitoba [22]. Similarly, a study in Saskatchewan also using administrative data showed that the prevalence of diabetes was four times higher among First Nations women than among non-First Nations women and 2.5 times higher among First Nations men than non-First Nations men (Fig. 13.2) [23]. According to administrative data from 2007, the prevalence of diabetes was 13.5 % in Indigenous peoples compared to 6 % in non-Indigenous peoples in the province of Alberta [24].

Over the past three decades, a limited number of more detailed studies using standardized oral glucose tolerance tests (OGTTs) have reported prevalence rates in Indigenous Canadians to be among the highest in the world (Fig. 13.3) [25, 26]. High prevalence rates were found in two Quebec communities, with a 48.6 % prevalence rate in Algonquin women of Lac Simon (aged 15 years and older) and a 16.3 % prevalence in women of River Desert (aged 15 years and older) [26]. According to a study in Sandy Lake First Nation, the age-standardized prevalence of type 2 DM was 26.1 % [25] over the age of 10.

Although the administrative data studies mentioned above have presented both incidence and prevalence rates of type 2 DM [22, 23], there are still relatively limited data on incidence of type 2 DM in Indigenous populations [23, 24]. In the Indigenous population of Alberta, the incidence of diabetes during 1995–2007 increased at a slower rate compared to the general population, even though the overall rates were higher among Indigenous people [24]. There has been one follow-up study using repeat OGTTs, which reported a 17 % diabetes conversion rate over 10 years [27].

In contrast to First Nations, data on diabetes prevalence and incidence among Métis and Inuit communities are sparser. According to the 2009–2010 Canadian Community Health Survey, age-standardized rates of self-reported diabetes among Métis were found to be 7.3 % compared to the non-Indigenous population which was 5 % (Fig. 13.1) [21]. In a recent report on a population-based study in Winnipeg, Manitoba, Métis aged 19 years and older were found to have age- and sex-adjusted diabetes rates that were higher (11.8 %) than compared to the provincial

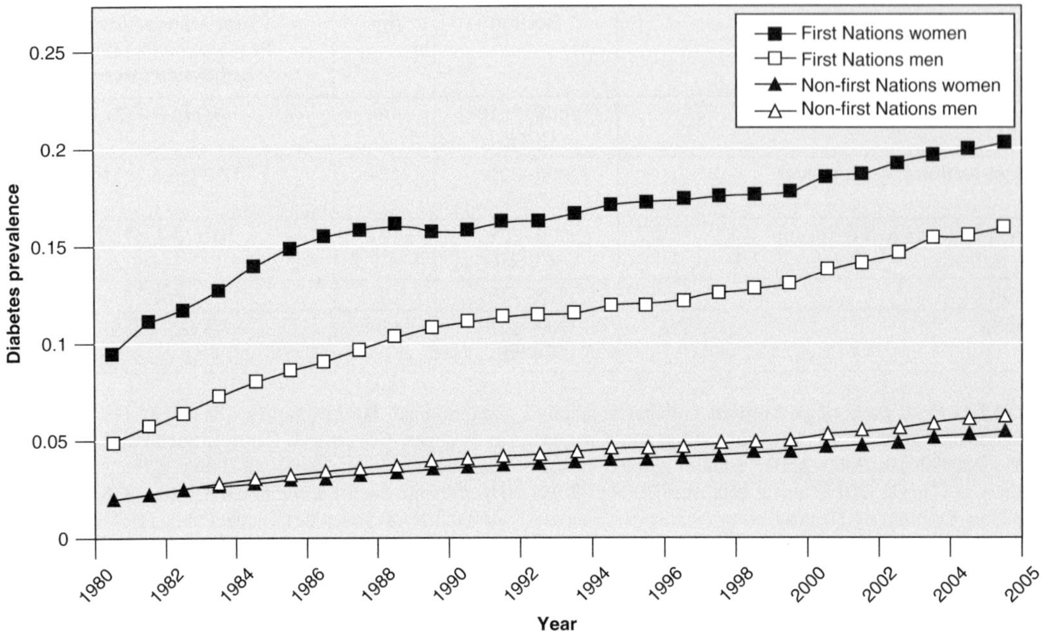

Fig. 13.2 Age-standardized diabetes prevalence in First Nations and non-First Nations men and women from 1990 to 2005 (Dyck et al. [23])

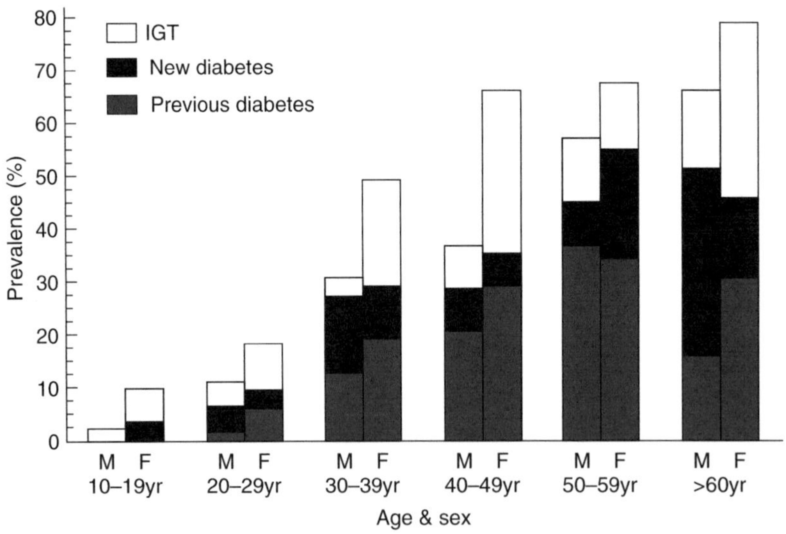

Fig. 13.3 Age- and sex-specific prevalence of impaired glucose intolerance, newly diagnosed diabetes, and previously diagnosed diabetes in Sandy Lake First Nation (Harris et al. [25])

prevalence (8.8 %) [28]. An evaluation of diabetes in 14,480 Métis people in Ontario found the age- and sex-standardized prevalence to be 11.2 % compared to the general population which was 9 % [29].

According to the 2006 Aboriginal Peoples Survey, the crude rate of self-reported type 2 DM in Inuit was 4 % compared to the non-general population which was 5 % (Fig. 13.1) [30]. Although the prevalence of diabetes in the Inuit population has previously been documented to be lower than the other Indigenous groups, recent evidence highlights that it has markedly increased and is now comparable to the general Canadian population [1, 31].

In addition to higher overall prevalence and incidence rates compared to the general population, rates of gestational diabetes mellitus (GDM) are two- to fourfold higher in Indigenous women. The onset of type 2 DM in Indigenous people in Canada occurs at a much earlier age than in most other populations [25], and pediatric type 2 DM is a major public health concern [32, 33]. The increasing incidence of early age of onset of type 2 DM in Indigenous youth over the past several decades is concomitant with increases in the prevalence of childhood obesity [34–39]. Potential risk factors of childhood obesity in Indigenous school-aged children have included physical activity, fitness levels, TV watching, and dietary factors [36, 38, 39]. According to a recent published report from a national surveillance study, the Indigenous Canadian population has the highest incidence rate and is the largest single ethnic group that contributes to new-onset type 2 DM [40, 41]. The report highlights that 100/227 new diabetes cases belong to Indigenous peoples, and 11 % of these cases account for children younger than age 10 years [40, 41]. This accelerated onset of both obesity and type 2 DM suggests that the origins of these disorders may be traced back to infancy and/or the intrauterine environment [42, 43]. The early life/intrauterine risk of type 2 DM will be covered in more detail below.

Complications

Indigenous peoples in Canada experience a heavier burden of diabetes-related comorbidities compared to non-Indigenous peoples [44]. Indigenous peoples are burdened with a higher prevalence of microvascular complications, such as end-stage renal disease [44, 45], lower extremity amputations [46], and retinopathy [46–48] than their non-Indigenous counterparts with type 2 DM. Additionally, higher prevalence rates of macrovascular complications, including atherosclerosis [49] and cardiovascular disease [50], are also evident among Indigenous Canadians compared to non-Indigenous Canadians with type 2 DM [51].

Complications of diabetes in Indigenous peoples are exacerbated by limited social and economic resources, including inadequate access to health services due to geographical barriers [10, 52, 53]. Moreover, complications are likely more prominent in Indigenous populations as a result of an earlier age of diabetes onset. This population also has a higher prevalence of cardiometabolic and lifestyle risk factors for other chronic diseases, including smoking, obesity, and hypertension [25, 54].

One of the most remarkable and worrisome aspects of the type 2 DM complication profile in the Indigenous Canadian population relates to the very heavy burden of kidney disease. A study of incidence rates of diabetic end-stage renal disease in First Nations in Saskatchewan found that even when the higher prevalence of diabetes was taken into account, First Nations with diabetes were still seven times as likely as non-First Nations with diabetes to have end-stage renal disease [45]. Between 1980 and 2000, there was an eightfold increase in the number of Indigenous patients with diabetic end-stage renal disease [55, 56]. Indigenous dialysis patients with end-stage renal disease are found to have reduced rate of kidney transplantation [57]. The remote location of Indigenous patients on dialysis does not explain the lower rate of kidney transplantation among this group [58]. Although referral rates for kidney transplantation assessment are the same for Indigenous patients as for non-Indigenous patients, completion of transplantation documents and wait-listing for transplantation are delayed in Indigenous patients [59].

Indigenous Canadians with end-stage renal disease are more likely to reside in rural or remote locations compared to other dialysis patients. As a result, access to hemodialysis units may not be as readily available. Therefore, peritoneal dialysis might be very helpful for Indigenous patients requiring dialysis as it provides the ability to undergo dialysis at home without visiting a medical facility with a hemodialysis unit [60]. However, data from three Canadian provinces show that there are less frequent Indigenous users of peritoneal dialysis compared to non-Indigenous patients in Canada [60]. Also, patients who were on peritoneal dialysis were more likely to experience technique failure, compared to non-Indigenous patients; however, adjusted risk for death was similar to non-Indigenous patients [60].

Modifiable Risk Factors

Individual

Obesity and Body Composition

Among the modifiable risk factors for type 2 DM, overweight and obesity are the most well documented. The standard measure of body weight in population studies is body mass index (BMI). According to the 2004 Canadian Community Health Survey, the prevalence of obesity (defined using BMI) was higher among Indigenous Canadians (37.8 %) when compared to non-Indigenous Canadians (22.6 %) [61]. The prevalence of obesity was also higher among Indigenous children and youth (15.8 %), when compared to their non-Indigenous counterparts [61, 62].

When determining the prevalence of overweight and obesity in Indigenous peoples, it is salient to consider that the body dimensions of this group, and the Inuit population in particular, are different than other populations [63]. The Inuit are shorter in height and have shorter legs [63]. As a result, in order to improve the assessment of obesity in Inuit people, measures of body fat distribution, such as waist circumference, waist-to-height, and waist-to-hip ratio, should be employed [64–66]. In fact, a meta-analysis of over 300,000 individuals from different populations around the world found that waist-to-hip ratio was a better predictor than waist circumference and BMI for diabetes risk [66]. In a study on First Nations in Ontario, the 10-year cumulative incidence of diabetes was associated with high adiposity (defined as higher body mass index, percent body fat, waist circumference, or waist-to-height ratio) [27].

Smoking

Cigarette smoking has been associated with an increased risk of type 2 DM in a meta-analysis of 25 prospective cohort studies [67]. According to the meta-analysis, the risk of type 2 DM was greater for those who smoked >20 cigarettes a day than those who smoked <20 cigarettes a day [67]. Smoking prevalence is high in Indigenous populations and has been associated with complications of type 2 DM [44]. According to national data from the 2009–2010 Canadian Community Health Survey, the prevalence rates of self-reported smoking among Indigenous peoples aged 18 years and older were twofold higher than the rates of the non-Indigenous population [21]. Moreover, rates of daily tobacco smoking in Indigenous peoples were also 2.2–2.8 times higher than non-Indigenous people [21]. According to the 2012 Aboriginal People's Survey, 52 % of Inuit aged 15 years and older smoked cigarettes daily, and another 9 % were occasional smokers [68].

In a study on First Nations in Ontario, former smoking was found to be associated with low beta-cell function, and current smoking was associated with high beta-cell function, independent of diabetes. Additionally, the association of smoking with insulin resistance varied depending on glycemic status [69]. In another First Nations population, smoking was found to increase incident diabetes risk in carriers of the *HNF1A* G319S allele. After stratification by baseline smoking status, *HNF1A* G319S carriers who were active smokers had increased risk of developing diabetes [70].

Diet

Research on the association of diet with type 2 DM has received considerable attention. Numerous dietary factors such as coffee, fiber, whole grains, and dairy products have been shown to have a protective effect on type 2 DM risk [71–74]. While some dietary factors including sugar-sweetened beverages and high consumption of fat have been associated with an increased risk for type 2 DM [75, 76]. Additionally, specific nutrients such as vitamin D have recently been investigated for their protective effects against the development of type 2 DM [77].

The nutritional habits of Indigenous peoples are of significant interest in the context of the management and prevention of type 2 DM [78]. Until relatively recently, Indigenous people of Canada were nomadic hunters and gatherers who had a traditional diet which consisted of large and small animals and birds (including the flesh and organs of moose, caribou, rabbit, ducks, geese, etc.), freshwater fish, marine fish and mammals, and some plant foods and, most notably, berries [79, 80]. In addition, the Iroquoian peoples of the Great Lakes and St. Lawrence River region farmed corn, beans, squash, and other crops. A significant body of research has documented a marked nutrition transition among Indigenous Canadians, in which the nutritional profile of Indigenous Canadians has changed from a traditional diet to a "market-foods" diet that is characterized by a higher intake in fat (especially saturated fat) and simple and high GI carbohydrates and low fiber [78, 81–84].

While the consumption of traditional foods has declined in general, Indigenous communities in some regions, most notably in the Northwest Territories and Yukon, have maintained a reasonably high degree of traditional food consumption [81, 85, 86]. Traditional food consumption is associated with beneficial impact on micronutrient intake. For instance, days with traditional food consumption are characterized by increased intakes of vitamins D, E, and B6, magnesium, and selenium. In addition, days when Indigenous participants consumed traditional food were characterized by higher intakes of energy as protein, whereas days when traditional food was not consumed were associated with a higher percentage of energy as carbohydrate, sucrose, and saturated and polyunsaturated fatty acids [81]. The potential benefits of high-fiber, high-fruit/vegetable/whole grain, low-fat, low-protein diets in the prevention of type DM among Indigenous Canadians have been studied [36, 38, 84, 87], and the findings have been largely consistent with those from other populations [88–90]. With regard to traditional foods, the consumption of seal oil and salmon has been found to be associated with a reduced risk of glucose intolerance in Indigenous people of Alaska [91]. In addition, in Cree from James Bay, higher traditional food consumption was associated with increased n-3 fatty acids [92]. Overall, however, very limited data are available regarding traditional food consumption and health outcomes among Indigenous peoples.

The transition to a market-foods diet has been accompanied by increasing prevalence of type 2 DM in Indigenous populations [10, 25]. A study in a First Nations community in Ontario found a high intake of total and saturated fat, and a diet high in GI foods was more common in people under 50 years of age, where rates of diabetes are showing their sharpest increase [83]. In another study in the same population, data was obtained using food frequency questionnaires to determine dietary patterns in the community. The intake of foods in the "junk foods" (chips/pop/candy/canned meat) category and fat (especially lard, consumed or used in preparation) category was associated with an increased risk of type 2 DM [84]. Similarly, a junk food dietary pattern (high-fat and high-sugar foods) identified in the Cree from Northern Quebec was associated with increased diabetes risk [92].

Another key public health nutrition problem affecting Indigenous communities is food insecurity. The prevalence of both individual and household food insecurity is much higher for Indigenous people compared to non-Indigenous people, with data from a national survey showing that 33 % of off-reserve Indigenous Canadians were food insecure compared to 9 % of non-Indigenous Canadians [93, 94]. After controlling for differences in household sociodemographic risk factors (including household income, highest level of education in household, household type, number of children, etc.), Indigenous households had two to six times greater odds for food insecurity compared to non-Indigenous households [93, 94]. In a recent national survey on Inuit, 41 % of Inuit aged 15 and older lived in households that experienced food insecurity [68].

Barriers to food security in Indigenous populations include income inadequacy and environmental pollution related to the impact of climate change on traditional food systems [86, 95]. A large number of Indigenous households rely on social assistance for income [93]. In fact, over 66 % of Indigenous households who received social assistance were food insecure [94]. In a study of access to traditional and market foods in 44 Indigenous communities across Arctic Canada, regional variation affected price and ability to purchase adequate food, with between 40 and 70 % of people saying they could afford enough food [96]. Additionally, Indigenous people reported inadequate access to fishing and hunting equipment, and 46 % of people could not afford to go hunting or fishing [96]. Changes in the local environment including changes in water levels have affected harvesting and traditional food acquirement in Indigenous communities [97]. Environmental contaminants in Indigenous traditional food resources such as heavy metals, radionuclides, and organochlorines put the health of Indigenous people at an increased risk [98]. In order to eradicate food insecurity among off-reserve Indigenous populations, government interventions must first address the great burden of poverty in this group by increasing income and social assistance funding for families [93, 95]. Overall, the considerable barriers to both traditional food and healthy market-food access discussed above have significant public health implications for both managing and preventing the type 2 DM epidemic currently being experienced by Indigenous communities in Canada.

Physical Activity

Engaging in physical activity has been well established to improve blood glucose control and has been identified as an important determinant in the prevention and management of type 2 DM [99–101]. A recent meta-analysis found that moderate intensity physical activity including brisk walking was negatively associated with the risk of type 2 DM [102].

Historically, Indigenous peoples engaged in activities such as hunting, fishing, and trapping to obtain sustenance [103]. However, as mentioned earlier, because of the nutrition transition, traditional activities are less prevalent, and this change has had a negative impact on the level of physical activity among Indigenous peoples and increasing the risk of type 2 DM and its complications [103]. According to a study in a First Nations community in Ontario, both physical activity and fitness were associated with lower insulin concentrations, suggesting that physical activity/fitness may be beneficial to the prevention of type 2 DM [104]. Television viewing was associated with childhood obesity in Mohawk children of Kahnawake [105]. Similarly, in First Nations people aged 10–19 years, 5 or more hours of television viewing/day was associated with a significantly higher risk of overweight than 2 or less hours of television viewing/day [36].

Intrauterine/Early Life Factors

High rates of youth-onset obesity and type 2 DM in Indigenous communities suggest that risk factors are operating very early in life, perhaps even in the intrauterine period. Recent research arising from the Developmental Origins of Health and Disease (DOHaD) paradigm has highlighted the importance to chronic disease etiology of a number of factors that have a significant importance in the context of type 2 DM in Indigenous Canadians [106], including high birth weight, gestational diabetes, and suboptimal breastfeeding.

High birth weight can have both immediate- and longer-term health consequences on infants, including shoulder dystocia, and an increased risk of type 2 DM [107, 108]. High birth weight appears to be closely associated with maternal diabetes and overweight. Consequently, as the prevalence of maternal obesity and gestational diabetes mellitus (GDM) continues to increase, higher birth weight babies will become increasingly prevalent as well [109].

There have been consistent observations of high birth weight in Indigenous Canadian babies [110, 111]. The prevalence of high birth weight in Cree was 34.3 % compared to 11 % in their non-Indigenous counterparts [112]. In a recent study on First Nations women in Northern and in Southern Quebec, First Nations women were more likely to have high birth weight babies than non-Indigenous women [113]. Similarly, a study reporting singleton births from Cree women living in rural or remote communities in Northern Quebec found prevalence rates of 2.4 % for low birth weight and 36.5 % for high birth weight. In the same study, infants who weighed >4500 g had a 14 % higher prevalence of birth injuries and were more likely born to women with GDM [114]. Another study on First Nations in Quebec reported a significant association between macrosomia and postnatal mortality [115].

Population Level

Environmental/Socioeconomic Risk Factors

Notwithstanding the importance of risk factors that occur at the level of the individual, it is increasingly being recognized that factors that characterize the local or broader social, environmental, and/or geographical environment are playing a critical role in the etiology of type 2 DM in Indigenous communities in Canada. These environmental risk factors for type 2 DM have emerged largely from historic policies of colonization unique to the Indigenous context [116]. In particular, the health and social conditions of Indigenous peoples vary significantly depending on residence on-reserve versus off-reserve and in rural versus urban areas [117]. Living in remote or rural areas may lead to limited opportunities for education and employment and reduced access to a safe and healthy food supply [20, 117]. Geographic and language barriers may also result in reduced access to health-care services [118]. As well, there is limited availability of culturally appropriate services in Indigenous communities [20, 119]. These limitations may potentially affect the prevalence and distribution of type 2 DM in Indigenous peoples by affecting the level of care and treatment available for type 2 DM and its complications [117].

Non-modifiable Risk Factors

Genetics

Genome-wide association studies (GWAS) of type 2 DM over the past several years have identified numerous susceptibility genes for type 2 DM [120–123]. Specific population groups have been shown to possess predisposing alleles to type 2 DM [124]. Indeed, high rates of type 2 DM in Indigenous communities in Canada suggest an inherited component. Early interest in the search for a single "Thrifty" gene [125] explaining the high type 2 DM burden in Indigenous Canadians was unsuccessful, due to the fact that type 2 DM in these communities is very likely caused by the cumulative small effects of multiple genes operating on the background of a detrimental environment [10, 126]. Nonetheless, a private mutation in the HNF1α gene (namely, G319S), restricted to the Oji-Cree population of Northwestern Ontario and Northeastern Manitoba, has been shown to be associated with an increased risk for type 2 DM [127]. In fact, by 50 years of age, HNF1α S319 has specificity (97 %) and positive predictive values (95 %) for the development of diabetes in the Oji-Cree population [106].

Clinical Care

For Indigenous people, health-care access and delivery depends on location, with urban and off-reserve Indigenous peoples accessing health care from provincially funded services. In contrast, as a part of the set of obligations arising from signed treaties with the federal government, health-care delivery on-reserves is delivered by federally operated nursing stations and health centers. The First Nations and Inuit Health Branch (FNIHB) provides health benefits to First Nations and Inuit that are noninsured by provincial insurance plans, including prescription drugs and dental and vision coverage [128, 129]. Physician services and hospital care are provided by the government of each province or territory [128]. The federal government's role in Indigenous health occurs primarily through public health and intervention strategies [128]. With regard to federal programs that specifically target diabetes, the Aboriginal Diabetes Initiative supports health promotion and type 2 DM prevention programs which are disseminated by community diabetes workers [129].

The current health-care delivery system in Indigenous communities consists predominately of acute and intermittent care management instead of coordinated chronic disease care [130]. As a result of geographical isolation, limited staff and other nonphysician health professionals provide clinical care in these communities [118]. Additionally, hospital admissions for ambulatory care conditions are much higher in Indigenous communities [131–133], and there is poor communication between provincially funded hospitals and federal nursing care centers in most Indigenous communities [33].

Research has documented suboptimal clinical care for diabetes among on-reserve First Nations peoples in Canada. These clinical care gaps are attributable to geographical isolation, limited health-care staff, poor chronic disease management, limited surveillance, and high staff turnover [134]. Despite the high burden of chronic disease in the Indigenous population, including type 2 DM, the use of primary health care is lower among Indigenous populations compared to the general population [132].

National data from the Western provinces (British Columbia, Alberta, Saskatchewan, and Manitoba) on type 2 DM burden and clinical care gaps found that the age-standardized hospital discharge rate was seven times higher in First Nations peoples living on- and off-reserve compared to the general population [119].

There is a higher mortality rate (19.5 per 100,000) due to type 2 DM in Indigenous Canadians compared to non-Indigenous Canadians (13.3 per 100,000) [135]. Although there is less frequent use of primary health services among Indigenous peoples in Northern or isolated communities [136], the per capita health-care costs of Indigenous populations with and without type 2 DM are much higher compared to non-Indigenous populations [137]. Particularly, health-care usage, including physician appointments, hospital visits, and dialysis, is 40–60% higher among First Nations in Saskatchewan with type 2 DM compared to the non-Indigenous population without type 2 DM [137].

Recently, a new program called the Trans formation of Indigenous Primary Healthcare Delivery (FORGE AHEAD) has been initiated in five First Nations communities across Canada to improve diabetes management through the development of community-based, culturally relevant primary health-care models. FORGE AHEAD also aims to develop appropriate access to services in First Nations communities [138].

Primary Prevention

There is a great necessity for Indigenous-specific diabetes prevention and intervention strategies that consider the unique cultures and traditions of First Nations, Métis, and Inuit people. Interventions which include tenets such as community involvement, face-to-face interventions, development of skills to promote behavior change, and the dissemination of educational and nutritional knowledge are required to alleviate the burden of type 2 DM in marginalized communities [139].

In the late 1990s, the government of Canada established the Aboriginal Diabetes Initiative to help improve the heavy burden of type 2 DM among First Nations, Inuit, and Métis [129]. The program has been delivered in three phases. The first phase, ADI Phase 1 (1999), allocated $115 M over 5 years for health promotion and primary prevention programming. The second phase, ADI Phase 2 (2005–2010), allocated $190 M over 5 years to strengthen community-based health promotion and diabetes prevention activities. The current phase, ADI Phase 3 (2010–2015), has allocated $275 M for continued support of health promotion and diabetes prevention activities and services.

Over the past 25 years, the Sandy Lake Health and Diabetes Project (SLHDP) has been addressing the high rates of type 2 DM in Sandy Lake First Nation in Ontario. The SLHDP has developed and implemented a number of community-wide interventions including community health promotion events, community surveys to track type 2 DM prevalence and risk factors, a grocery store program which aims to increase knowledge of healthy food choices, a community-wide walking trail to encourage physical activity, summer camps for youth, a diabetes radio program, and a school curriculum [140]. The Sandy Lake First

Nation school diabetes prevention program developed and evaluated a healthy diet and exercise curriculum for 1 year in children in grades 3–5 [141]. After 1 year, there were reductions in dietary fat, and increases in dietary fiber as well as an improvement in dietary knowledge, and an increase in confidence and intention to choose healthy foods [141].

The Kahnawake Schools Diabetes Prevention Program (KSDPP) is a community-based, primary diabetes prevention program based in Kahnawake Mohawk Territory, Canada, that aims to improve healthy eating and increase physical activity in school children. The school curriculum is delivered in ten 45-min sessions every year for all six grades. The curriculum focuses on lifestyle, nutrition, and diabetes education [142]. The program has also implemented a recreation path and a Community Advisory Board [142]. Results of 8 years of follow-up from the program showed early positive effects on a risk factor (skinfold thickness) for type 2 DM and a decrease in consumption of high-fat and high-sugar foods. Although physical activity, fitness, and television watching improved early on as well, they were not maintained at the 8-year follow-up date [143].

Recently, another school intervention in three remote First Nations communities in British Columbia promoted healthy eating and physical activity through "action plans" by teachers and administrators in Indigenous youth. Although the intervention did not find any changes in physical activity or overall cardiovascular risk, it did see an improvement in aerobic fitness [144].

Despite recent advances with community-based activities geared toward increasing physical activity and healthy eating practices in these communities, inadequate environmental and social support for physical activity and healthy eating practices remains an ongoing challenge. The results summarized above offer a reason for optimism regarding the impact and availability of type 2 DM interventions targeted for Indigenous populations. However, challenges include the need to implement these programs more broadly and support their sustainability. In this context, there is a greater need to support Indigenous populations with the necessary resources (health-care services, education, adequate funding), so they are able to prevent/control the occurrence of type 2 DM with a high-level of skill and independence.

Conclusions

Type 2 DM has been increasing dramatically in the Indigenous population of Canada over the past six decades and has reached epidemic levels in some communities. The high prevalence of type 2 DM and its complications among Indigenous populations is a major public health issue. Indigenous peoples also have a higher prevalence for cardiometabolic and lifestyle risk factors for other chronic diseases, including hypertension, obesity, unhealthy eating patterns, and smoking. Many of these occur on a background of the social determinants of health, including poverty, poor housing, low educational attainment, unemployment, and inadequate community resources. Clinical care for diabetes in Indigenous communities is also suboptimal. Despite recent advances with community-based interventions geared toward increasing physical activity and healthy eating practices in these communities, inadequate environmental and social support for physical activity and healthy eating practices remains an ongoing challenge. Moreover, there is an important need to increase the amount of high-quality interventions for prevention of type 2 DM in Indigenous peoples. Overall, in order to alleviate the heavy burden of type 2 DM and its complications among the Indigenous population, both culturally appropriate primary prevention programs and clinical care strategies that include the participation of community members are urgently required.

References

1. Public Health Agency of Canada. Diabetes in Canada: facts and figures from a public health perspective. Ottawa: Public Health Agency of Canada; 2011.
2. Friesen JW. Rediscovering the First Nations of Canada. Chicago: Detselig Enterprises Limited; 1997.

3. Statistics Canada. Aboriginal peoples in Canada: first nations people, Métis and Inuit: National Household Survey, 2011. Ottawa: Minister of Industry; 2011. 978-1-100-22203-5.
4. Lischke U, McNab DT. The long journey of a forgotten people: Métis identities and family histories. Waterloo: Wilfrid Laurier University Press; 2007.
5. Stern PR. Historical dictionary of the Inuit. Lanham: Scarecrow Press; 2013.
6. Langlois S, Turner A. In: Canada S, editor. Aboriginal languages in Canada. Ottawa: Minister of Industry; 2012.
7. Malenfant EC, Morency JD. Population projections by Aboriginal Identity in Canada, 2006 to 2031. Statistics Canada; 2011.
8. Statistics Canada. Aboriginal peoples in Canada: First nations people, Métis and Inuit: National household survey, 2011;99 - 011 - X2011001. Canada: Minister of Industry; 2013.
9. Reading CL, Wien F. Health inequalities and social determinants of aboriginal people's health. Prince George: National Collaborating Centre for Aboriginal Health; 2009.
10. Young TK, Reading J, Elias B, O'Neil JD. Type 2 diabetes mellitus in Canada's First nations: status of an epidemic in progress. CMAJ. 2000;163(5):561–6.
11. Reading J. The crisis of chronic disease among aboriginal peoples: a challenge for public health, population health and social policy. Victoria: Centre for Aboriginal Health Research: University of Victoria Press; 2009.
12. Chase LA. The trend of diabetes in Saskatchewan, 1905 to 1934. Can Med Assoc J. 1937;36(4):366–9.
13. Montour LT, Macaulay AC. High prevalence rates of diabetes mellitus and hypertension on a North American Indian reservation. Can Med Assoc J. 1985;132(10):1110, 2.
14. Evers S, McCracken E, Antone I, Deagle G. The prevalence of diabetes in Indians and Caucasians living in Southwestern Ontario. Can J Public Health. 1987;78(4):240–3.
15. Young TK, Szathmary EJ, Evers S, Wheatley B. Geographical distribution of diabetes among the native population of Canada: a national survey. Soc Sci Med. 1990;31(2):129–39.
16. Brassard P, Robinson E, Lavallée C. Prevalence of diabetes mellitus among the James Bay Cree of northern Quebec. CMAJ. 1993;149(3):303–7.
17. Pioro MP, Dyck RF, Gillis DC. Diabetes prevalence rates among First Nations adults on Saskatchewan reserves in 1990: comparison by tribal grouping, geography and with non-First Nations people. Can J Public Health. 1996;87(5):325–8.
18. Fox C, Harris S, Whalen-Brough E. Diabetes among Native Canadians in northwestern Ontario: 10 years later. Chron Dis Canada. 1994;15:92–6.
19. Office of the Auditor General of Canada. Chapter 4, Programs for First Nations on Reserves, of the 2011 Report of the Auditor General of Canada. In: Standing Committee on Public Accounts. Status Report of the Auditor General of Canada to the House of Commons. Report. Ottawa, Canada; 2011.
20. First Nations Information Governance Canada. First Nations regional longitudinal health survey (RHS) 2002/03: results for adults, youth and children living in first nations communities. Ottawa: Assembly of First Nations, First Nations Information Governance Centre; 2007.
21. Statistics Canada. Canadian Community Health Survey (CCHS); 2011.
22. Green C, Blanchard JF, Young TK, Griffith J. The epidemiology of diabetes in the Manitoba-registered First Nation population: current patterns and comparative trends. Diabetes Care. 2003;26(7):1993–8.
23. Dyck R, Osgood N, Lin TH, Gao A, Stang MR. Epidemiology of diabetes mellitus among First Nations and non-First Nations adults. CMAJ. 2010;182(3):249–56.
24. Oster RT, Johnson JA, Hemmelgarn BR, King M, Balko SU, Svenson LW, et al. Recent epidemiologic trends of diabetes mellitus among status Aboriginal adults. CMAJ. 2011;183(12):E803–8.
25. Harris SB, Gittelsohn J, Hanley A, Barnie A, Wolever TM, Gao J, et al. The prevalence of NIDDM and associated risk factors in native Canadians. Diabetes Care. 1997;20(2):185–7.
26. Delisle HF, Ekoé JM. Prevalence of non-insulin-dependent diabetes mellitus and impaired glucose tolerance in two Algonquin communities in Quebec. CMAJ. 1993;148(1):41–7.
27. Ley SH, Harris SB, Mamakeesick M, Noon T, Fiddler E, Gittelsohn J, et al. Metabolic syndrome and its components as predictors of incident type 2 diabetes mellitus in an Aboriginal community. CMAJ: Can Med Assoc J = J Assoc Med Can. 2009;180(6):617–24.
28. Martens P, Bartlett J, Burland E, Prior H, Burchill C, Huq S, et al. Métis health status and healthcare utilization in Manitoba: a population-based study. Winnipeg: Manitoba Centre for Health Policy; 2010.
29. Shah BR, Cauch-Dudek K, Pigeau L. Diabetes prevalence and care in the Métis population of Ontario, Canada. Diabetes Care. 2011;34(12):2555–6.
30. Aboriginal Peoples Survey, 2006: Inuit health and social conditions: supporting data tables. In: Statistics Canada, editor. Ottawa: Statistics Canada; 2008.
31. EgelandGM,CaoZ,YoungTK.Hypertriglyceridemic-waist phenotype and glucose intolerance among Canadian Inuit: the international polar year Inuit health survey for adults 2007–2008. CMAJ. 2011;183:E553–8.
32. Dean HJ, Mundy RL, Moffatt M. Non-insulin dependent diabetes mellitus in Indian children in Manitoba. Can Med Assoc J. 1992;147:52–7.
33. Harris SB, Perkins B, Whalen-Brough E. Non-insulin dependent diabetes mellitus among First Nations children: new entity among First Nations people of northwestern Ontario. Can Fam Phys. 1996;42:869–76.

34. Hannon TS, Rao G, Arslanian SA. Childhood obesity and type 2 diabetes mellitus. Pediatrics. 2005;116(2):473–80.
35. Zdravkovic V, Daneman D, Hamilton J. Presentation and course of Type 2 diabetes in youth in a large multi-ethnic city. Diabet Med. 2004;21(10):1144–8.
36. Hanley AJ, Harris SB, Gittelsohn J, Wolever TM, Saksvig B, Zinman B. Overweight among children and adolescents in a Native Canadian community: prevalence and associated factors. Am J Clin Nutr. 2000;71(3):693–700.
37. Willows ND, Johnson MS, Ball GD. Prevalence estimates of overweight and obesity in Cree preschool children in northern Quebec according to international and US reference criteria. Am J Public Health. 2007;97(2):311–6.
38. Bernard L, Lavallee C, Gray-Donald K, Delisle H. Overweight in Cree schoolchildren and adolescents associated with diet, low physical activity, and high television viewing. J Am Diet Assoc. 1995;95(7):800–2.
39. Willows ND. Overweight in Aboriginal children: prevalence, implications, and solutions. J Aborig Health. 2005;2:76–85.
40. Amed S, Dean HJ, Panagiotopoulos C, Sellers EA, Hadjiyannakis S, Laubscher TA, et al. Type 2 diabetes, medication-induced diabetes, and monogenic diabetes in Canadian children: a prospective national surveillance study. Diabetes Care. 2010;33(4):786–91.
41. Amed S, Hamilton JK, Sellers EA, Panagiotopoulos C, Hadjiyannakis S, Shah BR, et al. Differing clinical features in Aboriginal vs. non-Aboriginal children presenting with type 2 diabetes. Pediatr Diabetes. 2012;13(6):470–5.
42. Silverman BL, Rizzo TA, Cho NH, Metzger BE. Long-term effects of the intrauterine environment. The Northwestern University Diabetes in Pregnancy Center. Diabetes Care. 1998;21 Suppl 2:B142–9.
43. Druet C, Ong KK. Early childhood predictors of adult body composition. Best Pract Res Clin Endocrinol Metab. 2008;22(3):489–502.
44. Hanley AJ, Harris SB, Mamakeesick M, Goodwin K, Fiddler E, Hegele RA, et al. Complications of Type 2 diabetes among Aboriginal Canadians: prevalence and associated risk factors. Diabetes Care. 2005;28(8):2054–7.
45. Dyck RF, Tan L. Rates and outcomes of diabetic end-stage renal disease among registered native people in Saskatchewan. CMAJ. 1994;150(2):203–8.
46. McIntyre I, Boughen C, Trepman E, Embil JM. Foot and ankle problems of Aboriginal and non-Aboriginal diabetic patients with end-stage renal disease. Foot Ankle Int. 2007;28(6):674–86.
47. Maberley D, Walker H, Koushik A, Cruess A. Screening for diabetic retinopathy in James Bay, Ontario: a cost-effectiveness analysis. CMAJ. 2003;168(2):160–4.
48. Ross SA, McKenna A, Mozejko S, Fick GH. Diabetic retinopathy in native and nonnative Canadians. Exp Diabetes Res. 2007;2007:76271.
49. Macaulay AC, Montour LT, Adelson N. Prevalence of diabetic and atherosclerotic complications among Mohawk Indians of Kahnawake, PQ. CMAJ. 1988;139:221–4.
50. Shah BR, Hux JE, Zinman B. Increasing rates of ischemic heart disease in the native population of Ontario, Canada. Arch Intern Med. 2000;160(12):1862–6.
51. Naqshbandi M, Harris SB, Esler JB, Antwi-Nsiah F. Global complication rates of type 2 diabetes in indigenous peoples: a comprehensive review. Diabetes Res Clin Pract. 2008;82(1):1–17.
52. Health Canada. Diabetes among Aboriginal people in Canada: the evidence. Ottawa: Health Canada; 2001.
53. Martens PJ, Martin BD, O'Neil JD, MacKinnon M. Diabetes and adverse outcomes in a First Nations population: associations with healthcare access, and socioeconomic and geographical factors. Can J Diabetes. 2007;31(3):223–32.
54. Oster RT, Toth EL. Differences in the prevalence of diabetes risk-factors among First Nation, Métis and non-Aboriginal adults attending screening clinics in rural Alberta, Canada. Rural Remote Health. 2009;9(2):1170.
55. Dyck RF. Mechanisms of renal disease in indigenous populations: influences at work in Canadian indigenous peoples. Nephrology. 2001;6:3–7.
56. Register COR. Annual report. vol. 1: dialysis and renal transplantation. Ottawa: Canadian Institute for Health Information; 2001.
57. Yeates KE. Aboriginal patients on the road to kidney transplantation: is residence location a barrier? Kidney Int. 2006;70(5):826–8.
58. Tonelli M, Hemmelgarn B, Kim AK, Bertazzon S, Klarenbach S, Manns B, et al. Association between residence location and likelihood of kidney transplantation in Aboriginal patients treated with dialysis in Canada. Kidney Int. 2006;70(5):924–30.
59. Tonelli M, Chou S, Gourishankar S, Jhangri GS, Bradley J, Hemmelgarn B, et al. Wait-listing for kidney transplantation among Aboriginal hemodialysis patients. Am J Kidney Dis. 2005;46(6):1117–23.
60. Tonelli M, Hemmelgarn B, Manns B, Davison S, Bohm C, Gourishankar S, et al. Use and outcomes of peritoneal dialysis among Aboriginal people in Canada. J Am Soc Nephrol. 2005;16(2):482–8.
61. Statistics Canada. Canadian community health survey, nutrition: general health component, public use microdata file guide. Ottawa: Health Statistics Division, Statistics Canada; 2005.
62. Katzmarzyk PT. Obesity and physical activity among Aboriginal Canadians. Obesity (Silver Spring). 2008;16(1):184–90.
63. Charbonneau-Roberts G, Saudny-Unterberger H, Kuhnlein HV, Egeland GM. Body mass index may

overestimate the prevalence of overweight and obesity among the Inuitd. Int J Circumpolar Health. 2005;64(4):163–9.
64. Weyer C, Funahashi T, Tanaka S, Hotta K, Matsuzawa Y, Pratley RE, et al. Hypoadiponectinemia in obesity and type 2 diabetes: close association with insulin resistance and hyperinsulinemia. J Clin Endocrinol Metab. 2001;86(5):1930–5.
65. Warne DK, Charles MA, Hanson RL, Jacobsson LT, McCance DR, Knowler WC, et al. Comparison of body size measurements as predictors of NIDDM in Pima Indians. Diabetes Care. 1995;18(4):435–9.
66. Ashwell M, Gunn P, Gibson S. Waist-to-height ratio is a better screening tool than waist circumference and BMI for adult cardiometabolic risk factors: systematic review and meta-analysis. Obes Rev Off J Int Assoc Study Obes. 2012;13(3):275–86.
67. Willi C, Bodenmann P, Ghali WA, Faris PD, Cornuz J. Active smoking and the risk of type 2 diabetes: a systematic review and meta-analysis. JAMA: J Am Med Assoc U S. 2007;298:2654–64.
68. Wallace S. Inuit health: selected findings from the 2012 Aboriginal peoples survey. Statistics Canada. 2014 89-653-X-003.
69. Daniel M, Cargo MD. Association between smoking, insulin resistance and beta-cell function in a Northwestern First Nation. Diabet Med. 2004;21(2): 188–93.
70. Ley SH, Hegele RA, Harris SB, Mamakeesick M, Cao H, Connelly PW, et al. HNF1A G319S variant, active cigarette smoking and incident type 2 diabetes in Aboriginal Canadians: a population-based epidemiological study. BMC Med Genet. 2011;12:1.
71. Wolever TM. Dietary carbohydrates and insulin action in humans. Br J Nutr. 2000;83 Suppl 1:S97–102.
72. Wolfram T, Ismail-Beigi F. Efficacy of high-fiber diets in the management of type 2 diabetes mellitus. Endocr Pract Off J Am Coll Endocrinol Am Assoc Clin Endocrinol. 2011;17(1):132–42.
73. Tunnicliffe JM, Shearer J. Coffee, glucose homeostasis, and insulin resistance: physiological mechanisms and mediators. Appl Phys Nutr Metab = Physiol Appl Nutr Metab. 2008;33(6):1290–300.
74. Tong X, Dong JY, Wu ZW, Li W, Qin LQ. Dairy consumption and risk of type 2 diabetes mellitus: a meta-analysis of cohort studies. Eur J Clin Nutr. 2011;65(9):1027–31.
75. Malik VS, Schulze MB, Hu FBCPCN. Intake of sugar-sweetened beverages and weight gain: a systematic review. Am J Clin Nutr. 2006;84:274–88.
76. Bray GA, Popkin BM. Dietary fat intake does affect obesity! Am J Clin Nutr. 1998;68(6):1157–73.
77. Mansuri S, Badawi A, Kayaniyil S, Cole DE, Harris SB, Mamakeesick M, et al. Associations of circulating 25(OH)D with cardiometabolic disorders underlying type 2 diabetes mellitus in an Aboriginal Canadian community. Diabetes Res Clin Pract. 2015;109(2):440–9.
78. Kuhnlein HV, Receveur O, Soueida R, Berti PR. Unique patterns of dietary adequacy in three cultures of Canadian Arctic indigenous peoples. Public Health Nutr. 2008;11(4):349–60.
79. Johnson-Down L, Egeland GM. Adequate nutrient intakes are associated with traditional food consumption in nunavut Inuit children aged 3–5 years. J Nutr. 2010;140(7):1311–6.
80. Receveur O, Kuhnlein HV. Benefits of traditional food in Dene/Métis communities. Int J Circumpolar Health. 1998;57 Suppl 1:219–21.
81. Kuhnlein HV, Receveur O, Soueida R, Egeland GM. Arctic indigenous peoples experience the nutrition transition with changing dietary patterns and obesity. J Nutr. 2004;134(6):1447–53.
82. Sharma S, Cao X, Roache C, Buchan A, Reid R, Gittelsohn J. Assessing dietary intake in a population undergoing a rapid transition in diet and lifestyle: the Arctic Inuit in Nunavut, Canada. Br J Nutr. 2010;103(5):749–59.
83. Wolever TMS, Hamad S, Gittelsohn J, Hanley AJG, Logan A, Harris SB, et al. Nutrient intake and food use in an Ojibwa-Cree community in Northern Ontario assessed by 24h dietary recall. Nutr Res. 1997;17:603–18.
84. Gittelsohn J, Wolever TM, Harris SB, Harris-Giraldo R, Hanley AJ, Zinman B. Specific patterns of food consumption and preparation are associated with diabetes and obesity in a Native Canadian community. J Nutr. 1998;128:541–7.
85. Batal M, Gray-Donald K, Kuhnlein HV, Receveur O. Estimation of traditional food intake in indigenous communities in Denendeh and the Yukon. Int J Circumpolar Health. 2005;64(1):46–54.
86. Receveur O, Boulay M, Kuhnlein HV. Decreasing traditional food use affects diet quality for adult Dene/Métis in 16 communities of the Canadian Northwest Territories. J Nutr. 1997;127(11):2179–86.
87. Wolever TM, Hamad S, Gittelsohn J, Gao J, Hanley AJ, Harris SB, et al. Low dietary fiber and high protein intakes associated with newly diagnosed diabetes in a remote aboriginal community. Am J Clin Nutr. 1997;66(6):1470–4.
88. Costacou T, Mayer-Davis EJ. Nutrition and prevention of type 2 diabetes. Annu Rev Nutr. 2003;23:147–70.
89. Schulze MB, Hu FB. Primary prevention of diabetes: what can be done and how much can be prevented? Annu Rev Public Health. 2005;26: 445–67.
90. Parillo M, Riccardi G. Diet composition and the risk of type 2 diabetes: epidemiological and clinical evidence. Br J Nutr. 2004;92(1):7–19.
91. Adler AI, Boyko EJ, Schraer CD, Murphy NJ. Lower prevalence of impaired glucose tolerance and diabetes associated with daily seal oil or salmon consumption among Alaska Natives. Diabetes Care. 1994; 17(12):1498–501.
92. Johnson-Down L, Labonte ME, Martin ID, Tsuji LJ, Nieboer E, Dewailly E, et al. Quality of diet is associated with insulin resistance in the Cree (Eeyouch) indigenous population of northern Quebec. Nutr Metab Cardiovasc Dis. 2015;25(1):85–92

93. Willows ND, Veugelers P, Raine K, Kuhle S. Prevalence and sociodemographic risk factors related to household food security in Aboriginal peoples in Canada. Public Health Nutr. 2009;12(8):1150–6.
94. Office of Nutrition Policy and Promotion and Health Canada. Canadian Community Health Survey Cycle 2.2, Nutrition (2004): Income-Related Household Food Security in Canada. Health Canada: Ottawa, ON, 2007.
95. Power EM. Conceptualizing food security or aboriginal people in Canada. Can J Public Health. 2008;99:95–7.
96. Lambden J, Receveur O, Marshall J, Kuhnlein HV. Traditional and market food access in Arctic Canada is affected by economic factors. Int J Circumpolar Health. 2006;65(4):331–40.
97. Guyot M, Dickson C, Paci M, Furgal F, Chan HM. Local observations of climate change and impacts on traditional food security in two northern Aboriginal communities. Int J Circumpolar Health. 2006;65:403–15.
98. Kuhnlein HV, Chan HM. Environment and contaminants in traditional food systems of northern indigenous peoples. Annu Rev Nutr. 2000;20:595–626.
99. Hu FB, Manson JE, Stampfer MJ, Colditz G, Liu S, Solomon CG, et al. Diet, lifestyle, and the risk of type 2 diabetes mellitus in women. N Engl J Med. 2001;345(11):790–7.
100. Hu FB, Li TY, Colditz GA, Willett WC, Manson JE. Television watching and other sedentary behaviors in relation to risk of obesity and type 2 diabetes mellitus in women. JAMA. 2003;289(14):1785–91.
101. Colberg SR, Sigal RJ, Fernhall B, Regensteiner JG, Blissmer BJ, Rubin RR, et al. Exercise and type 2 diabetes: the American College of Sports Medicine and the American Diabetes Association: joint position statement executive summary. Diabetes Care. 2010;33(12):2692–6.
102. Jeon CY, Lokken RP, Hu FB, van Dam RM. Physical activity of moderate intensity and risk of type 2 diabetes: a systematic review. Diabetes Care. 2007;30(3):744–52.
103. Reading J. Confronting the growing crisis of cardiovascular disease and heart health among Aboriginal peoples in Canada. Can J Cardiol. 2015;31(9):1077–80.
104. Kriska AM, Hanley AJ, Harris SB, Zinman B. Physical activity, physical fitness, and insulin and glucose concentrations in an isolated Native Canadian population experiencing rapid lifestyle change. Diabetes Care. 2001;24(10):1787–92.
105. Horn OK, Paradis G, Potvin L, Macaulay AC, Desrosiers S. Correlates and predictors of adiposity among Mohawk children. Prev Med. 2001;33(4):274–81.
106. Hegele RA. Genes and environment in type 2 diabetes and atherosclerosis in aboriginal Canadians. Curr Atheroscler Rep. 2001;3(3):216–21.
107. Group HSCR, Metzger BE, Lowe LP, Dyer AR, Trimble ER, Chaovarindr U, et al. Hyperglycemia and adverse pregnancy outcomes. N Engl J Med. 2008;358(19):1991–2002.
108. Boney CM, Verma A, Tucker R, Vohr BR. Metabolic syndrome in childhood: association with birth weight, maternal obesity, and gestational diabetes mellitus. Pediatrics. 2005;115(3):e290–6.
109. Dyck R, Klomp H, Tan LK, Turnell RW, Boctor MA. A comparison of rates, risk factors, and outcomes of gestational diabetes between aboriginal and non-aboriginal women in the Saskatoon health district. Diabetes Care. 2002;25(3):487–93.
110. Munroe M, Shah CP, Badgley R, Bain HW. Birth weight, length, head circumference and bilirubin level in Indian newborns in the Sioux Lookout Zone, northwestern Ontario. Can Med Assoc J. 1984;131(5):453–6.
111. Thomson M. Heavy birth weight in Native Indians of British Columbia. Can J Public Health. 1990;81(6):443–6.
112. Rodrigues S, Robinson EJ, Kramer MS, Gray-Donald K. High rates of infant macrosomia: a comparison of a Canadian native and a non-native population. J Nutr. 2000;130(4):806–12.
113. Luo ZC, Wilkins R, Heaman M, Smylie J, Martens PJ, McHugh NG, et al. Birth outcomes and infant mortality among First Nations Inuit, and non-indigenous women by northern versus southern residence, Quebec. J Epidemiol Community Health. 2012;66(4):328–33.
114. Willows ND, Sanou D, Bell RC. Assessment of Canadian Cree infants' birth size using the WHO Child Growth Standards. Am J Hum Biol. 2011;23(1):126–31.
115. Wassimi S, Wilkins R, McHugh NG, Xiao L, Simonet F, Luo ZC. Association of macrosomia with perinatal and postneonatal mortality among First Nations people in Quebec. CMAJ. 2011;183(3):322–6.
116. Kirmayer LJ, Brass GM, Tait CL. The mental health of Aboriginal peoples: transformations of identity and community. Can J Psychiatry. 2000;45(7):607–16.
117. Tjepkema M. The health of the off-reserve Aboriginal population. In: Canada S, editor. Supplement to health reports. Ottawa: Statistics Canada; 2002.
118. Health Canada. Rural health in rural hands: strategic directions for rural, remote, northern and aboriginal communities. Health Canada, 2002. [cited 2000 July 20]. Available from http://publications.gc.ca/pub?id=9.689374&sl=0.
119. Carriere G, Garner R, Sanmartin C, LHAD. Acute-care hospitalizations and aboriginal identity in Canada, 2001/2001. Ottawa: Statistics Canada; 2010.
120. Imamura M, Maeda S. Genetics of type 2 diabetes: the GWAS era and future perspectives. Rev Endocr J. 2011;58(9):723–39.

121. Billings LK, Florez JC. The genetics of type 2 diabetes: what have we learned from GWAS? Ann N Y Acad Sci. 2010;1212:59–77.
122. Lyssenko V, Laakso M. Genetic screening for the risk of type 2 diabetes: worthless or valuable? Diabetes Care. 2013;36 Suppl 2:S120–6.
123. Medici F, Hawa M, Ianari A, Pyke DA, Leslie RD. Concordance rate for type II diabetes mellitus in monozygotic twins: actuarial analysis. Diabetologia. 1999;42(2):146–50.
124. Chen R, Corona E, Sikora M, Dudley JT, Morgan AA, Moreno-Estrada A, et al. Type 2 diabetes risk alleles demonstrate extreme directional differentiation among human populations, compared to other diseases. PLoS Genet. 2012;8(4):e1002621.
125. Neel JV. Diabetes mellitus: a "thrifty" genotype rendered detrimental by "progress"? Am J Hum Genet. 1962;14:353–62.
126. Hegele RA, Cao H, Harris SB, Hanley AJ, Zinman B. The hepatic nuclear factor-1alpha G319S variant is associated with early-onset type 2 diabetes in Canadian Oji-Cree. J Clin Endocrinol Metab. 1999;84(3):1077–82.
127. Pollex RL, Hanley AJ, Zinman B, Harris SB, Hegele RA. Clinical and genetic associations with hypertriglyceridemic waist in a Canadian aboriginal population. Int J Obes (2005). 2006;30(3):484–91.
128. Health Canada. Fact sheet- First Nations and Inuit health branch health Canada website 2008 (updated 2008; cited 26 Feb 2016). Available from http://www.hc-sc.gc.ca/ahc-asc/branch-dirgen/fnihb-dgspni/fact-fiche-eng.php.
129. Health Canada. Aboriginal diabetes initiative 2010–2015 (updated 2011; cited 26 Feb 2016) 2016. Available from http://www.hc-sc.gc.ca/fniah-spnia/pubs/diseases-maladies/_diabete/2010-2015-frame-cadre/indexeng.php.
130. Minore B, Boone M, Katt M, Kinch P, Birch S. Facilitating the continuity of care for first nation clients within a regional context. 2001.
131. King M, Smith A, Gracey M. Indigenous health part 2: the underlying causes of the health gap. Lancet. 2009;374(9683):76–85.
132. Shah BR, Gunraj N, Hux JE. Markers of access to and quality of primary care for aboriginal people in Ontario, Canada. Am J Public Health. 2003;93(5):798–802.
133. Lavoie JG, Forget EL, Prakash T, Dahl M, Martens P, O'Neil JD. Have investments in on-reserve health services and initiatives promoting community control improved First Nations' health in Manitoba? Soc Sci Med. 2010;71(4):717–24.
134. Gracey M, King M. Indigenous health part 1: determinants and disease patterns. Lancet. 2009;374(9683):65–75.
135. Bramley D, Hebert P, Tuzzio L, Chassin M. Disparities in indigenous health: a cross-country comparison between New Zealand and the United States. Am J Public Health. 2005;95(5):844–50.
136. Bhattacharyya OK, Rasooly IR, Naqshbandi M, Estey EA, Esler J, Toth E, et al. Challenges to the provision of diabetes care in first nations communities: results from a national survey of healthcare providers in Canada. BMC Health Serv Res. 2011;11:283.
137. Pohar SL, Johnson JA. Health care utilization and costs in Saskatchewan's registered Indian population with diabetes. BMC Health Serv Res. 2007;7:126.
138. FORGE AHEAD program description London, ON: the national diabetes management strategy. 2011 [cited 7 Mar 2016]. Available from http://tndms.ca/forgeahead/index.html.
139. Glazier RH, Bajcar J, Kennie NR, Willson K. A systematic review of interventions to improve diabetes care in socially disadvantaged populations. Diabetes Care. 2006;29(7):1675–88.
140. Kakekagumick KE, Naqshbandi Hayward M, Harris SB, Saksvig B, Gittelsohn J, Manokeesic G, et al. Sandy lake health and diabetes project: a community-based intervention targeting type 2 diabetes and its risk factors in a first nations community. Front Endocrinol. 2013;4:170.
141. Saksvig BI, Gittelsohn J, Harris SB, Hanley AJ, Valente TW, Zinman B. A pilot school-based healthy eating and physical activity intervention improves diet, food knowledge, and self-efficacy for native Canadian children. J Nutr. 2005;135(10):2392–8.
142. Macaulay AC, Paradis G, Potvin L, Cross EJ, Saad-Haddad C, McComber A, et al. The Kahnawake Schools Diabetes Prevention Project: intervention, evaluation, and baseline results of a diabetes primary prevention program with a native community in Canada. Prev Med. 1997;26(6):779–90.
143. Paradis G, Levesque L, Macaulay AC, Cargo M, McComber A, Kirby R, et al. Impact of a diabetes prevention program on body size, physical activity, and diet among Kanien'keha:ka (Mohawk) children 6 to 11 years old: 8-year results from the Kahnawake Schools Diabetes Prevention Project. Pediatrics. 2005;115(2):333–9.
144. Tomlin D, Naylor PJ, McKay H, Zorzi A, Mitchell M, Panagiotopoulos C. The impact of Action Schools! BC on the health of Aboriginal children and youth living in rural and remote communities in British Columbia. Int J Circumpolar Health. 2012;71:17999.

14 Diabetes in Native Populations and Underserved Communities in the USA

Joshua J. Joseph and Sherita Hill Golden

Epidemiology, Classification, and Unique Pathophysiological Aspects of Diabetes Mellitus in Minority Populations in the USA

In the USA roughly 25.8 million individuals (8.3 % of US population) have type 2 diabetes mellitus (diabetes) [1]. While 18.8 million are diagnosed, another 7 million remain undiagnosed [1]. The prevalence of diagnosed diabetes in adults over 20 years of age is highest among non-Hispanic blacks (NHBs) (12.6 %), Mexican Americans (13.3 %), Puerto Rican Americans (13.8 %), and Native Americans (16.1 %) [1]. The prevalence of diagnosed diabetes is similar among non-Hispanic whites (NHWs), Cuban Americans, Central Americans, and South Americans. It is important to note that diabetes prevalence in Hispanic Americans is influenced by the country of origin and primarily driven by the high prevalence in people of Mexican and Puerto Rican descent [2]. Similarly, diabetes prevalence is lowest in Alaska Natives (5.5 %) but very high in American Indians (approaching 33 %) [1]. Estimates based only on physician diagnosis may underestimate diabetes in certain racial/ethnic groups.

As of 2010, approximately 1.9 million individuals over 20 years of age in the USA developed incident diabetes [1]. Compared to NHWs, the risk of incident diabetes was 18 % higher in Asian Americans, 66 % higher in Hispanic Americans, and 77 % higher in NHBs [1]. Compared to NHWs, the diabetes incidence was significantly higher among Mexican Americans (87 %) and Puerto Rican Americans (94 %), whereas the risk was similar in Cuban Americans, Central Americans, and South Americans [1]. The most recent data examining trends for incidence of type 1 and type 2 diabetes in the USA are from the National Health Interview Survey (NHIS), where data from 664,969 adults was analyzed from 1980 to 2012 [3]. The incidence per 1,000 persons was 3.2 in 1990, 8.8 in 2008, and 7.1 in 2012, suggesting that the diabetes incidence has reached a plateau. However, diabetes incidence rates in NHBs and Hispanic Americans continue to rise significantly more than for NHWs.

NHIS contains the only estimates of the prevalence of diabetes in Asian Americans in the USA. It revealed that there is significant ethnic variation in the prevalence of diabetes, which is highest among Asian Indians (close to 15 %) and Filipinos (close to 10 %) and lowest among Koreans, Vietnamese, and Chinese (3–7 %) in the

J.J. Joseph, MD • S.H. Golden, MD, MHS (✉)
Division of Endocrinology, Diabetes, and Metabolism, Department of Medicine, Johns Hopkins University School of Medicine,
1830 E. Monument Street, Suite# 333, Baltimore, MD 21287, USA
e-mail: sahill@jhmi.edu

S. Dagogo-Jack (ed.), *Diabetes Mellitus in Developing Countries and Underserved Communities*,
DOI 10.1007/978-3-319-41559-8_14

USA [4], consistent with the known higher diabetes prevalence in individuals living in India, South Asia, and the Philippines [5]. In the Diabetes Study of Northern California, diabetes incidence was highest among Pacific Islanders, South Asians, and Filipinos (19.9, 17.2, and 14.7 per 1,000 person-years) compared to other racial/ethnic groups, including other minorities (NHBs, Latinos, and Native Americans) [6].

Race/Ethnic Differences in Biological Factors

Obesity and Fat Distribution

Obesity is one of the strongest risk factors for developing diabetes. Racial/ethnic differences in obesity contribute to the higher risk of diabetes in NHBs and Mexican Americans; however, NHB women have greater subcutaneous compared to visceral fat than NHW women at a given body mass index (BMI) and waist circumference and may therefore develop diabetes at a higher BMI than NHW women. Among Asian Americans, there is variation in the prevalence of overweight and obesity depending on the country of origin (Table 14.1). Differences in body fat distribution are important contributors to diabetes risk in certain Asian populations, for instance, Japanese Americans and Filipinos have more visceral fat at similar levels of BMI and waist circumference compared to NHWs [4].

Table 14.1 Age-adjusted prevalence of overweight and obesity by Asian American ethnicity from the National Health Interview Survey [4]

Race/ethnic group	Age-adjusted overweight prevalence (%)	Age-adjusted obesity prevalence (%)
Chinese	21.8	4.2
Filipino	33.0	14.1
Asian Indian	34.4	6.0
Japanese	25.9	8.7
Vietnamese	19.1	5.3
Korean	27.3	2.8
Other Asian and Native Hawaiian or other Pacific Islander	29.2	12.5

Golden et al. [1]

Glucose Metabolism and Insulin Resistance

Insulin resistance is a key contributor to diabetes risk in NHB, Mexican American, Asian American, and Native American populations. Compared to their NHW counterparts and independent of adiposity, NHBs, Mexican Americans, Asian Americans, and Native Americans have greater insulin resistance [7]. Studies in non-Mexican Hispanic Americans have yielded conflicting results. Glucose metabolic features differ among Hispanic Americans from different countries of origin. This may explain the higher prevalence of diabetes in Mexican Americans compared to those of Cuban American and South American descent. Asian Americans have lower beta-cell insulin secretion compared to NHWs [7]. The reduced beta-cell function in Asian Americans may also explain why they are at high risk for diabetes at lower levels of BMI [8].

Individual Racial/Ethnic Differences in Nonbiological Factors

Acculturation

Acculturation in Hispanic American immigrants results in an increase in dietary habits that promote obesity [9]. The association of acculturation with diabetes, however, is mixed and inconsistent. Even though acculturation appears to promote obesity, its association with diabetes may be offset by its positive influence on physical activity and access to care, in that screening and intervention occur sooner [9]. Japanese immigrants to the USA have a threefold higher rate of diabetes compared to their native Japanese counterparts [7].

Health Behaviors

Physical inactivity is an important risk factor for diabetes. NHBs, Native Americans, and Alaska Natives report less leisure-time physical activity than NHWs [10]. Mexican American women report less leisure-time physical activity than NHW and NHB women [10]. There are sparse data currently on physical activity in Asian American populations [4].

Smoking has also been identified as a risk factor for diabetes, independent of adiposity. Native Americans and Alaska Natives have a higher prevalence of smoking than NHWs [10]. NHBs and NHWs have similar smoking rates, while Mexican Americans have significantly lower smoking rates. In Asian Americans there is variation in rates of smoking, with the highest prevalence among Korean men and the lowest prevalence among Asian Indian men [4].

Genomic and Epigenetic Landscape of Diabetes

Results of several genome-wide association studies (GWAS) have linked the following common gene variants with a 15–20% increased risk of diabetes: reduced insulin secretion via reduce beta-cell mass (CDKAL1, CDKN2A, CDKN2B) and beta-cell dysfunction (MTNR1B, TCF7L2, KCNJ11) and increased insulin resistance related to obesity (FTO) and unrelated to obesity (IRS1, PPARG) [11]. While most of the early studies focused on individuals of European descent, several recent studies have demonstrated that these susceptibility loci are also present and associated with increased diabetes risk in ethnic minority populations. The limited amount of data in non-European ancestry populations does not suggest that the genetic architecture of diabetes differs across race/ethnic groups. Until recently, there were no GWAS analyses in non-European populations; however, several studies have identified novel diabetes-associated SNPs in specific race/ethnic groups that are being further evaluated (see Table 14.2).

Epigenetics represents the interface of environmental and biological factors and has implications in the predisposition of NHBs to developing diabetes. Low birth weight, fetal undernutrition, and maternal-fetal stress appear to be unique contributors to elevated diabetes and metabolic risk in NHBs. NHBs have lower birth weight than NHWs, which may be related to maternal conditions during pregnancy, including stressful life events, depressive and anxiety symptoms, economic inequality (e.g., lower income and education, less access to healthcare in NHBs), racial discrimination, residential segregation, neighborhood-level poverty, and maternal hypertension [15]. Smaller birth weight is linked to insulin resistance and diabetes, abdominal pattern of fat distribution, higher blood pressure, abnormal lipid profiles, and increased cardiovascular disease risk [15]. Studies have also linked low birth weight with elevated cortisol reactivity in childhood and adolescence [15]. And chronic cortisol exposure can contribute to abdominal adiposity and insulin resistance [16]. Maternal psychological stress and fetal overexposure to cortisol lead to the same metabolic abnormalities as fetal undernutrition [15].

Epigenetic changes in the pattern of cellular gene expression may influence how a fetus adapts to an adverse intrauterine environment which may increase survival in utero but predispose that individual to enhanced metabolic risk later in life [15]. Further studies are needed to determine how epigenetic changes contribute to the role of the fetal environment in racial/ethnic differences in future risk of obesity and diabetes [17].

Diagnosis of Diabetes and Prediabetes

In 2010 the American Diabetes Association (ADA) updated its clinical practice guidelines to include HbA1c criteria for the diagnosis of diabetes and prediabetes. In the context of using HbA1c as a diagnostic criteria in nondiabetic individuals, recent studies have suggested that non-glycemic factors may contribute to the higher HbA1c at similar levels of fasting glucose seen in NHBs, Hispanic Americans, Asian Americans, and Native Americans, compared to NHWs [18]. Suggested factors include variations in erythrocyte membrane permeability to glucose, regulation of glucose transport across the erythrocyte membrane, glycolytic rates, differences in nonenzymatic glycosylation reactions, and deglycation [18].

Two recent studies have examined the effect glycemia has on HbA1c differences in NHBs and NHWs with diabetes [19, 20]. One study

Table 14.2 Novel GWAS-identified loci associated with type 2 diabetes in non-European populations [1]

Population	New identified SNP	Chromosome	Associated gene(s)	Associated physiological function
South Asians [12]	Rs3923113	2	GRB14	Associated with insulin sensitivity
	Rs16861329	3	ST6GAL1	Associated with pancreatic beta-cell function
	Rs1802295	10	VPS26A	
	Rs7178572	15	HMC20A	
	Rs2028299	15	AP3S2	
	Rs4812829	20	HNF4A	Associated with pancreatic beta-cell function
East Asians [13]				
Loci with strong associations	Rs6815464	4	MAEA	
	Rs7041847	9	GLIS3	Associated with pancreatic beta-cell development, insulin gene expression, and glucose
	Rs6017317	20	FITM2-R3HDML-HNF4A	
	Rs6467136	7	GCC1-PAX4	
	Rs831581	3	PSMD6	
	Rs9470794	6	ZFAND3	
	Rs3786897	19	PEPD	
	Rs1535500	6	KCNK16	May regulate glucose-independent insulin secretion in the pancreas
Loci with moderate associations	Rs16955379	16	CMIP	
	Rs17797882	16	WWOX	
NHBs [14]				
Loci with strong associations	Rs7560163	2	RBM43	
			RND3	
Loci with nominal associations	Rs7542900		SLC44A3	
			F3	
	Rs4659485	2	RYR2	
			MTR	
	Rs2722769	11	GALNTL4	
			LOC729013	
	Rs7107217	11	TMEM45B	
			BARX2	

Golden et al. [1]
SNP single nucleotide polymorphism

used data from National Health and Nutrition Examination Survey III and the Screening for Impaired Glucose Tolerance Studies and found that NHBs with diabetes had significantly higher HbA1c than NHWs with diabetes, which persisted following adjustment for plasma glucose [19]. A subsequent study, using data from the Atherosclerosis Risk in Communities Study, however, came to a different conclusion [20]. This study attributed the higher HbA1c in NHBs with diabetes (compared with NHWs with diabetes) to higher fasting glucose and other covariates [20]. In addition, nontraditional glycemic markers, glycated albumin, and fructosamine, which are not subject to the effects of erythrocyte turnover and hemoglobin glycation, were also significantly elevated in NHBs with diabetes, compared to NHWs with diabetes [20]. Thus, these data support more hyperglycemia in NHBs with diabetes. As conflicting evidence is evolving about the contribution of non-glycemic factors to HbA1c levels in minorities with diabetes, caution should be used in applying HbA1c as the only measure to assess diagnosis of prediabetes and/or diabetes.

Diabetes Complications

Overall, ethnic minorities appear to be disproportionately affected by microvascular complications and mortality associated with diabetes, likely related to poorer glycemic and cardiovascular disease risk factor control; however, there are some notable paradoxes. NHBs with diabetes have a lower incidence of cardiovascular disease than NHWs with diabetes; however, once they have cardiovascular disease, they are more likely to die. NHBs have a higher rate of ESRD secondary to diabetic nephropathy but are less likely to die on dialysis than NHWs. NHBs, Native Americans and Alaska Natives, and Hispanic Americans are 2.3, 1.9, and 1.5 times more likely to die from diabetes than NHWs [21]. And while Asian Americans, overall, are 20 % less likely to die from diabetes than NHWs, there are variations among subgroups, such that Native Hawaiians and Filipinos living in Hawaii are 5.7 and 3.0 times more likely to die from diabetes than NHWs living in Hawaii [21].

Race/Ethnic Differences in Biological Factors Contributing to Complications

Glycemic Control

Several systematic reviews and meta-analyses have shown that ethnic minorities with diabetes have worse glycemic control than NHWs, which likely contributes to the higher risk of microvascular complications seen in these populations [22–24]. The proportion of diabetic ethnic minorities with poor glycemic control, defined as glycemia above a specific threshold, was significantly higher among NHBs, Hispanic Americans, Native Americans, and Asian Americans and Pacific Islanders [22]. Although discussed more in the context of using HbA1c as a diagnostic criteria for diabetes, recent studies have suggested that non-glycemic factors may contribute to the higher HbA1c at similar levels of fasting glucose seen in NHBs, Hispanic Americans, Asian Americans, and Native Americans, compared to NHWs [18]. However, HbA1c is similarly associated with prevalence and risk of microvascular and macrovascular complications, and mortality, among NHB and NHWs with diabetes [25–27], lending credence to true differences in glycemia between the two race/ethnic groups.

Cardiovascular Risk Factors

Hypertension is an important risk factor for diabetic nephropathy/end-stage renal disease (ESRD) and peripheral arterial disease and likely contributes to the higher prevalence of these complications in certain ethnic groups. NHBs have a higher prevalence of hypertension than NHWs [10]. Mexican American women have a higher prevalence of hypertension than NHW women; however, the prevalence of hypertension is similar among men in the two race/ethnic groups [10]. Native Americans and Alaska Natives have a lower prevalence of hypertension compared to NHWs and NHBs; however, there are regional differences [10]. Studies of blood pressure control and hypertension prevalence comparing NHWs to Native Americans and Asian Americans with diabetes are lacking. Research to date from clinical trials indicates that control of reversible risk factors, including hypertension, is equally effective in lowering the risk of nephropathy and cardiovascular disease in minority and NHW populations [28].

In a prior systematic review comparing low-density lipoprotein cholesterol between minority populations and NHWs with diabetes, Hispanic Americans had slightly lower low-density lipoprotein cholesterol than NHBs and NHWs. In this review, there were no studies comparing lipid control in NHWs with Native Americans and Asian Americans with diabetes [29]. While NHBs have lower triglycerides than NHWs [25], which may explain their lower risk of macrovascular disease, they generally have a higher prevalence of low high-density lipoprotein cholesterol, a strong cardiovascular risk factor [30].

Individual Race/Ethnic Differences in Nonbiological Factors (Health Behaviors) Contributing to Complications

Self-Monitoring of Blood Glucose (SMBG)

While some studies have shown no differences in SMBG by race/ethnicity, several have shown lower rates among NHBs, Hispanic Americans, and Asian Americans, compared to NHWs. Two studies found no difference in SMBG frequency in Native Americans compared to NHWs [31]. There are several barriers to SMBG, including inconvenience and intrusiveness, pain, lower socioeconomic position, education level, social class, and living in a high poverty area, many of which are disproportionately prevalent in ethnic minority groups [31].

Physical Activity and Smoking

As summarized above, ethnic minorities are less likely to engage in leisure-time physical activity, which can contribute to worse glycemic control and a propensity to developing microvascular complications [10].

Native Americans and Alaska Natives have a higher prevalence of smoking that NHWs [10], which can contribute to their higher risk of peripheral arterial disease and amputations. NHBs and NHWs have similar smoking rates, while Mexican Americans have significantly lower smoking rates. Therefore, smoking may not explain ethnic differences in peripheral arterial disease in these populations.

Coordination and Delivery of Diabetes Care Services: Health System Interventions Targeting Minority and Underserved Patients with Poorly Controlled Type 2 Diabetes

Evidence-Based General Diabetes Quality Improvement Interventions

Quality improvement strategies can target several areas—health systems (case management, team changes, electronic patient registry, facilitated relay of information to clinicians, continuous QI), healthcare providers (audit and feedback, clinician education, clinician reminders, financial incentives), or patients (patient education, promotion of self-management, reminder systems) [32]. Several prior meta-analyses have examined the impact of these intervention approaches on glycemic control and other metabolic control indices in patients with diabetes [32–34]. Shojania et al. performed a systematic review and meta-analysis of 58 studies of 66 distinct trials. These studies utilized a median of three quality improvement strategies and had a median follow-up of 13 months. The mean post-intervention HbA1c difference, compared to pre-intervention, was –0.42 % with greater reductions if baseline HbA1c was ≥8 % [33]. Strategies associated with at least a 0.5 % reduction in HbA1c after controlling for baseline HbA1c ≥8 % and study size included team changes (−0.67 %) and case management (−0.52 %). In comparative analyses, interventions that included case management reduced HbA1c significantly more than interventions that did not include case management, and of these types of interventions, the most effective case management interventions were those in which the interventionists could make independent medication changes [33]. This was confirmed in a subsequent meta-analysis of randomized controlled trials of disease management programs improving glycemic control in adults with type 1 and type 2 diabetes [34]. This same study suggested that interventions with high-frequency patient contact (several times/month) were more effective than those with low-frequency contact intervention [34].

Similarly, interventions that included team changes reduced HbA1c significantly more than interventions that did not include team changes, particularly those that included multidisciplinary, interactive teams [34]. Interventions with team changes remained significant after controlling for the presence of case management [33]. In those studies, adding a new team member alone was not effective, but rather, adding a team member with shared care between specialists and primary care providers or new team members with an expanded role were most effective.

A more recent meta-analysis expanded on Shojania's prior study by including process outcome measures (proportion taking aspirin, statins, and antihypertensives and the proportion screened for retinopathy, foot abnormalities, and renal dysfunction) and additional non-glycemic outcome measures (LDL cholesterol, blood pressure, and proportion with controlled hypertension or quitting smoking) to evaluate the additional impact of multicomponent diabetes quality improvement interventions [32]. Overall, interventions resulted in lower HbA1c, LDL cholesterol, and blood pressure in those receiving compared to those not receiving the interventions [32]. These strategies also improved the likelihood that patients received aspirin therapy, antihypertensives, and screening for diabetic complications. Statin use, blood pressure control, and smoking cessation were unchanged. For patients with HbA1c ≥8 % intervention strategies that lower HbA1c ≥0.5 % included team changes, case management, patient education, and promotion of self-management; however, for patients with HbA1c<8 %, facilitated relay was more effective in lowering HbA1c≥0.5 % [32]. The only intervention strategy that was not effective in lowering HbA1c was clinician education [32]. These data suggest that greater improvements in HbA1c can be achieved utilizing QI intervention strategies that target the healthcare system and patients.

Diabetes Quality Improvement Interventions Among Underserved and Minority Populations

Glazier et al. conducted a systematic review of 17 studies examining the effectiveness of patient, provider, and health system interventions among patients with type 1 or type 2 diabetes in socially disadvantaged populations, defined as those of low socioeconomic status, or belonging to an ethnic/racial minority group [35]. Eight of 13 studies showed improvements in HbA1c but less impact on body weight, lipids, and blood pressure (see Table 14.3).

Features of effective interventions included cultural and health literacy tailoring, led by community educators or lay people; 1:1 (versus group) interventions with individualized assessment/reassessment; incorporation of treatment algorithms, focusing on behavior-related tasks and providing feedback; and high intensity interventions over a long duration [35]. With one exception, interventions targeting racial/ethnic minorities specifically did not involve endocrinology subspecialty input on the care team. One study of NHBs and Latinos involved nurse implementation of a detailed protocol and algorithm with endocrinologist supervision which resulted in a significant 3.5 % reduction in HbA1c and improvement in 8/10 ADA process measures [36]. Components of successful interventions from this review are summarized in Table 14.4.

Table 14.3 Improvement in diabetes-related metabolic and process measures in response to patient, provider, and health system quality improvement interventions in socially disadvantaged populations [35]

Metabolic or process measure	# of studies with improvement/total # of studies examining measure
HbA1c	8/13
Weight/body mass index	2/9
Lipids	2/7
Blood pressure	2/4
Adherence to annual eye exam	3/3
Achievement of ADA care indicators	2/3
Adherence to exercise recommendations	1/3
Improved diabetes knowledge	2/2
Improved physician trust	1/1

Table 14.4 Summary of components of successful diabetes quality improvement interventions in socially disadvantaged populations

Intervention level	Successful components
Patient	Interpersonal
	Utilize social networks
	Culturally tailored
Provider	In-person feedback (compared to computerized decision support)
Health system	Utilize on-site nurse case managers
	Utilize community health workers
	Provide medical assistance programs for prescriptions

Interventions specifically targeting NHBs and Latino Americans with diabetes were recently summarized in two systematic reviews and meta-analyses [37, 38]. Table 14.5 below summarizes the types of interventions employed in these studies and the effect on process measures and clinical outcomes.

Patient Interventions Within Healthcare Organization

In Peek's review of 17 studies of patient interventions within the healthcare organization that sought to improve dietary habits, physical activity, and self-management activities, those that were culturally tailored were more effective in

Table 14.5 Quality improvement intervention components in studies of predominantly minority populations

Intervention target(s)	Intervention component(s)	Summary of outcomes
General patient level interventions		
Basch (1999) [39] (100 % NHB)	Education and counseling	↑ Receipt of dilated eye exam
Clancy (2003) [40] (78 % NHB)	Education and stress management (MD and RN group visits)	Improvement in testing of HbA1c, LDL, microalbumin; use of ACE inhibitors, ASA, statins, vaccinations, and eye and foot exams
		Increased physician trust
Gerber (2005) [41] (66 % Latino, 29 % NHB)	Computer training on skills and self-management support in waiting room kiosk	No significant change in HbA1c, BP, weight, knowledge, self-efficacy
Erdman (2002) [42] (91 % NHB)	Self-management, lifestyle counseling	↓ HbA1c, total cholesterol, LDL (due to statins)
		↑ HDL
Ziemer (2003) [43] (90 % NHB)	Diet counseling	↓ HbA1c
Anderson (2003) [44] (100 % NHB)	Patient reminders to schedule eye exam	↑ Returning for annual diabetes retinal exam
D'Eramo-Melkus (2004) [45] (100 % NHB)	Culturally tailored CBT and monthly nurse practitioner visits	↓ HbA1c, weight, BMI, diabetes-related emotional distress
Tang (2005) [46] (100 % NHB)	Patient-centered DSME	↓ BMI, dyslipidemia
		Improved self-management behaviors, quality of life, difficulty with diet, difficulty with exercise
Amoak (2008) [47] (100 % NHB)	Phone calls focusing on aspects of experience with diabetes administered by geriatric NP	Improved psychological adjustment and exercise
Skelly (2009) [48] (100 % NHB)	Teaching and counseling modules delivered by RN in patient's home	No change
Tang (2010) [49] (100 % NHB)	DSME groups	↓ HbA1c, BMI, dyslipidemia
Walker (2010) [50] (100 % NHB)	Educational sessions with patient navigator follow-up	Improved diabetes knowledge
Carter (2011) [51] (100 % NHB)	Online DSM	↓ Weight, BMI, HbA1c
		Improved diabetes knowledge, diabetes management practices, physical health status, mental health status
Ellish (2011) [52] (100 % NHB)	Eye exam newsletter	No change
Tang (2012) [53] (100 % NHB)	Empowerment-based DSM support	↓ Blood pressure, serum cholesterol
		Improved self-management behaviors, quality of life

Table 14.5 (continued)

Intervention target(s)	Intervention component(s)	Summary of outcomes
Culturally tailored patient level interventions		
Agurs-Collins (1997) [54] (100 % NHB)	Dieticians and medical staff support for weight loss	↓ HbA1c, weight, blood pressure
Anderson-Loftin (2005) [55] (100 % NHB)	Nutrition counseling by RN and DM educator	↓ BMI, improved food habits
Brown and Hanis (1999), Brown (2002) [56, 57] (>90 % Mexican American)	DSM education and support group by bilingual Mexican American nurses, dietitians, and CHWs	↓ HbA1c
Brown (2005) [58] (100 % Mexican American)	Extended DSM education support/education (vs. compressed education/support)	No difference in HbA1c
Corkery (1997) [59] (75 % Puerto Rican; 25 % other Latinos)	Diabetes education via bicultural CHWs and diabetes RN educator (vs. diabetes RN educator)	Better program completion rate
		No difference in knowledge, behaviors, or HbA1c
Keyserling (2002) [60] (100 % NHB)	CHW/peer counselors + nutritionist	↑ Physical activity and diabetes knowledge
Mayer-Davis (2001, 2004) [61, 62] (82 %NHB)	Diet and physical activity intervention	↓ Weight, BMI, fasting blood glucose (2001)
McNabb (1993) (100 % NHB) [63]	Diet and exercise education	↓ Weight
Rosal (2005) [64] (80 % Puerto Rican low-income, Spanish speaking)	Diet, physical activity, DSME education led by DM nurse, nutritionist, and CHW	↓ HbA1c
		Non-sustained ↓ depressive symptoms
		No change in physical activity
		↑ Self-monitoring
Two Feathers (2005) [65] (64 % NHB; 36 % Latino)	CHW lifestyle interventions	Improved dietary knowledge and behaviors and physical activity knowledge
		↓ HbA1c
Vazquez (1998) [66] (100 % Caribbean American Latinos)	Nutrition program with nutritionists and psychologists	↓ Caloric, total fat, total saturated fat, total energy intake
		↑ Carbohydrate intake
Anderson (2005) [67] (100 % NHB)	Self-management experiments, problem-solving, discussing emotional experience living with diabetes delivered by RN and dietician	↓ HbA1c, serum cholesterol, LDL, triglycerides, weight
		↑ HDL, SMBG
		Improved perceived understanding of diabetes, diabetes empowerment, attitudes toward seriousness of diabetes, positive attitudes
Murrok (2009) [68] (100 % NHB)	Dance classes choreographed to gospel music	↓ Body fat and blood pressure
Bogner (2010) [69] (100 % NHB)	Individualized program to improve adherence to oral hypoglycemic and |antidepressants (recognizing social and cultural context)	↓ HbA1c
		Improved adherence to oral hypoglycemics
D'Eramo (2010) [70] (100 % NHB)	Culturally relevant group DSME training, coping skills training, and diabetes care intervention	↓ HbA1c, blood pressure, dyslipidemia
		Improved quality of life, vitality, role physical, bodily pain, perceived provider support for diet, exercise, diabetes-related emotional distress

(continued)

Table 14.5 (continued)

Intervention target(s)	Intervention component(s)	Summary of outcomes
Hill-Briggs (2011) [71] (100 % NHB)	Problem-based DSM training	↓ HbA1c Improved knowledge, problem-solving, self-management behavior
Provider level interventions		
Benjamin (1999) [72] (40 % NHB, 36 % Latino)	Provide based learning methods to increase MD use of practice guidelines	Improvement in annual eye and microalbumin exams Trends of improvements in annual lipids, influenza vaccines, and diet/diabetes education ↓ HbA1c
Din-Dzietham (2004) [73] (100 % NHB)	CME and guideline distribution (continuous QI program targeting providers)	Positive change in prevalence in selected patterns of care
Fox and Mahoney (1998) [74] (100 % NHB)	Chart audit and feedback	Improvement in HbA1c, self-management behavior, eye exams, and vaccinations
Phillips (2002, 2005) [75, 76] (100 % NHB)	Computerized decision-support reminders, bimonthly in-person individualized feedback	↓ HbA1c
Thaler (1999) [77] (100 % NHB)	Rapid turnaround HbA1c in one group; both groups seen by nurse practitioner and endocrinologist	↓ Fasting or random plasma glucose ↑ Frequency of therapy intensification by treatment modality
Ziemer (2006) [78] (100 % NHB)	Computerized reminders to intensify medications, reminders	Improvement in medication titration by providers; therapy intensification associated with ↓ HbA1c
Health system		
Thaler (1999) [77] (100 % NHB)	Rapid turnaround HbA1c in one group; both groups seen by nurse practitioner and endocrinologist	↓ Fasting or random plasma glucose ↑ Frequency of therapy intensification by treatment modality
Bray and Thompson (2005), Bray and Roupe (2005) [79, 80] (72 % NHB)	RN case management, DM registry, visit reminders	↓ HbA1c
Davidson (2003) [36] (86 % Latino)	RN-directed care with treatment algorithms	Improved HbA1c, lipid, annual eye exams, renal tests, foot exams, education, diet counseling ↓ HbA1c
Fanning (2004) [81] (100 % NHB)	RN case management (university and community settings)	↓ HbA1c, LDL, blood pressure
Gary (2004) [82] (100 % NHB)	RN case management, CHW	↓ Blood pressure, lipid profile
Hopper (1984) [83] (75 % NHB)	Home health aide	↓ Fasting blood sugar (among those offered aides) ↑ Eye clinic visits among those who accepted aides
Hosler (2002) [84] (45 % NHB, 25 % Latino, 7 % Native American)	Evidence-based guidelines, multidisciplinary DM team, minority outreach, community partnerships (CHWs, patient incentives)	Improved assessment of HbA1c, lipids, eye exam, and SMBG, exercise, and diet assessment
Jaber (1996) [85] (100 % NHB)	Pharmacist-led education	↓ HbA1c and fasting glucose
Miller (2003) [86] (100 % NHB)	Rapid turnaround HbA1c	↓ HbA1c ↑ Frequency of pharmacological diabetes therapy

Table 14.5 (continued)

Intervention target(s)	Intervention component(s)	Summary of outcomes
Philis-Tsimikas (2004) [87] (72 % Latino)	RN case management with treatment algorithms + CHW	100 % compliance with ADA standards for performing HbA1c, lipids, foot exams, and urine microalbumin
		↓ HbA1c, cholesterol, blood pressure
		Improved DM knowledge and self-efficacy
Multi-target interventions (patients and healthcare system)		
Cook (1999) [88] (88 % NHB)	Patient education, nurse case management, multidisciplinary diabetes team (including endocrinologist), treatment algorithms	↓ HbA1c
		↑ BMI
Anderson-Loftin (2002) [55] (100 % NHB)	Culturally competent, dietary self-management intervention with dietician and nurse case manager	↓ HbA1c, fasting blood glucose, frequency of acute care visits
		Improved dietary habits
Bray and Thompson (2005) [79] (100 % NHB)	RN case management (APN) with supervising physician (unclear if endocrinologist), DM registry, visit reminders, patient education and self-management support, provider decision-support tools	↓ HbA1c
Mahotiere (2006) [89] (100 % NHB)	Provider QI interventions focused on system changes surrounding the physician visit combined with patient interventions	↑ proportion of beneficiaries with diabetes receiving biennial lipid profile
Gary (2009) [90] (100 % NHB)	Nurse case management and CHW using evidence-based clinical algorithms with feedback to PCPs	↓ ED visits and blood pressure
		↑ HDL
Thaler (1999) [77] (100 % NHB)	Rapid turnaround HbA1c in one group; both groups seen by nurse practitioner and endocrinologist	↓ Fasting or random plasma glucose
		↑ Frequency of therapy intensification by treatment modality
Rith-Najarian (1998) [91] (100 % NHB)	Podiatric screening and patient education, provider guidelines, multidisciplinary team, DM registry and tracking system, flow sheets	↓ Amputations

lowering HbA1c than general QI interventions (–0.69 % versus –0.1 %) [37]. Also, peer support and 1:1 interventions were more effective than online and computer-based approaches. In a systematic review and meta-analysis looking exclusively at randomized controlled trials of patient interventions targeting NHBs, most of which were culturally adapted and included peer providers, two of 22 increased patient attendance at screening visits, and 20 of 22 promoted diabetes self-management [38]. In a meta-analysis of eight studies, interventions resulted in a significant 0.83 % reduction in HbA1c [38].

Provider Interventions

In Peek's review, provider interventions including education, continuing medical education, computerized decision support, in-person feedback, and problem-based learning improved process measures [37]. The majority of these studies were conducted in NHBs with diabetes. Interventions involving computerized decision-support reminders and chart audit and individual's feedback resulted in improved HbA1c and treatment modification [74–76, 92].

Healthcare Organization Interventions

Healthcare organization interventions in minority populations have included systems for rapid turnaround HbA1c, circumscribed appointments, support staff (e.g., nurse case management, community health worker, pharmacist), and increased follow-up through home visits or telephone/mail contact [37, 38]. In Peek's review, 14 studies with interventions targeting the healthcare organization resulted in a mean HbA1c reduction of 0.34 %. Ricci-Cabello et al. included five healthcare system intervention trials in NHBs in their systematic review and meta-analysis and found the two most highly effective interventions in improving HbA1c, and frequency of therapy intensification included rapid turnaround HbA1c [77, 86].

Multi-target Interventions

Multi-target interventions target all aspects and components of healthcare delivery, including patients, providers, and the healthcare system. Five of these studies have targeted NHBs with diabetes and used various approaches. Three studies showed an improvement in HbA1c [55, 79, 88]. All of these interventions included patient education and self-management support and nurse case management, two included treatment algorithms [79, 88], and two involved collaboration with a physician in treatment decisions (one an endocrinologist [88] and one an unspecified physician [79]). While two additional multi-target interventions showed improvement in process measures and non-glycemic clinical outcomes [89, 90], they did not improve glycemic control. One study involved patient interventions and provider-focused QI interventions focusing on system changes surrounding the physician visit [89] and the other involved nurse case management and community health workers using evidence-based clinical algorithms with feedback to primary care physicians [90]. Finally, one study focusing exclusively on Native Americans in the Indian Health Service included provider guidelines, a multidisciplinary team, diabetes registry/tracking system, and flow sheets [91]. Compared to podiatric screening and patient education, the multi-target intervention resulted in a significant reduction in amputation rate [91].

Non-pharmacological Management of Diabetes in Minority and Underserved Populations

Lifestyle intervention is the mainstay of non-pharmacological management of diabetes. The American Diabetes Association recommends initial management of diabetes with 6 months of diabetes self-management education (DSME) to support lifestyle modifications to achieve modest weight loss. The physical activity and dietary recommendations are >150 min of moderate-intensity physical activity, and medical nutrition therapy emphasizing a variety of nutrient-dense foods in appropriate portion sizes focused on reduced energy intake for individuals with a BMI ≥25 kg/m^2 with proper macronutrient distribution [93]. In addition to physical activity and dietary management, novel factors for diabetes management have emerged including dietary patterns, dietary composition, intensity of physical activity, and weight loss with both nonsurgical and surgical approaches.

Dietary Patterns

Mediterranean Diet

The largest analysis of the Mediterranean diet was the Prevention with Mediterranean Diet (PREDIMED) study. The trial enrolled 7,447 persons in Spain at high cardiovascular risk with either diabetes or three cardiovascular risk factors. Participants were randomized to one of three diets: a Mediterranean diet supplemented with extra-virgin olive oil, a Mediterranean diet supplemented with mixed nuts, or a control diet (advise to reduce dietary fat) and were followed for 4.8 years for the development of the primary end point of major cardiovascular events. Mediterranean diet with extra-virgin olive oil and Mediterranean diet with nuts were associated with 30 and 28 % reductions in major cardiovascular events [94]. Among participants with diabetes in the Mediterranean diet groups compared to control, there was a 29 % reduction in major cardiovascular events. The Mediterranean diet also reduces HbA1c. In 215 overweight Italian individuals with newly diagnosed diabetes, Mediterranean diet vs. low-fat diet was associated with a 0.6 % and 0.4 % lower HbA1c at 1 and 4 years, respectively, with a 37 % reduction in antidiabetic medication use [95]. In 259 Israeli participants, a low-carbohydrate Mediterranean diet versus a traditional Mediterranean diet or American Diabetes Association diet was associated with greater reductions in HbA1c and cardiovascular risk factors [96]. Notably, the majority of the improved glucometabolic findings with the Mediterranean diet remained significant with adjustment for weight loss. Although, the Mediterranean diet has not been assessed in a clinical trial among US ethnic minorities, observational findings in the Multiethnic Study of Atherosclerosis (MESA) (42 % white (NHW), 12 % Chinese American (CA), 26 % NHB, 21 % Hispanic American) reveal that participants with greater adherence to a Mediterranean dietary pattern had lower insulin and glucose independent of racial/ethnic group [97]. These results suggest a likely beneficial effect of the Mediterranean diet on improved glucose metabolism among US racial/ethnic minorities with diabetes, although intervention trials in these populations are needed.

Vegetarian Diet

The Adventist Health Study 2 assessed the role of vegan and vegetarian diets in the USA. Among 73,308 NHB and NHW participants with no history of cancer or cardiovascular disease, there was a 12 % reduction in all-cause mortality over 5.8 years [98], 30–50 % lower diabetes prevalence [99], and 40–60 % lower diabetes incidence in the vegetarian versus non-vegetarian groups [100]. These findings lend credence to improved glucose metabolism with vegetarian dietary patterns. In individuals with diabetes, a small ($n = 99$) multiethnic (NHW 44 %, NHB 44 %, Hispanic American 4 %, and Asian American 8 %) clinical trial of a low-fat vegan diet or American Diabetes Association diet for 72 weeks revealed greater reductions in HbA1c and cardiovascular risk factors in the low-fat vegan group [101].

DASH Diet

The Dietary Approaches to Stop Hypertension (DASH) diet encourages the intake of fruits, vegetables, whole grains, and low-fat dairy products in combination with sodium restriction [102]. The DASH diet was initially studied in a multiethnic trial with 65 % ethnic minorities (35 % NHW, 60 % NHB, 5 % other minority groups) and significantly lowered blood pressure among all participants with twofold greater reductions among racial/ethnic minorities [102]. Further studies revealed that components of the DASH diet may also improve insulin sensitivity [103]. The DASH diet is recommended for all Americans including those with diabetes [93].

Dietary Composition

Glycemic Index/Glycemic Load

Carbohydrates are the chief dietary component influencing insulin secretion and postprandial glycemia [104]. The glycemic index measures the effect of carbohydrates on postprandial blood glucose, and the glycemic load takes into account the glycemic index and the amount of carbohydrate consumed. Several studies with multiethnic participants using low-glycemic index eating patterns have demonstrated HbA1c decreases (0.2–0.5 %), but these are not unanimous [105]. One difficulty is that fiber intake was not consistently controlled, thereby causing difficulty in interpretation. Results of low-glycemic index/glycemic load diets on cardiovascular disease risk factors including low-density lipoprotein and total cholesterol are mixed [105].

Low-Carbohydrate/Low-Fat Dietary Approaches

Low-carbohydrate versus low-fat diets have been extensively examined in diabetes management. A 2012 meta-analysis of 23 clinical trials of low-carbohydrate versus low-fat diets including studies of participants with and without diabetes revealed that both diets reduced glucose in a similar manner [106]. We will focus on data from two recent low-carbohydrate versus low-fat diet trials in overweight or obese patients with diabetes. First, a 12-month multiethnic trial (59 % NHB, 3 % Hispanic American, 38 % NHW) of obese (BMI ≥35 kg/m2) adults was randomized to low-carbohydrate (LC) (<30 g/day) or a calorie-restricted low-fat diet (LF) (500 calorie reduction with <30 % calories from fat). Among 54 participants with diabetes, HbA1c decreased by 0.7 % in the LC group versus 0.1 % in the LF group ($p=0.02$) with no significant weight-loss differences [107]. Second, a 12-month multiethnic trial (64 % NHB, 16 % Hispanic American, 15 % NHW, and 3 % Asian) of 105 overweight participants with diabetes randomized to a LC versus LF diet revealed no significant difference in weight (–3.4 %) or HbA1c change (−0.02 % LC versus 0.24 % LF, nonsignificant) [108]. A major strength of these studies is the inclusion of ethnic minorities, but a weakness is the inability to stratify by race due to power limitations, so it is unclear whether there are racial/ethnic differences. Based on these studies, the potentially greater HbA1c reduction with LC vs. LF diets appears to be independent of weight loss.

Physical Activity and Exercise

Exercise interventions improve glycemic control in diabetes in majority of NHW studies [109]. A meta-analysis examining the effects of exercise interventions (mean 3.4 sessions/week with 49 min/session) on glycemic control in individuals with diabetes revealed mean HbA1c reduction of 0.66 % ($p<0.001$) in people with diabetes, even with no significant change in BMI [109]. Higher levels of exercise intensity are associated with greater improvements in HbA1c and fitness [110]. Clinical trials have provided strong evidence for the HbA1c lowering value of resistance training in NHW older adults with type 2 diabetes [111]. There are limited data on glycemia in response to exercise in NHB, Hispanic Americans, and Native Americans with diabetes. Among individuals without diabetes in the HERITAGE Family Study, a 20-week trial of thrice weekly exercise in NHB and NHW, NHB had a greater increase in fasting glucose with exercise compared to NHW, although there were reductions in fasting insulin in both groups [112]. A multiethnic (52.7 NHW, 43.5 % NHB, 3.8 % Hispanic American) randomized clinical trial examining the effect of aerobic exercise, resistance training or combined aerobic exercise, and resistance training on HbA1c levels in 221 participants with diabetes found that aerobic exercise alone or resistance training alone had no effect on HbA1c, only the combined group revealed significant reductions in HbA1c (−0.34 %, $p=0.03$) and improvements in cardiorespiratory fitness over 9 months [113]. They lacked the power to examine racial/ethnic differences. Potential components of improved glucose metabolism with physical activity are skeletal muscle mitochondrial mass, mitochondrial function, and aerobic capacity [114, 115]. The racial/ethnic differences of aerobic capacity with physical activity were tested in a 6-month trial of aerobic exercise training in NHB and NHW postmenopausal women. The NHW women had a greater increase in cardiorespiratory fitness with sustained resting metabolic rate, whereas in NHB women, resting metabolic rate declined over the course of the trial, suggesting a perturbation in mitochondrial function [116, 117]. A study of exercise capacity and all-cause mortality in NHB and NHW men with diabetes found that exercise capacity is a stronger and more graded predictor of mortality for NHW than for NHB men [118]. The high-fit compared to low-fit NHW and NHB men had a 67 % and 46 % reduction in mortality risk, respectively [118]. These studies reveal that there is a benefit to physical activity in US racial/ethnic minorities, but the type (aerobic vs. resistance) and intensity of the physical activity need to be further characterized. A recent meta-analysis of step counters to improve physical activity and HbA1c in individuals with diabetes underscores this point. Data from 11 randomized clinical trials using step counters (pedometers) revealed that step counter use is associated with a significant increase in physical activity (1,822 steps/day), but no change in HbA1c [119].

Weight Reduction: Bariatric Surgery/ Lifestyle Interventions

Elevated body mass index and adiposity are the most important predictors of diabetes [120–122]. Obesity is also an independent predictor of clinical cardiovascular disease [123–125]. Mortality for diabetes, myocardial infarction, and stroke was similar for each of these conditions, but when any two are combined, the risk is multiplicative [126], reinforcing the importance of improving weight in individuals with elevated weight. The underlying relationship between obesity, cardiovascular disease, and diabetes has been reviewed and is potentially mediated through the adipokines released from visceral fat [127–130]. In this section we will review the data on nonsurgical and surgical interventions to promote weight loss in diabetes and improve glycemia with the goal of long-term reduction in morbidity and mortality.

Lifestyle, Diet, and Behavioral Interventions

The largest analysis of a lifestyle intervention in individuals with diabetes was Look AHEAD [131], a multiethnic (63 % NHW, 16 % NHB, 13 % Hispanic American, 5 % Native American, 1 % Asian or Pacific Islander, and 2 % other minorities) randomized controlled lifestyle intervention trial with 5,145 overweight or obese participants. Participants were randomized to either intensive lifestyle intervention that promoted weight loss through decreased caloric intake and increased physical activity (intervention group) or received diabetes support and education (control group) and followed a median of 9.6 years for the development of the primary outcome of a composite of death from cardiovascular causes, nonfatal myocardial infarction, nonfatal stroke, or hospitalization for angina. They found no association between the lifestyle intervention and primary outcome (HR: 0.95, $p=0.51$). Notably, the hazard ratios for Hispanic Americans, NHBs, NHWs, and Native Americans were 0.66 (95 % CI: 0.41–1.05), 1.34 (95 % CI: 0.91–1.96), 0.94 (95 % CI: 0.80–1.11), and 0.74 (95 % CI: 0.31–1.76), suggesting possible variance by race/ethnicity, especially for Hispanic Americans (HA) compared to NHBs. The authors and others note that differences in rates of cardioprotective medication use and power issues due to lower than expected cardiovascular disease event rates may account for the null finding. There was also a suggestion of heterogeneity of response to intervention based on the history of cardiovascular disease at baseline ($p=0.06$). There were a number of positive outcomes of the study including reduced hepatic steatosis, body weight, healthcare costs, and microvascular outcomes including diabetic nephropathy and retinopathy, as well as increased physical fitness, physical function, glucose control, and quality of life [132–134]. Given the benefit in these secondary outcomes from a diabetes management perspective, there are many important reasons to encourage overweight and obese individuals with diabetes to enroll in a lifestyle intervention program with the goal of weight loss [134].

In a multiethnic (59 % NHB, 32 % NHW, 2 % Hispanic American) randomized comparison of a commercially available portion-controlled weight-loss intervention with a diabetes self-management education program, the portion-controlled group lost greater weight (7.3 kg vs. 2.2 kg) with a larger reduction in HbA1c (0.7 % vs. 0.4 %) [135]. Finally, a recent systematic review and network meta-analysis of 33 studies (4,774 participants) evaluating behavioral programs in diabetes management revealed that in comparison with usual care among ethnic minority participants, behavioral programs lowered HbA1c by 0.42 % compared to usual care [136].

Surgical Interventions

Bariatric Surgery for Individuals with BMI ≥35 kg/m²

Bariatric surgery procedures are associated with diabetes remission due to hormonal changes and weight loss [137]. Hormonal changes include reduction in ghrelin and increases in glucagon-like peptide-1 (GLP-1) and glucose-dependent insulinotropic peptide (GIP). Lower levels of ghrelin postsurgically decrease appetite stimulation through a decrease in stimulation of orexigenic neurons neuropeptide Y/agouti-related peptide. Postsurgically levels of glucagon-like peptide-1 and glucose-dependent insulinotropic peptide increase exerting effects on the enteroinsular axis with potent insulinotropic activity. The long-term weight loss occurs due to decreased food (energy) consumption caused by the reduction in appetite and anatomical constraints. The surgical procedures currently performed include laparoscopic adjustable gastric banding (LAGB), laparoscopic vertical sleeve gastrectomy (LVSG), Roux-en-Y gastric bypass (RYGB), biliopancreatic diversion, and biliopancreatic diversion with duodenal switch (Fig. 14.1). In the USA, RYGB was the most commonly performed procedure but with wide adoption of LVSG; LVSG has surpassed RYGB and is performed in one half of bariatric surgical procedures [139]. The type of procedure is important for individuals with diabetes as diabetes remission varies greatly across procedures. Meta-analyses and reviews report remission rates of 48 % (29–67 %) for LAGB, 84 % (77–90 %) for RYGB, 72 % (55–88 %) for LVSG, and 99 % (97–100 %) for biliopancreatic diversion with duodenal switch [140, 141]. Recent analysis of the two most popular procedures have shown diabetes remission rates ranging from 27 to 75 % for LVSG versus 42–93 % for RYGB [142]. In the STAMPEDE trial, diabetes remission rates at 1 and 3 years of follow-up were 12 and 5 % with intensive medical therapy alone, 42 and 38 % in RYGB group, and 37 and 24 % in the LVSG group (Table 14.6). The diminishing rates of diabetes remission over time noted in STAMPEDE are also seen in other studies of LVSG and RYGB at a rate of 7–15 % per year [137]. Given the current popularity of LVSG, longer-term comparative effectiveness data on LVSG are needed. However, bariatric surgery experts believe the effect of LVSG on weight loss and comorbidity improvements seems to be somewhere between those of RYGB and LAGB [151]. Five-year outcomes from RYGB among mostly NHW participants found that shorter diabetes duration, lower HbA1c, younger age, higher serum insulin levels, and nonuse of insulin were associated with higher remission rates [152].

Bariatric Surgery for Individuals with BMI <35 kg/m²

Controversy exists regarding bariatric surgery for treatment of diabetes with BMI <35 kg/m². There are limited data to assess the benefit of bariatric surgery for individuals with BMI 30–35 kg/m². Short-term data from the STAMPEDE trial in the 36 % of the participants having a BMI <35 kg/m² revealed similar benefits as participants with BMI ≥35 kg/m² [143], and two systematic reviews draw similar conclusions [153, 154], but there remain no high-quality longer-term data on remission rates and complications. Thus, the current ADA guidelines do not recommend bariatric surgery treatment for individuals with diabetes and BMI <35 kg/m² [155]. The complication rates are important including near-term (30-day) and longer-term mortality rates which vary depending on procedure, center, and surgical expertise. Morbidities of bariatric surgery including vitamin deficiencies, mineral deficiencies, and post-bariatric surgery hypoglycemia secondary to insulin hypersecretion require long-term management [156]. Further understanding of non-trial-based 1-year complication rates (morbidity and mortality) are important as part of the risk/benefit criteria for all individuals with diabetes regardless of BMI.

Morbidity and Mortality

While glycemia is important in diabetes, the goal in diabetes management is to maximize longevity and quality of life. This involves control of

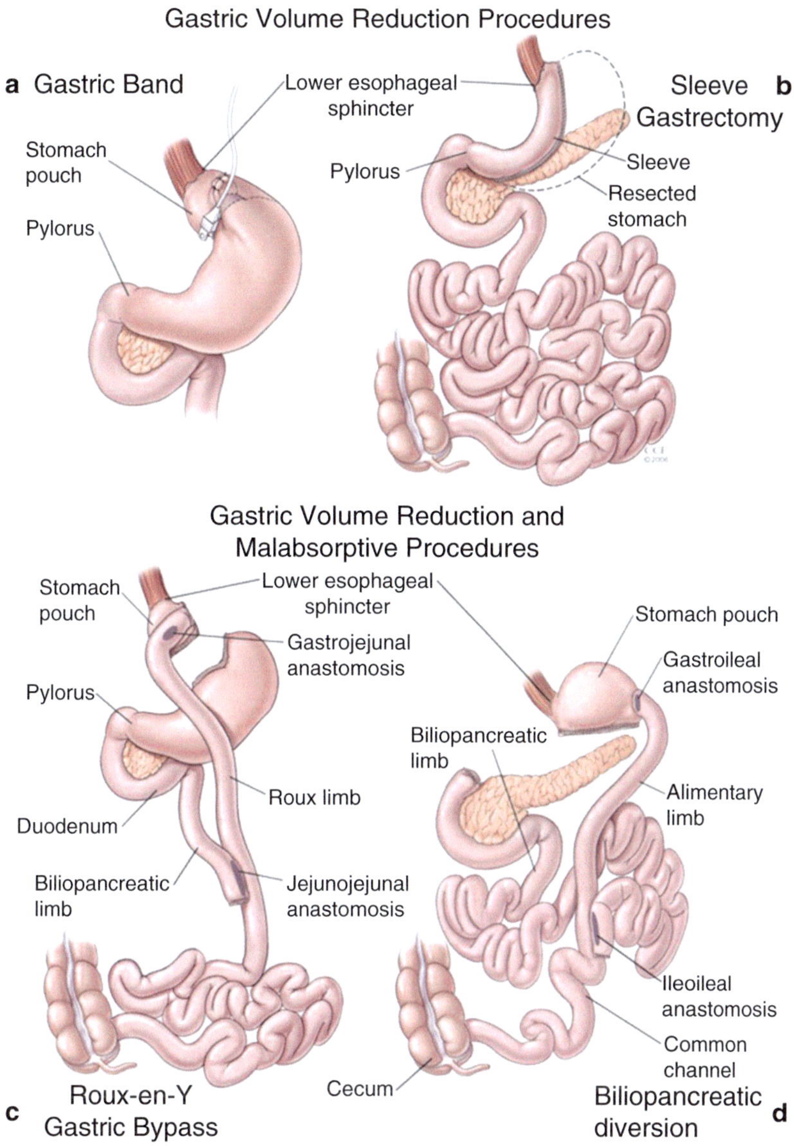

Fig. 14.1 Anatomic modifications as created in the four most common bariatric surgery procedures. (**a**) Gastric banding involves placement of an adjustable gastric band around the proximal part of the stomach. The band is fixed in position by inserting plication sutures anteriorly. The band can be adjusted/tightened over time by injecting fluid into the subcutaneous port connected to the band. (**b**) Sleeve gastrectomy involves reducing gastric volume by 75–80 % by resecting the stomach alongside a 30 F endoscope beginning 3 cm from the pylorus and ending at the angle of His. (**c**) The Roux-en-Y gastric bypass involves creation of a 15- to 20-mL gastric pouch, a 150-cm Roux limb, and a 50-cm biliopancreatic limb. (**d**) The biliopancreatic diversion procedure includes a distal gastrectomy with long Roux-en-Y reconstruction, where the enteroenterostomy is placed ≈50 cm proximal to the ileocecal valve. Both the volume of the gastric remnant and the length of the alimentary limb can be modified to suit the patient's weight loss goal (Vest et al. [138])

glycemia, but also cardiovascular risk factors with a focus on blood pressure and lipids. In the multiethnic Diabetes Surgery Substudy, participants randomized to intensive lifestyle medical treatment (ILMT) plus RYGB versus ILMT alone had a twofold greater achievement of the primary composite outcome of HbA1C <7 %, LDL <100 mg/dl, and systolic BP <130 mmHg at

Table 14.6 Glycemia, diabetes remission, cardiovascular risk factors, and cardiovascular events in diabetes bariatric surgery studies

Publication year	Study/site/size	Population characteristics/ethnicity	Study design/interventions	Summary of primary findings
2012, 2014	STAMPEDE trial [143, 144]	Uncontrolled type 2 diabetes (HbA1c 9.7 %) and moderate obesity (BMI 36.6 kg/m^2 (27–43 kg/m^2)) with a diabetes duration of 8.5 years	Randomized in a non-blinded fashion to intensive medical therapy (IMT) alone, IMT plus Roux-en-Y gastric bypass (RYGB) or IMT plus laporoscopic vertical sleeve gastrectomy (LVSG) and followed for a primary end point of HbA1C <6 %	The primary end point at years 1 and 3 was reached in 12 and 5 % IMT alone group (HbA1c 7.5 and 8.4 %) vs. 42 and 38 % in gastric bypass group (HbA1c 6.4 and 6.7 %) and 37 and 24 % in the LVSG group (HbA1c 6.6 and 7.0 %)
	USA	74 % NHW		
	150 and 137 participants (years 1 and 3)			
2013	STAMPEDE trial substudy [145]	Subset of participants with a diabetes duration of 8.4 years and BMI ≈36 kg/m^2	Evaluated at 1 and 2 years for assessment of beta-cell function (mixed-meal tolerance testing) and body composition	At 2 years, HbA1c was 8.4 % for IMT vs. 6.7 % for RYGB and 7.1 % for LVSG with greater insulin sensitivity, beta-cell function, and reduction in truncal fat in the RYGB group, but not in the LVSG group
	USA	72 % NHW		
	60 participants			
2012	Prospective Utah Obesity Study [146]	Secondary outcome: BMI ≥35 kg/m^2 and diabetes (FBG <126 mg/dl, HbA1c <6.5 % and no use of antidiabetic medication)	RYGB surgery (n = 88)	Diabetes remission rates at years 2 and 6 were 75 and 62 % in RYGB and 7 and 8 % in control group 1, and 6 and 6 % in control group 2. Of note, 13 % of participants in control groups underwent bariatric surgery over the 6 years of follow-up
	USA	96 % NHW	Control group 1 (n = 93): sought but did not have surgery Control group 2 (n = 88): randomly selected from a population-based sample not seeking weight-loss surgery. Diabetes remission: FBG <126 mg/dl, HbA1c <6.5 %, and no use of antidiabetic medication	
	269 participants			
2013	The Longitudinal Assessment of Bariatric Surgery (LABS) [147]	BMI ≥35 kg/m^2	Observational cohort study assessing RYGB or laparoscopic adjustable gastric banding (LAGB) at 3 years for weight loss and diabetes remission	Among participants who had diabetes at baseline, 216 RYGB participants (67.5 %) and 28 LAGB participants (28.6 %) experienced remission at 3 years
	USA	NHW: 86 %	Diabetes remission:	
	774 participants (33 % of total cohort)	NHB: 11 %	FBG <126 mg/dL or HbA1c <6.5 % both without use of antidiabetic medication	
		Hispanic American: 5 %		

Table 14.6 (continued)

Publication year	Study/site/size	Population characteristics/ ethnicity	Study design/interventions	Summary of primary findings
2014	Courcoulas et al. (2014) [148]	Diabetes and BMI 30–40 kg/m^2	Participants were randomized to RYGB ($n=24$), LAGB ($n=22$), or lifestyle weight-loss program groups (LWLI) ($n=22$)	Partial and complete remission of diabetes were 50 % and 17 %, respectively, in the RYGB group and 27 % and 23 %, respectively, in the LAGB group ($P<.001$ and $P=.047$ between groups for partial and complete remission), with no remission in the LWLI group. Significant reductions in use of antidiabetic medications occurred in both surgical groups
	USA	NHB:	Partial diabetes remission: subdiabetic hyperglycemia (HbA1c <6.5 % and fasting glucose 100–125 mg/dl with no antidiabetic medications	
	69 participants	33 % RYGB	Complete diabetes remission: normal HbA1c and FBG with no antidiabetic medications	
		14 % LAGB		
		17 % LWLI		
		Diabetes duration:		
		RYGB: 7.4 years		
		LAGB: 6.1 years		
		LWLI: 5.7 years		
2015	Ng et al. (2015) [149]	593 patients with diabetes	Retrospective analysis of weight change and comorbidities outcomes with LAGB and RYGB in a prospective database over 1 year	NHB patients showed less % expected weight loss than Caucasian and Hispanic patients. DM remission rates did not vary by ethnicity ≈70 % (RYGB) and 50 % (LAGB)
	USA	BMI 46.2 kg/m^2		
	1,684 patients	8 % NHB (37 % diabetes)		
		68 % NHW (36 % diabetes)		
		14 % Hispanic American (30 % diabetes)		
2013	Diabetes Surgery Study [150]	HbA1c ≥8 % and BMI 30–39.9 kg/m^2	Subjects underwent ILMT plus RYGB ($n=60$) versus ILMT alone ($n=60$) with a primary composite outcome of HbA1c <7 %, LDL <100 mg/dl and systolic BP <130	At 1 year the primary end point occurred in 49 % of subjects in the surgery/ ILMT vs. 19 % in the ILMT group
	USA and Taiwan	52 % NHW		
	120 participants	28 % East Asian		
		9 % NHB		
		7 % Hispanic American		
		3 % Native American		

Surgical Treatment and Medications Potentially Eradicate Diabetes Efficiently trial (STAMPEDE) trial

1 year (Table 14.6). This finding suggests improved cardiovascular risk factor control with RYGB. Prospective data on cardiovascular events in participants with diabetes are limited to the Swedish outcome study, with a 44 % reduction in CHD events at 13 years. Both retrospective analyses including analysis by Adams et al. [157] and prospective analysis in the SOS [158] have shown long-term reductions in mortality, but these analyses are underpowered to report mortality among diabetes participants alone. No studies have focused on cardiovascular events and mortality in racial/ethnic minorities.

Ethnic Differences

Limited data are available to assess the effects of bariatric surgery in US racial/ethnic minorities. The major US trials STAMPEDE, Diabetes

Surgery Study, LABS, and Courcoulas et al. (Table 14.6) were multiethnic but lacked the power to examine racial/ethnic differences in diabetes remission. There is conflicting data regarding weight-loss post-bariatric surgery in NHW versus racial/ethnic minorities with some studies showing greater weight loss in NHW and a smaller number of studies showing equivalent weight loss [149]. Some of the variation in findings may be due to majority/minority status of participants or variations in African or Hispanic origins. A study in South Florida, USA (a majority Hispanic region) with NHBs, Hispanic Americans (less Mexican Americans), and NHWs revealed similar outcomes for weight-loss post-RYGB and LAGB among HA and NHWs, with decreased weight loss among NHBs [159]. A retrospective analysis by Ng et al. (Table 14.6) revealed NHB patients had less % excess weight loss than NHW and HA patients [149]. Among 539 patients with diabetes, diabetes remission rates did not vary by ethnicity [149]. A second retrospective analysis examining metabolic effects of bariatric surgery in 4,088 nondiabetic multiethnic adults (17 % NHB, 23 % Hispanic American) in the Kaiser-Permanente system (USA) showed racial/ethnic variation with decreased metabolic syndrome remission in NHB or Hispanic American vs. NHW participants independent of weight loss [160]. Racial/ethnic differences in response to bariatric surgery remain a high-priority area for further research given the potential for improved diabetes control and remission.

Rational Selection of Antidiabetes Medications in Minority and Underserved Populations

Pharmacokinetics and pharmacodynamics of drugs are potentially affected by race/ethnicity, thus resulting in variability in response to drug therapy. One of the most important sources of variability in drug exposure is potentially genetic differences in variant alleles effecting the expression of enzymes that metabolize or transport drugs or in the expression of targets of drug therapy [161]. The emerging fields of pharmacogenomics and precision medicine have the potential to transform the specificity of medication selection based on genetic alterations. An example of the potential clinical utility of this approach is found in maturity-onset diabetes of the young (MODY) caused by HNF1-alpha mutations. Individuals with MODY are often misdiagnosed with type 1 or type 2 diabetes, but the diagnosis is clinically important because patients can often be managed with sulfonylurea treatment alone [162]. Other monogenic forms of MODY and neonatal diabetes have been identified and have resulted in targeted treatment or did not require treatment with excellent long-term outcomes [163].

Repaglinide

Antidiabetic medication metabolism may be affected by variant alleles. Cytochrome P450 superfamily member CYP2C8 is an enzyme involved in the metabolic inactivation of several drugs. The *CYP2C8**2 is a common variant allele in NHB, with a frequency of 18 % vs. 0.4 % in whites. This common variant allele causes reduced CYP2C8 function and thus has the potential to alter therapeutic levels of repaglinide [161, 164]. It is currently unclear which other antidiabetic medications are affected by similar mechanisms.

Metformin

Recently, a large retrospective analysis of electronic health record database revealed a greater HbA1c response to metformin among NHB patients (−0.90 %) when compared with European American patients (−0.42 %) irrespective of baseline HbA1c [165]. Genetic ancestry explains only a small proportion of the variation in HbA1c levels among NHB, and HbA1c is similarly predictive of cardiovascular events among NHB and NHW, so the response may translate into improvement in clinical outcomes [165]. Further evidence comes from a US Veteran Affairs study where NHB patients treated with metformin had a trend toward lower all-cause mortality (HR 0.89, $p=0.29$) compared to NHW [166].

Sodium-Glucose Co-transporter 2 (SGLT2) Inhibitors

Racial/ethnic minorities have worse control of cardiovascular risk factors in diabetes [167]. NHB compared to NHW has a higher prevalence of hypertension, poorer rates of control, and higher long-term morbidity and mortality associated with hypertension [168]. HA, particularly Mexican Americans, also has poorer rates of blood pressure control compared to NHW [169, 170]. Thus, antidiabetic medications that lower blood pressure may be of greater benefit in racial/ethnic minorities. The sodium-glucose co-transporter 2 (SGLT2) inhibitors lower blood glucose by preventing reabsorption of glucose in the proximal tubule of the nephron, which leads to elimination of glucose and an osmotic diuresis. The osmotic diuresis results in lower systolic (3–6 mmHg) and diastolic blood pressures (1–3 mmHg) and mild weight loss (1–3 kg) [171]. These changes in blood pressure and weight could potentially help to ameliorate the disparities in blood pressure control. Long-term follow-up of SGLT2 inhibitor trials are ongoing to evaluate the effect of SGLT2 inhibitors on cardiovascular events.

GLP-1 Receptor Agonists

Racial/ethnic disparities exist in obesity prevalence in the USA with NHBs and Hispanic Americans having a higher prevalence of overweight (BMI ≥25 kg/m^2) and obese (BMI ≥30 kg/m^2) individuals compared to NHWs [172]. Asian Americans have a lower prevalence of overweight (BMI ≥25 kg/m^2) and obese (BMI ≥30 kg/m^2) individuals compared to NHWs [172], but this is confounded by evidence that Asian Americans have increased risk of diabetes at a lower BMI due to greater visceral adiposity [155]. Given these disparities medications that lower blood glucose and promote significant weight loss may be an attractive option specifically among NHBs, Hispanic Americans, and Native Americans. In a multinational study (92 % white and 6 % black (includes some NHBs)), liraglutide and exenatide reduced weight by 3 kg at 26 weeks with reductions in HbA1c of 1.12 and 0.79 %, respectively [173]. They have also been associated with reductions in blood pressure [174]. Unfortunately, these medications have been understudied in US racial/ethnic minority populations [175], where they may be of even greater benefit.

Weight-Loss Medications

Currently, less than 2 % of patients with obesity use anti-obesity drugs [176]. Even though the rates of obesity are higher in US racial/ethnic minorities [172], visits made to physician offices by NHW patients compared to nonwhites (OR,1.55; 95 % CI, 1.08–2.24) were more likely to involve an anti-obesity drug prescription [176]. This differs from earlier trends showing the highest usage among Hispanic American women [177]. Pharmacological agents approved for weight management can be useful adjuncts to lifestyle change for patients who have been unsuccessful with diet and exercise alone and have been recently reviewed by Apovian et al. [178]. See Table 14.7 for 1-year weight loss among patients that complete therapy.

Table 14.7 Odds of reducing body weight by % categories at 1 year with lifestyle intervention and adjunctive medication among those who complete treatment

Medication	>5 % Weight loss	>10 % Weight loss
Phentermine/topiramate 7.5/46 mg daily	74.5 %	49.1 %
Phentermine/topiramate 15/92 mg daily	85.1 %	64.3 %
Lorcaserin 10 mg twice daily	65.8 %	35.2 %
Naltrexone/bupropion 32/360 mg daily	65 %	39 %
Liraglutide 3.0 mg daily	73 %	41 %

Translating Primary Prevention of Type 2 Diabetes in Minority and Underserved Populations

Prevention is important for the individual person, as well as for the US healthcare system. Diabetes is associated with higher lifetime medical expenditures despite being associated with reduced life expectancy with twofold greater annual per capita medical spending than for nondiabetic individuals which accounts for 20 % of US healthcare dollars [179]. The American Diabetes Association recommends patients with prediabetes be referred to an intensive diet and physical activity behavioral counseling program targeting 7 % weight loss and increasing moderate-intensity physical activity (such as brisk walking) to at least 150 min/week. They also recommend metformin especially for individuals with BMI >35 kg/m^2, aged <60 years, and women with prior gestational diabetes mellitus [93]. These recommendations are based on randomized controlled diabetes prevention trials [180, 181]. Clinical trials of lifestyle intervention including the Diabetes Prevention Program (DPP) (physical activity/dietary modification) aimed at reducing incident diabetes in at-risk individuals have proved successful in US racial/ethnic minorities [180]. The DPP [180] compared standard lifestyle recommendations plus placebo twice daily to standard lifestyle recommendations plus metformin at a dose of 850 mg twice daily or an intensive program of lifestyle modification (aimed for 7 % weight loss through a low-calorie low-fat diet and at least 150 min of physical activity per week) in overweight (BMI >24 kg/m^2) individuals at risk for diabetes (impaired fasting glucose and 2-h post 75-g glucose load). The program had a 16-lesson curriculum covering diet, exercise, and behavior modification designed to help the participants achieve these goals. The curriculum was taught by case managers on a one-to-one basis during the first 24 weeks after enrollment and was flexible, culturally sensitive, and individualized. The mean body mass index was 34.0 kg/m^2 at baseline, and the trial contained 45 % racial/ethnic minority participants (20 % NHBs, 16 % Hispanic American, 5 % American Indian, 4 % Asian American). Over the course of 2.8 years, the lifestyle intervention and metformin intervention reduced diabetes risk by 58 % and 31 %, respectively, compared to placebo [180]. For every kilogram of weight loss, there was a 16 % reduction in risk, adjusted for changes in diet and activity [182]. Study participants are being followed long term in the DPP Outcomes Study, in which the original lifestyle intervention group was offered lifestyle reinforcement semiannually and the metformin group received unmasked metformin. At 10 years of follow-up, progression to diabetes was reduced by 34 % in the lifestyle group and 18 % in the metformin group compared with placebo [183]. At 15 years of follow-up, diabetes incidence was reduced by 27 % in the lifestyle intervention group and by 18 % in the metformin group with cumulative incidences of diabetes of 55 % for lifestyle, 56 % metformin, and 62 % placebo [184]. There were no overall differences in an aggregate microvascular outcome between treatment groups, although those whom did not develop diabetes had a 28 % lower prevalence of microvascular complications [184].

Current Landscape

Given the initial short-term success of the DPP [180], funding agencies have sponsored many culturally specific interventions using the DPP as a general guide. A systematic review and meta-analysis of twenty-eight US-based studies applying the findings of the DPP revealed an average 4 % weight loss at 12 months [185]. Change in weight was similar regardless of whether the intervention was delivered by clinically trained professionals or lay educators. Additional analyses limited to 17 studies with a 9-month or greater follow-up assessment showed similar weight change. Every additional lifestyle session attended increased weight loss by 0.26 %. The authors conclude that costs associated with diabetes prevention can be lowered without sacrificing effectiveness by using nonmedical personnel and motivating higher attendance at program sessions [185]. The effectiveness on community-based interventions based on the DPP is controversial, and the long-term impact of these interventions given the lower magnitude of weight loss compared to the DPP remains unknown [186].

Non-Hispanic Blacks

Twenty-one DPP translations focused on NHBs led to half of the weight loss reported in the DPP immediately post-intervention [187]. A YMCA translation of the DPP lifestyle intervention among multiethnic (57 % NHB, 35 % NHW, 3 % Hispanic American, 2 % others) low-income nondiabetic adults found that persons attending nine or more lessons had a 5.3 kg (95 % CI = 2.8, 7.9 kg) greater weight loss at 12 months than did those with standard care alone [188]. Interestingly, this study found no difference in cardiovascular risk factor control [188]. A 24-month lifestyle weight-loss program (75 % NHW, 25 % NHB) delivered by community health workers with a goal of 7 % weight loss vs. usual care found that the intervention group experienced significantly greater decreases in fasting glucose (4.35 mg/dL), insulin (3.01 U/ml), insulin resistance (0.97), body weight (4.19 kg), waist circumference (3.23 cm), and BMI (1.40) over 2 years [189]. Other interventions including a community health advisor-based diabetes prevention intervention in urban NHB communities have not shown weight reduction at 1 year [190].

Hispanic American

In Project HEED (Help Educate to Eliminate Diabetes), participants were randomized to a peer-led lifestyle intervention (8–1.5 h sessions) versus control for 12 months. The participants were majority Hispanic American (90 %), low-income undereducated women. The intervention group lost more weight than the control group and maintained weight loss at 12 months (7.2 versus 2.4 lb, $P<0.01$) [191]. Unfortunately, one quarter of participants progressed to diabetes at 1 year [191]. Promotora Effectiveness Versus Metformin Trial (PREVENT-DM) is a randomized comparative effectiveness trial of a lifestyle intervention based on the DPP delivered by community health workers (or promotoras), metformin, and standard care in Hispanic women [192]. This trial will be the first US study to test the comparative effectiveness of metformin and lifestyle intervention versus standard care among prediabetic Hispanic adults in a "real-world" setting [192].

American Indian/Native Alaskan

The Special Diabetes Program for Indians Diabetes Prevention (SDPI-DP) demonstration project implemented the DPP lifestyle intervention among 36 healthcare programs serving 80 American Indian/Alaskan Native tribes [193]. With similar eligibility criteria, the crude diabetes incidence of SDPI-DP (4.0 % per year) was close to that of the American Indians in the lifestyle intervention group of the DPP clinical trial (4.7 % per year) and lower than that of the American Indians in the placebo group of DPP (12.9 % per year), strongly suggesting the feasibility of translating the DPP intervention across a wide range of Native American communities [193].

Asian American

Efforts to translate the DPP findings with Asian American populations are limited to short-term pilot studies in different ethnic subgroups that were generally associated with weight loss [194–197].

In summary, a recent US report revealed that while most diabetes prevention programs were moderately successful at reducing the risk for developing diabetes consistent with prior analyses [198], only four studied primarily NHB or Hispanic American subjects [199]. These four analyses are constrained by lack of standardization in the implementation and documentation making it difficult to assess their costs and long-term effectiveness [199]. The results of the SDPI-DP study in American Indian and Native

Alaskan tribes are promising, but the lack of a comparison group and high loss to follow-up temper conclusions about its long-term effectiveness [200]. Further research in all racial/ethnic subgroups is critical to determine the most efficacious and cost-effective community-based translations for diabetes prevention.

Research Gaps and Future Directions

Approaches to Healthcare Delivery in Minority and Underserved Populations

A high level of evidence supports the effectiveness of culturally tailored patient-targeted interventions in lowering HbA1c in minority populations with diabetes; however, there is less evidence for the role of healthcare system and multi-target interventions in improving the quality of diabetes care in this population [38]. A recent study observed a trend since 2001 for most interventions to occur in primary care settings and since 2008, for many to occur in non-clinical settings [34]; however, endocrinologists are an integral part of the clinical management of patients with diabetes and may not be integrated into these care settings. In reviewing general diabetes QI interventions not specific to minority populations, many successful diabetes QI interventions involved endocrinologists who assisted with medical management either within an endocrinology clinic [201, 202] or outside of an endocrinology clinic [203–209]. Among studies of diabetes disease management programs, several have included endocrinology input/consultation as part of the care management team [206, 209–212].

Minority and socially disadvantaged patients with diabetes have less access to subspecialty care than majority and more socioeconomically advantaged patients. In one study, diabetic adults with only a primary or secondary education had more contacts with their general practitioner and dieticians but fewer visits with endocrinologists or diabetes nurses [213]. While management of specialty referrals through a gatekeeper may lead to more appropriate referral patterns [202, 214], restrictions on specialist referrals differentially applied to patients who are poor, uneducated, or have low literacy can adversely affect health outcomes [1]. Therefore, incorporating endocrinology subspecialty care into the infrastructure of multi-target diabetes QI interventions may improve the clinic outcomes for minority and underserved patients with diabetes.

Surgical Interventions for Non-pharmacological Management of Diabetes

Given the high prevalence of diabetes among racial/ethnic minorities, there remains a critical need for further research to understand differences in weight loss and metabolic effects including diabetes remission post-bariatric surgery in an appropriately powered prospective manner. Given the variance in prevalent diabetes rates within ethnicities based on ancestry, there will need to be significant consideration given to the size of prospective trials. For instance, within Hispanic Americans, the prevalence is lower among Cubans (9.3 %) and Central and South Americans (8.5 %), whereas the prevalence is higher in Mexican Americans (13.9 %) and Puerto Ricans (14.8 %), suggesting possible differences in etiology or risk factors which may limit the generalizability of subgroup findings to the whole. The same is true for Native American populations with an overall prevalence of 15.9 %, ranging from 6.0 % among Alaskan tribes to 24.1 % among those living in Southern Arizona [175].

Diabetes Prevention

Significant barriers remain to primary prevention of diabetes in the US racial/ethnic minorities including US work and leisure-time culture. Americans work long hours, and for those in lower SES groups, they often are required to work more than one job in order to make enough money to support themselves and family. Among low socioeconomic status groups, there is a link between longer working hours and incident diabetes [215]. Americans live far from their workplaces, and physically active modes of transportation (biking, walking) are uncommon (<4 % of Americans) [216]. During the work commute, Americans are exposed to fast-food restaurants that prioritize food calorie-dense food [217]. Neighborhood fast-food exposure is associated with poorer diets [218] and increased energy intake [219]. Predominantly racial/ethnic minority neighborhoods have greater fast-food restaurant density compared to predominantly NHW neighborhoods [220]. Long work hours and commutes may leave less time for sleep and other health-restorative behaviors. Poor sleep quality and sleep insufficiency occur with greater frequency in NHB [221–223] and have been associated with insulin resistance [224, 225], hyperglycemia, and incident diabetes in NHW populations [226, 227]. In the Insulin Resistance and Atherosclerosis Study, short sleep duration showed a nonsignificant protective effect on incident diabetes in NHBs [228]. This finding is contrary to findings in NHWs and Hispanic Americans in the same study which showed a significant association between short sleep duration and incident diabetes, consistent with the prevailing literature [228]. Leisure-time activities are becoming increasingly sedentary involving sitting, television viewing, and screen time [229].

In the face of these barriers, instituting healthful habits for diabetes prevention remains difficult. Primary prevention of diabetes in US racial/ethnic minorities would benefit from being multilevel and multifaceted and requires buy-in from multiple stakeholders. An attractive model is the chronic care model promoting self-management skills and tracking systems in the individual patient and coordination/promotion of care partnerships between health systems, community resources, and public policy [230]. In this model all the pieces are equally important from the patient to public service officials. Examples of this include a patient being educated regarding diabetes prevention in the office and then being supported in the community by a diabetes prevention program, which is bolstered by a tax on soda, which serves to increase public awareness of the caloric/glycemic content of soda.

In most trials, participants lose weight for the first 6 months and then begin slow and steady weight regain. Notably, in trials this sometimes corresponds to a decrease in intensity of the intervention as well. Clearly, the nexus of cost versus length/intensity of interventions is important. Interventions need to be long enough and transmissible enough so that participants can develop and commit to lifelong healthy habits for diabetes prevention and improved cardiometabolic health. Currently in the USA, there is a large degree of short-term dieting and meal replacements, but in our opinion the most effective approach is education surrounding healthy dietary choices and food preparation. Understanding methods to promote further weight loss beyond 6 months remains important and may lead to further long-term reductions in diabetes incidence. Second, "type 2 diabetes" is likely inclusive of more specific diseases with polygenetic inheritance, gene environment, and environment interactions. The genetic influence may be different among various ethnicities, which may change how we consider not only targeted interventions but also translation of targeted interventions. The Human Genome Project and the current trends toward personalized medicine using genomic and pharmacogenomic data may cause large shifts in how we categorize, diagnose, and treat diabetes. It is possible that for populations where the key issue is genetic or epigenetic, changes causing insulin resistance, physical activity, or metformin may be an excellent option, whereas for someone with insulin secretory deficits, these may not represent promising options, and a sulfonylurea or early provision of insulin may be efficacious. On the individual patient level, we have already seen the success of these approaches with MODY, as discussed previously. Given the rising incidence of diabetes in minority and underserved populations, it will be critical to identify and implement the most effective treatment and healthcare delivery interventions to improve outcomes in these high-risk populations in the USA.

References

1. Golden SH, Brown A, Cauley JA, Chin MH, Gary-Webb TL, Kim C, et al. Health disparities in endocrine disorders: biological, clinical, and nonclinical factors – an Endocrine Society scientific statement. J Clin Endocrinol Metab. 2012;97(9):E1579–639.
2. Daviglus ML, Talavera GA, Avilés-Santa ML, Allison M, Cai J, Criqui MH, et al. Prevalence of major cardiovascular risk factors and cardiovascular diseases among Hispanic/Latino individuals of diverse backgrounds in the United States. JAMA. 2012;308(17):1775.
3. Geiss LS, Wang J, Cheng YJ, Thompson TJ, Barker L, Li Y, et al. Prevalence and incidence trends for diagnosed diabetes among adults aged 20 to 79 years, United States, 1980–2012. JAMA. 2014; 312(12):1218.
4. Narayan KMV, Aviles-Santa L, Oza-Frank R, Pandey M, Curb JD, McNeely M, et al. Report of a National Heart, Lung, And Blood Institute Workshop: heterogeneity in cardiometabolic risk in Asian Americans in the U.S. Opportunities for research. J Am Coll Cardiol. 2010;55(10):966–73.
5. Chien AT, Chin MH, Davis AM, Casalino LP. Pay for performance, public reporting, and racial disparities in health care: how are programs being designed? Med Care Res Rev MCRR. 2007;64(5 Suppl):283S–304.
6. Karter AJ, Schillinger D, Adams AS, Moffet HH, Liu J, Adler NE, et al. Elevated rates of diabetes in Pacific Islanders and Asian subgroups: the Diabetes Study of Northern California (DISTANCE). Diabetes Care. 2013;36(3):574–9.
7. Dagogo-Jack S. Ethnic disparities in type 2 diabetes: pathophysiology and implications for prevention and management. J Natl Med Assoc. 2003;95(9):774. 779–89.
8. Torrens J. Ethnic differences in insulin sensitivity and beta-cell function in premenopausal or early perimenopausal women without diabetes: the Study of Women's Health Across the Nation (SWAN). Diabetes Care. 2004;27(2 SRC - GoogleScholar): 354–61.
9. Perez-Escamilla RJ. Acculturation, nutrition, and health disparities in Latinos. Am Nutr P S. 2011;93(5 SRC - GoogleScholar):1163S–7.
10. Kurian AK, Cardarelli KM. Racial and ethnic differences in cardiovascular disease risk factors: a systematic review. Ethn Dis. 2007;17(1):143–52.
11. McCarthy MI. Genomics, type 2 diabetes, and obesity. N Engl J Med. 2010;363(24):2339–50.
12. Kooner JS, Saleheen D, Sim X, Sehmi J, Zhang W, Frossard P, et al. Genome-wide association study in individuals of South Asian ancestry identifies six new type 2 diabetes susceptibility loci. Nat Genet. 2011;43(10):984–9.
13. Cho YS, Chen C-H, Hu C, Long J, Hee Ong RT, Sim X, et al. Meta-analysis of genome-wide association studies identifies eight new loci for type 2 diabetes in east Asians. Nat Genet. 2011;44(1):67–72.
14. Palmer ND, McDonough CW, Hicks PJ, Roh BH, Wing MR, An SS, et al. A genome-wide association search for type 2 diabetes genes in African Americans. PLoS One. 2012;7(1):e29202.
15. Kuzawa CW, Sweet E. Epigenetics and the embodiment of race: developmental origins of US racial disparities in cardiovascular health. Am J Hum Biol Off J Hum Biol Counc. 2009;21(1):2–15.
16. Anagnostis P, Athyros VG, Tziomalos K, Karagiannis A, Mikhailidis DP. The pathogenetic role of cortisol in the metabolic syndrome: a hypothesis. J Clin Endocrinol Metab. 2009;94(8): 2692–701.
17. Slomko H, Heo HJ, Einstein FH. Minireview: epigenetics of obesity and diabetes in humans. Endocrinology. 2012;153(3):1025–30.
18. Dagogo-Jack S. Pitfalls in the use of $HbA_1(c)$ as a diagnostic test: the ethnic conundrum. Nat Rev Endocrinol. 2010;6(10):589–93.
19. Ziemer DC, Kolm P, Weintraub WS, Vaccarino V, Rhee MK, Twombly JG, et al. Glucose-independent, black-white differences in hemoglobin A1c levels: a cross-sectional analysis of 2 studies. Ann Intern Med. 2010;152(12):770–7.
20. Selvin E, Steffes MW, Ballantyne CM, Hoogeveen RC, Coresh J, Brancati FL. Racial differences in glycemic markers: a cross-sectional analysis of community-based data. Ann Intern Med. 2011;154(5): 303–9.
21. Minority H. Office of Office of Minority Health. 2012.
22. Kirk JK, Bell RA, Bertoni AG, Arcury TA, Quandt SA, Goff DC, et al. Ethnic disparities: control of glycemia, blood pressure, and LDL cholesterol among US adults with type 2 diabetes. Ann Pharmacother. 2005;39(9):1489–501.
23. Kirk JK. Disparities in HbA1c levels between African-American and Non-Hispanic white adults with diabetes: a meta-analysis. Diabetes Care. 2006;29(9):2130–6.
24. Kirk JK, Passmore LV, Bell RA, Narayan K, D'Agostino RB, Arcury TA, et al. Disparities in A1c levels between Hispanic and non-Hispanic White adults with diabetes. Diabetes Care. 2008;31(2): 240.
25. Selvin E, Ning Y, Steffes MW, Bash LD, Klein R, Wong TY, et al. Glycated hemoglobin and the risk of kidney disease and retinopathy in adults with and without diabetes. Diabetes. 2011;60(1):298–305.
26. Selvin E, Steffes MW, Zhu H, Matsushita K, Wagenknecht L, Pankow J, et al. Glycated hemoglobin, diabetes, and cardiovascular risk in nondiabetic adults. N Engl J Med. 2010;362(9):800–11.
27. Matsushita K, Blecker S, Pazin-Filho A, Bertoni A, Chang PP, Coresh J, et al. The association of hemoglobin a1c with incident heart failure among people without diabetes: the atherosclerosis risk in communities study. Diabetes. 2010;59(8):2020–6.

28. Lakkis J, Weir MR. Pharmacological strategies for kidney function preservation: are there differences by ethnicity? Adv Ren Replace Ther. 2004;11(1):24–40.
29. Lopes AA. End-stage renal disease due to diabetes in racial/ethnic minorities and disadvantaged populations. Ethn Dis. 2009;19(1 Suppl 1):S1–47.
30. Sumner AE, Zhou J, Doumatey A, Imoisili OE, Amoah A, Acheampong J, et al. Low HDL-cholesterol with normal triglyceride levels is the most common lipid pattern in west Africans and African Americans with metabolic syndrome: implications for cardiovascular disease prevention. CVD Prev Control. 2010;5(3):75–80.
31. Kirk JK, Graves DE, Bell RA, Hildebrandt CA, Narayan KMV. Racial and ethnic disparities in self-monitoring of blood glucose among US adults: a qualitative review. Ethn Dis. 2007;17(1):135–42.
32. Tricco AC, Ivers NM, Grimshaw JM, Moher D, Turner L, Galipeau J, et al. Effectiveness of quality improvement strategies on the management of diabetes: a systematic review and meta-analysis. Lancet Lond Engl. 2012;379(9833):2252–61.
33. Shojania KG, Ranji SR, McDonald KM, Grimshaw JM, Sundaram V, Rushakoff RJ, et al. Effects of quality improvement strategies for type 2 diabetes on glycemic control: a meta-regression analysis. JAMA. 2006;296(4):427–40.
34. Pimouguet C, Le Goff M, Thiébaut R, Dartigues JF, Helmer C. Effectiveness of disease-management programs for improving diabetes care: a meta-analysis. CMAJ Can Med Assoc J J Assoc Med Can. 2011;183(2):E115–27.
35. Glazier RH, Bajcar J, Kennie NR, Willson K. A systematic review of interventions to improve diabetes care in socially disadvantaged populations. Diabetes Care. 2006;29(7):1675–88.
36. Davidson MB. Effect of nurse-directed diabetes care in a minority population. Diabetes Care. 2003;26(8):2281–7.
37. Peek ME, Cargill A, Huang ES. Diabetes health disparities: a systematic review of health care interventions. Med Care Res Rev. 2007;64(5 suppl):101S–56.
38. Ricci-Cabello I, Ruiz-Pérez I, Olry de Labry-Lima A, Márquez-Calderón S. Do social inequalities exist in terms of the prevention, diagnosis, treatment, control and monitoring of diabetes? A systematic review. Health Soc Care Community. 2010;18(6):572–87.
39. Basch CE, Walker EA, Howard CJ, Shamoon H, Zybert P. The effect of health education on the rate of ophthalmic examinations among African Americans with diabetes mellitus. Am J Public Health. 1999;89(12):1878–82.
40. Clancy DE, Cope DW, Magruder KM, Huang P, Salter KH, Fields AW. Evaluating group visits in an uninsured or inadequately insured patient population with uncontrolled type 2 diabetes. Diabetes Educ. 2003;29(2):292–302.
41. Gerber BS, Brodsky IG, Lawless KA, Smolin LI, Arozullah AM, Smith EV, et al. Implementation and evaluation of a low-literacy diabetes education computer multimedia application. Diabetes Care. 2005;28(7):1574–80.
42. Erdman DM, Cook CB, Greenlund KJ, Giles WH, El-Kebbi I, Ryan GJ, et al. The impact of outpatient diabetes management on serum lipids in urban African-Americans with type 2 diabetes. Diabetes Care. 2002;25(1):9–15.
43. Ziemer DC, Berkowitz KJ, Panayioto RM, El-Kebbi IM, Musey VC, Anderson LA, et al. A simple meal plan emphasizing healthy food choices is as effective as an exchange-based meal plan for urban African Americans with type 2 diabetes. Diabetes Care. 2003;26(6):1719–24.
44. Anderson RM, Musch DC, Nwankwo RB, Wolf FM, Gillard ML, Oh MS, et al. Personalized follow-up increases return rate at urban eye disease screening clinics for African Americans with diabetes: results of a randomized trial. Ethn Dis. 2003;13(1):40–6.
45. D'Eramo-Melkus G, Spollett G, Jefferson V, Chyun D, Tuohy B, Robinson T, et al. A culturally competent intervention of education and care for black women with type 2 diabetes. Appl Nurs Res ANR. 2004;17(1):10–20.
46. Tang TS, Gillard ML, Funnell MM, Nwankwo R, Parker E, Spurlock D, et al. Developing a new generation of ongoing: diabetes self-management support interventions: a preliminary report. Diabetes Educ. 2005;31(1):91–7.
47. Amoako E, Skelly AH, Rossen EK. Outcomes of an intervention to reduce uncertainty among African American women with diabetes. West J Nurs Res. 2008;30(8):928–42.
48. Skelly AH, Carlson J, Leeman J, Soward A, Burns D. Controlled trial of nursing interventions to improve health outcomes of older African American women with type 2 diabetes. Nurs Res. 2009;58(6):410–8.
49. Tang TS, Funnell MM, Brown MB, Kurlander JE. Self-management support in "real-world" settings: an empowerment-based intervention. Patient Educ Couns. 2010;79(2):178–84.
50. Walker EA, Stevens KA, Persaud S. Promoting diabetes self-management among African Americans: an educational intervention. J Health Care Poor Underserved. 2010;21(3 Suppl):169–86.
51. Carter EL, Nunlee-Bland G, Callender C. A patient-centric, provider-assisted diabetes telehealth self-management intervention for urban minorities. Perspect Health Inf Manag AHIMA Am Health Inf Manag Assoc. 2011;8:1b.
52. Ellish NJ, Royak-Schaler R, Higginbotham EJ. Tailored and targeted interventions to encourage dilated fundus examinations in older African Americans. Arch Ophthalmol Chic Ill 1960. 2011;129(12):1592–8.

53. Tang TS, Funnell MM, Noorulla S, Oh M, Brown MB. Sustaining short-term improvements over the long-term: results from a 2-year diabetes self-management support (DSMS) intervention. Diabetes Res Clin Pract. 2012;95(1):85–92.
54. Agurs-Collins TD, Kumanyika SK, Ten Have TR, Adams-Campbell LL. A randomized controlled trial of weight reduction and exercise for diabetes management in older African-American subjects. Diabetes Care. 1997;20(10):1503–11.
55. Anderson-Loftin W, Barnett S, Sullivan P, Bunn PS, Tavakoli A. Culturally competent dietary education for southern rural African Americans with diabetes. Diabetes Educ. 2002;28(2):245–57.
56. Brown SA, Hanis CL. Culturally competent diabetes education for Mexican Americans: the Starr County Study. Diabetes Educ. 1999;25(2):226–36.
57. Brown SA, Garcia AA, Kouzekanani K, Hanis CL. Culturally competent diabetes self-management education for Mexican Americans: the Starr County border health initiative. Diabetes Care. 2002;25(2):259–68.
58. Brown SA, Blozis SA, Kouzekanani K, Garcia AA, Winchell M, Hanis CL. Dosage effects of diabetes self-management education for Mexican Americans: the Starr County Border Health Initiative. Diabetes Care. 2005;28(3):527–32.
59. Corkery E, Palmer C, Foley ME, Schechter CB, Frisher L, Roman SH. Effect of a bicultural community health worker on completion of diabetes education in a Hispanic population. Diabetes Care. 1997;20(3):254–7.
60. Keyserling TC, Samuel-Hodge CD, Ammerman AS, Ainsworth BE, Henríquez-Roldán CF, Elasy TA, et al. A randomized trial of an intervention to improve self-care behaviors of African-American women with type 2 diabetes: impact on physical activity. Diabetes Care. 2002;25(9):1576–83.
61. Mayer-Davis EJ, D'Antonio A, Martin M, Wandersman A, Parra-Medina D, Schulz R. Pilot study of strategies for effective weight management in type 2 diabetes: Pounds Off with Empowerment (POWER). Fam Community Health. 2001;24(2):27–35.
62. Mayer-Davis EJ, D'Antonio AM, Smith SM, Kirkner G, Levin Martin S, Parra-Medina D, et al. Pounds off with empowerment (POWER): a clinical trial of weight management strategies for black and white adults with diabetes who live in medically underserved rural communities. Am J Public Health. 2004;94(10):1736–42.
63. McNabb WL, Quinn MT, Rosing L. Weight loss program for inner-city black women with non-insulin-dependent diabetes mellitus: PATHWAYS. J Am Diet Assoc. 1993;93(1):75–7.
64. Rosal MC, Olendzki B, Reed GW, Gumieniak O, Scavron J, Ockene I. Diabetes self-management among low-income Spanish-speaking patients: a pilot study. Ann Behav Med Publ Soc Behav Med. 2005;29(3):225–35.
65. Feathers J. Racial and Ethnic Approaches to Community Health (REACH) detroit partnership: improving diabetes-related outcomes among African American and Latino adults. Am J Publ Health P. 2005;95(9 SRC - GoogleScholar):1552–60.
66. Vazquez IM, Millen B, Bissett L, Levenson SM, Chipkin SR. Buena Alimentacion, Buena Salud: a preventive nutrition intervention in Caribbean Latinos with type 2 diabetes. Am J Health Promot AJHP. 1998;13(2):116–9.
67. Anderson RM, Funnell MM, Nwankwo R, Gillard ML, Oh M, Fitzgerald JT, et al. Evaluating a problem-based empowerment program for African Americans with diabetes: results of a randomized controlled trial. Ethn Dis. 2005;15(4):671.
68. Murrock CJ, Higgins PA, Killion C. Dance and peer support to improve diabetes outcomes in African American women. Diabetes Educ. 2009;35(6):995–1003.
69. Bogner HR, de Vries HF. Integrating type 2 diabetes mellitus and depression treatment among African Americans: a randomized controlled pilot trial. Diabetes Educ. 2010;36(2):284–92.
70. D'Eramo MG. The effect of a diabetes education, coping skills training, and care intervention on physiological and psychosocial outcomes in black women with type 2 diabetes. Biol Res Nurs P. 2010;12(1 SRC - GoogleScholar):7–19.
71. Hill-Briggs F, Lazo M, Peyrot M, Doswell A, Chang Y-T, Hill MN, et al. Effect of problem-solving-based diabetes self-management training on diabetes control in a low income patient sample. J Gen Intern Med. 2011;26(9):972–8.
72. Benjamin EM, Schneider MS, Hinchey KT. Implementing practice guidelines for diabetes care using problem-based learning. A prospective controlled trial using firm systems. Diabetes Care. 1999;22(10):1672–8.
73. Din-Dziethan R, Porterfield DS, Cohen SJ, Reaves J, Burrus B, Lamb BM. Quality care improvement program in a community-based participatory research project: example of Project DIRECT. J Natl Med Assoc. 2004;96(10):1310–21.
74. Fox CH, Mahoney MC. Improving diabetes preventive care in a family practice residency program: a case study in continuous quality improvement. Fam Med. 1998;30(6):441–5.
75. Phillips LS, Hertzberg VS, Cook CB, El-Kebbi IM, Gallina DL, Ziemer DC, et al. The Improving Primary Care of African Americans with Diabetes (IPCAAD) project: rationale and design. Control Clin Trials. 2002;23(5):554–69.
76. Phillips LS, Ziemer DC, Doyle JP, Barnes CS, Kolm P, Branch WT, et al. An endocrinologist-supported intervention aimed at providers improves diabetes management in a primary care site: improving primary care of African Americans with diabetes (IPCAAD) 7. Diabetes Care. 2005;28(10):2352–60.
77. Thaler LM, Ziemer DC, Gallina DL, Cook CB, Dunbar VG, Phillips LS, et al. Diabetes in urban

African-Americans. XVII. Availability of rapid HbA1c measurements enhances clinical decision-making. Diabetes Care. 1999;22(9):1415–21.
78. Ziemer DC, Doyle JP, Barnes CS, Branch WT, Cook CB, El-Kebbi IM, et al. An intervention to overcome clinical inertia and improve diabetes mellitus control in a primary care setting: Improving Primary Care of African Americans with Diabetes (IPCAAD) 8. Arch Intern Med. 2006;166(5):507–13.
79. Bray P, Thompson D, Wynn JD, Cummings DM, Whetstone L. Confronting disparities in diabetes care: the clinical effectiveness of redesigning care management for minority patients in rural primary care practices. J Rural Health Off J Am Rural Health Assoc Natl Rural Health Care Assoc. 2005;21(4): 317–21.
80. Bray P, Roupe M, Young S, Harrell J, Cummings DM, Whetstone LM. Feasibility and effectiveness of system redesign for diabetes care management in rural areas: the eastern North Carolina experience. Diabetes Educ. 2005;31(5):712–8.
81. Fanning EL, Selwyn BJ, Larme AC, DeFronzo RA. Improving efficacy of diabetes management using treatment algorithms in a mainly Hispanic population. Diabetes Care. 2004;27(7):1638–46.
82. Gary TL, Batts-Turner M, Bone LR, Yeh H-C, Wang N-Y, Hill-Briggs F, et al. A randomized controlled trial of the effects of nurse case manager and community health worker team interventions in urban African-Americans with type 2 diabetes. Control Clin Trials. 2004;25(1):53–66.
83. Hopper SV, Miller JP, Birge C, Swift J. A randomized study of the impact of home health aides on diabetic control and utilization patterns. Am J Public Health. 1984;74(6):600–2.
84. Hosler AS, Godley K, Rowland DH. An initiative to improve diabetes care standards in healthcare organizations serving minorities. Diabetes Educ. 2002;28(4):581–9.
85. Jaber LA, Halapy H, Fernet M, Tummalapalli S, Diwakaran H. Evaluation of a pharmaceutical care model on diabetes management. Ann Pharmacother. 1996;30(3):238–43.
86. Miller CD, Barnes CS, Phillips LS, Ziemer DC, Gallina DL, Cook CB, et al. Rapid A1c availability improves clinical decision-making in an urban primary care clinic. Diabetes Care. 2003;26(4):1158–63.
87. Philis-Tsimikas A, Walker C, Rivard L, Talavera G, Reimann JOF, Salmon M, et al. Improvement in diabetes care of underinsured patients enrolled in project dulce: a community-based, culturally appropriate, nurse case management and peer education diabetes care model. Diabetes Care. 2004;27(1):110–5.
88. Cook CB, Penman A, Cobb AB, Miller D, Murphy T, Horn T. Outpatient diabetes management of medicare beneficiaries in four Mississippi fee-for-service primary care clinics. J Miss State Med Assoc. 1999;40(1):8–13.
89. Mahotiere TJ. A program to reduce the disparity in the rate of biennial lipid profiles between African-American and white Medicare beneficiaries with diabetes mellitus in New York City. Health P. 2006;31(4 SRC - GoogleScholar):263–88.
90. Gary TL, Batts-Turner M, Yeh H-C, Hill-Briggs F, Bone LR, Wang N-Y, et al. The effects of a nurse case manager and a community health worker team on diabetic control, emergency department visits, and hospitalizations among urban African Americans with type 2 diabetes mellitus: a randomized controlled trial. Arch Intern Med. 2009;169(19): 1788–94.
91. Rith-Najarian S, Branchaud C, Beaulieu O, Gohdes D, Simonson G, Mazze R. Reducing lower-extremity amputations due to diabetes. Application of the staged diabetes management approach in a primary care setting. J Fam Pract. 1998;47(2):127–32.
92. Ziemer DC, Tsui C, Caudle J, Barnes CS, Dames F, Phillips LS. An informatics-supported intervention improves diabetes control in a primary care setting. AMIA Annu Symp Proc AMIA Symp AMIA Symp. 2006:1160.
93. American Diabetes Association. Standards of medical care in diabetes – 2014. Diabetes Care. 2014;37 Suppl 1:S14–80.
94. Estruch R, Ros E, Salas-Salvadó J, Covas M-I, Corella D, Arós F, et al. Primary prevention of cardiovascular disease with a Mediterranean diet. N Engl J Med. 2013;368(14):1279–90.
95. Esposito K, Maiorino MI, Ciotola M, Di Palo C, Scognamiglio P, Gicchino M, et al. Effects of a Mediterranean-style diet on the need for antihyperglycemic drug therapy in patients with newly diagnosed type 2 diabetes: a randomized trial. Ann Intern Med. 2009;151(5):306–14.
96. Elhayany A, Lustman A, Abel R, Attal-Singer J, Vinker S. A low carbohydrate Mediterranean diet improves cardiovascular risk factors and diabetes control among overweight patients with type 2 diabetes mellitus: a 1-year prospective randomized intervention study. Diabetes Obes Metab. 2010;12(3):204–9.
97. Abiemo EE, Alonso A, Nettleton JA, Steffen LM, Bertoni AG, Jain A, et al. Relationships of the Mediterranean dietary pattern with insulin resistance and diabetes incidence in the Multi-Ethnic Study of Atherosclerosis (MESA). Br J Nutr. 2013;109(08): 1490–7.
98. Orlich MJ. Vegetarian dietary patterns and mortality in adventist health study 2. JAMA Intern Med. 2013;173(13):1230.
99. Tonstad S, Butler T, Yan R, Fraser GE. Type of vegetarian diet, body weight, and prevalence of type 2 diabetes. Diabetes Care. 2009;32(5):791–6.
100. Tonstad S, Stewart K, Oda K, Batech M, Herring RP, Fraser GE. Vegetarian diets and incidence of diabetes in the Adventist Health Study-2. Nutr Metab Cardiovasc Dis. 2013;23(4):292–9.
101. Barnard ND, Cohen J, Jenkins DJ, Turner-McGrievy G, Gloede L, Green A, et al. A low-fat vegan diet and a conventional diabetes diet in the treatment of

type 2 diabetes: a randomized, controlled, 74-wk clinical trial. Am J Clin Nutr. 2009;89(5): 1588S–96.
102. Appel LJ, Moore TJ, Obarzanek E, Vollmer WM, Svetkey LP, Sacks FM, et al. A clinical trial of the effects of dietary patterns on blood pressure. N Engl J Med. 1997;336(16):1117–24.
103. Shirani F, Salehi-Abargouei A, Azadbakht L. Effects of Dietary Approaches to Stop Hypertension (DASH) diet on some risk for developing type 2 diabetes: a systematic review and meta-analysis on controlled clinical trials. Nutrition. 2013;29(7-8): 939–47.
104. Brand-Miller JC. Postprandial glycemia, glycemic index, and the prevention of type 2 diabetes. Am J Clin Nutr. 2004;80(2):243–4.
105. Evert AB, Boucher JL, Cypress M, Dunbar SA, Franz MJ, Mayer-Davis EJ, et al. Nutrition therapy recommendations for the management of adults with diabetes. Diabetes Care. 2014;37(Supplement_1): S120–43.
106. Hu T, Mills KT, Yao L, Demanelis K, Eloustaz M, Yancy WS, et al. Effects of low-carbohydrate diets versus low-fat diets on metabolic risk factors: a meta-analysis of randomized controlled clinical trials. Am J Epidemiol. 2012;176 suppl 7:S44–54.
107. Stern L, Iqbal N, Seshadri P, Chicano KL, Daily DA, McGrory J, et al. The effects of low-carbohydrate versus conventional weight loss diets in severely obese adults: one-year follow-up of a randomized trial. Ann Intern Med. 2004;140(10):778–85.
108. Davis NJ, Tomuta N, Schechter C, Isasi CR, Segal-Isaacson CJ, Stein D, et al. Comparative study of the effects of a 1-year dietary intervention of a Low-carbohydrate diet versus a low-fat diet on weight and glycemic control in type 2 diabetes. Diabetes Care. 2009;32(7):1147–52.
109. Boulé NG, Haddad E, Kenny GP, Wells GA, Sigal RJ. Effects of exercise on glycemic control and body mass in type 2 diabetes mellitus: a meta-analysis of controlled clinical trials. JAMA. 2001;286(10):1218.
110. Haddad E, Wells GA, Sigal RJ, Boulé NG, Kenny GP. Meta-analysis of the effect of structured exercise training on cardiorespiratory fitness in Type 2 diabetes mellitus. Diabetologia. 2003;46(8):1071–81.
111. Colberg SR, Sigal RJ, Fernhall B, Regensteiner JG, Blissmer BJ, Rubin RR, et al. Exercise and type 2 diabetes: the American College of Sports Medicine and the American Diabetes Association: joint position statement. Diabetes Care. 2010;33(12): e147–67.
112. Boulé NG, Weisnagel SJ, Lakka TA, Tremblay A, Bergman RN, Rankinen T, et al. Effects of exercise training on glucose homeostasis: the HERITAGE Family Study. Diabetes Care. 2005;28(1):108–14.
113. Church TS, Blair SN, Cocreham S, Johannsen N, Johnson W, Kramer K, et al. Effects of aerobic and resistance training on hemoglobin A1c levels in patients with type 2 diabetes. JAMA J Am Med Assoc. 2010;304(20):2253.
114. Petersen KF, Dufour S, Befroy D, Garcia R, Shulman GI. Impaired mitochondrial activity in the insulin-resistant offspring of patients with type 2 diabetes. N Engl J Med. 2004;350(7):664–71.
115. Kelley DE, He J, Menshikova EV, Ritov VB. Dysfunction of mitochondria in human skeletal muscle in type 2 diabetes. Diabetes. 2002;51(10): 2944–50.
116. Swift DL, Johannsen NM, Lavie CJ, Earnest CP, Johnson WD, Blair SN, et al. Racial differences in the response of cardiorespiratory fitness to aerobic exercise training in Caucasian and African American postmenopausal women. J Appl Physiol. 2013;114(10):1375–82.
117. Santa-Clara H, Szymanski L, Ordille T, Fernhall B. Effects of exercise training on resting metabolic rate in postmenopausal African American and Caucasian women. Metabolism. 2006;55(10): 1358–64.
118. Kokkinos P, Myers J, Nylen E, Panagiotakos DB, Manolis A, Pittaras A, et al. Exercise capacity and all-cause mortality in African American and Caucasian men with type 2 diabetes. Diabetes Care. 2009;32(4):623–8.
119. Qiu S, Cai X, Chen X, Yang B, Sun Z. Step counter use in type 2 diabetes: a meta-analysis of randomized controlled trials. BMC Med. 2014;12(1):36.
120. Hu FB, Manson JE, Stampfer MJ, Colditz G, Liu S, Solomon CG, et al. Diet, lifestyle, and the risk of type 2 diabetes mellitus in women. N Engl J Med. 2001;345(11):790–7.
121. Narayan KMV, Boyle JP, Thompson TJ, Gregg EW, Williamson DF. Effect of BMI on lifetime risk for diabetes in the U.S. Diabetes Care. 2007;30(6): 1562–6.
122. Neeland IJ, Turer AT, Ayers MCR, Powell-Wiley TM, Vega GL, Farzaneh-Far R, et al. Dysfunctional adiposity and the risk of prediabetes and type 2 diabetes in obese adults. JAMA J Am Med Assoc. 2012;308(11):1150.
123. Rabkin SW, Mathewson FA, Hsu P-H. Relation of body weight to development of ischemic heart disease in a cohort of young North American men after a 26 year observation period: the Manitoba Study. Am J Cardiol. 1977;39(3):452–8.
124. Hubert HB, Feinleib M, McNamara PM, Castelli WP. Obesity as an independent risk factor for cardiovascular disease: a 26- year follow-up of participants in the Framingham Heart Study. Circulation. 1983;67(5):968–77.
125. Wilson PWF, D'Agostino RB, Sullivan L, Parise H, Kannel WB. Overweight and obesity as determinants of cardiovascular risk: the Framingham experience. Arch Intern Med. 2002;162(16):1867–72.
126. Di Angelantonio E, Kaptoge S, Wormser D, Willeit P, Butterworth AS, Bansal N, et al. Association of cardiometabolic multimorbidity with mortality. JAMA. 2015;314(1):52.
127. Després J-P, Lemieux I. Abdominal obesity and metabolic syndrome. Nature. 2006;444(7121):881–7.

128. Kahn SE, Hull RL, Utzschneider KM. Mechanisms linking obesity to insulin resistance and type 2 diabetes. Nature. 2006;444(7121):840–6.
129. Rosen ED, Spiegelman BM. Adipocytes as regulators of energy balance and glucose homeostasis. Nature. 2006;444(7121):847–53.
130. Lau DCW. Adipokines: molecular links between obesity and atherosclerosis. AJP Heart Circ Physiol. 2005;288(5):H2031–41.
131. The Look AHEAD Research Group. Cardiovascular effects of intensive lifestyle intervention in type 2 diabetes. N Engl J Med. 2013;369(2):145–54.
132. Lazo M, Solga SF, Horska A, Bonekamp S, Diehl AM, Brancati FL, et al. Effect of a 12-month intensive lifestyle intervention on hepatic steatosis in adults with type 2 diabetes. Diabetes Care. 2010;33(10):2156–63.
133. Group LAR, et al. Effect of a long-term behavioural weight loss intervention on nephropathy in overweight or obese adults with type 2 diabetes: a secondary analysis of the Look AHEAD randomised clinical trial. Lancet Diabetes Endocrinol. 2014;2(10):801–9.
134. Wing RR. Implications of Look AHEAD for clinical trials and clinical practice. Diabetes Obes Metab. 2014;16(12):1183–91.
135. Foster GD, Wadden TA, LaGrotte CA, Vander Veur SS, Hesson LA, Homko CJ, et al. A randomized comparison of a commercially available portion-controlled weight-loss intervention with a diabetes self-management education program. Nutr Diabetes. 2013;3(3):e63.
136. Pillay J, Armstrong MJ, Butalia S, Donovan LE, Sigal RJ, Vandermeer B, et al. Behavioral programs for type 2 diabetes mellitus: a systematic review and network meta-analysis. Ann Intern Med. 2015;163(11):848.
137. Malkani S. An update on the role of bariatric surgery in diabetes management. Curr Opin Endocrinol Diabetes Obes. 2015;22(2):98–105.
138. Vest AR, Heneghan HM, Schauer PR, Young JB. Surgical management of obesity and the relationship to cardiovascular disease. Circulation. 2013;127(8):945–59. doi: 10.1161/CIRCULATIONAHA.112.103275.
139. Spaniolas K, Kasten KR, Brinkley J, Sippey ME, Mozer A, Chapman WH, et al. The changing bariatric surgery landscape in the USA. Obes Surg. 2015;25(8):1544–6.
140. Buchwald H, Avidor Y, Braunwald E, Jensen MD, Pories W, Fahrbach K, et al. Bariatric surgery: a systematic review and meta-analysis. JAMA. 2004;292(14):1724–37.
141. Tice JA, Karliner L, Walsh J, Petersen AJ, Feldman MD. Gastric banding or bypass? A systematic review comparing the two most popular bariatric procedures. Am J Med. 2008;121(10):885–93.
142. Trastulli S, Desiderio J, Guarino S, Cirocchi R, Scalercio V, Noya G, et al. Laparoscopic sleeve gastrectomy compared with other bariatric surgical procedures: a systematic review of randomized trials. Surg Obes Relat Dis. 2013;9(5):816–29.
143. Schauer PR, Bhatt DL, Kirwan JP, Wolski K, Brethauer SA, Navaneethan SD, et al. Bariatric surgery versus intensive medical therapy for diabetes—3-year outcomes. N Engl J Med. 2014;370(21):2002–13.
144. Schauer PR, Kashyap SR, Wolski K, Brethauer SA, Kirwan JP, Pothier CE, et al. Bariatric surgery versus intensive medical therapy in obese patients with diabetes. N Engl J Med. 2012;366(17):1567–76.
145. Kashyap SR, Bhatt DL, Wolski K, Watanabe RM, Abdul-Ghani M, Abood B, et al. Metabolic effects of bariatric surgery in patients with moderate obesity and type 2 diabetes: analysis of a randomized control trial comparing surgery with intensive medical treatment. Diabetes Care. 2013;36(8):2175–82.
146. Adams TD, Davidson LE, Litwin SE, Kolotkin RL, LaMonte MJ, Pendleton RC, et al. Health benefits of gastric bypass surgery after 6 years. JAMA. 2012;308(11):1122.
147. Courcoulas AP. Weight change and health outcomes at 3 years after bariatric surgery among individuals with severe obesity. JAMA [Internet]. 2013 [cited 5 Dec 2015]. Available from: http://jama.jamanetwork.com/article.aspx?. doi:10.1001/jama.2013.280928.
148. Courcoulas AP, Goodpaster BH, Eagleton JK, Belle SH, Kalarchian MA, Lang W, et al. Surgical vs medical treatments for type 2 diabetes mellitus: a randomized clinical trial. JAMA Surg. 2014;149(7):707.
149. Ng J, Seip R, Stone A, Ruano G, Tishler D, Papasavas P. Ethnic variation in weight loss, but not co-morbidity remission, after laparoscopic gastric banding and Roux-en-Y gastric bypass. Surg Obes Relat Dis. 2015;11(1):94–100.
150. Ikramuddin S, Korner J, Lee W-J, Connett JE, Inabnet WB, Billington CJ, et al. Roux-en-Y gastric bypass vs intensive medical management for the control of type 2 diabetes, hypertension and hyperlipidemia. JAMA. 2013;309(21):2240–9.
151. Hutter MM, Schirmer BD, Jones DB, Ko CY, Cohen ME, Merkow RP, et al. First Report from the American College of Surgeons Bariatric Surgery Center Network: laparoscopic sleeve gastrectomy has morbidity and effectiveness positioned between the band and the bypass. Ann Surg. 2011;254(3):410–22.
152. Still CD, Wood GC, Benotti P, Petrick AT, Gabrielsen J, Strodel WE, et al. Preoperative prediction of type 2 diabetes remission after Roux-en-Y gastric bypass surgery: a retrospective cohort study. Lancet Diabetes Endocrinol. 2014;2(1):38–45.
153. Maggard-Gibbons M, Maglione M, Livhits M, Ewing B, Maher AR, Hu J, et al. Bariatric surgery for weight loss and glycemic control in nonmorbidly obese adults with diabetes. JAMA. 2013;309(21):2250–61.
154. Parikh M, Issa R, Vieira D, McMacken M, Saunders JK, Ude-Welcome A, et al. Role of bariatric surgery as treatment for type 2 diabetes in patients who do not meet current NIH criteria: a systematic review and meta-analysis. J Am Coll Surg. 2013;217(3):527–32.

155. American Diabetes Association. Standards of medical care in diabetes – 2015. Diabetes Care. 2015;38(Supplement_1):S1–2.
156. Lee CJ, Clark JM, Schweitzer M, Magnuson T, Steele K, Koerner O, et al. Prevalence of and risk factors for hypoglycemic symptoms after gastric bypass and sleeve gastrectomy: postsurgical hypoglycemic symptoms. Obesity. 2015;23(5): 1079–84.
157. Adams TD, Gress RE, Smith SC, Halverson RC, Simper SC, Rosamond WD, et al. Long-term mortality after gastric bypass surgery. N Engl J Med. 2007;357(8):753–61.
158. Sjöström L, Narbro K, Sjöström CD, Karason K, Larsson B, Wedel H, et al. Effects of bariatric surgery on mortality in Swedish obese subjects. N Engl J Med. 2007;357(8):741–52.
159. Khorgami Z, Arheart KL, Zhang C, Messiah SE, de la Cruz-Muñoz N. Effect of ethnicity on weight loss after bariatric surgery. Obes Surg. 2015;25(5): 769–76.
160. Coleman KJ, Huang Y-C, Koebnick C, Reynolds K, Xiang AH, Black MH, et al. Metabolic syndrome is less likely to resolve in hispanics and non-hispanic blacks after bariatric surgery. Ann Surg. 2014;259(2): 279–85.
161. Yasuda S, Zhang L, Huang S-M. The role of ethnicity in variability in response to drugs: focus on clinical pharmacology studies. Clin Pharmacol Ther. 2008;84(3):417–23. 38.
162. Pearson ER, Starkey BJ, Powell RJ, Gribble FM, Clark PM, Hattersley AT. Genetic cause of hyperglycaemia and response to treatment in diabetes. Lancet Lond Engl. 2003;362(9392):1275–81.
163. Fajans SS, Bell GI. MODY: history, genetics, pathophysiology, and clinical decision making. Diabetes Care. 2011;34(8):1878–84.
164. García-Martín E, Martínez C, Ladero JM, Agúndez JA. Interethnic and intraethnic variability of CYP2C8 and CYP2C9 polymorphisms in healthy individuals. Mol Diagn Ther. 2006;10(1):29–40.
165. Williams LK, Padhukasahasram B, Ahmedani BK, Peterson EL, Wells KE, González Burchard E, et al. Differing effects of metformin on glycemic control by race-ethnicity. J Clin Endocrinol Metab. 2014;99(9):3160–8.
166. Gosmanova EO, MANGOLD TA, RAWLS WN, WALL BM, et al. Effect of metformin-containing antidiabetic regimens on all-cause mortality in veterans with type 2 diabetes mellitus. Am J Med Sci. 2008;336(3):241–7.
167. Ford ES. Trends in the control of risk factors for cardiovascular disease among adults with diagnosed diabetes: findings from the National Health and Nutrition Examination Survey 1999–2008*: cardiovascular risk factor control. J Diabetes. 2011;3(4): 337–47.
168. Lackland DT. Racial differences in hypertension: implications for high blood pressure management. Am J Med Sci. 2014;348(2):135–8.
169. Egan BM, Zhao Y, Axon RN. US trends in prevalence, awareness, treatment, and control of hypertension, 1988–2008. JAMA. 2010;303(20):2043–50.
170. Guo F, He D, Zhang W, Walton RG. Trends in prevalence, awareness, management, and control of hypertension among United States adults, 1999 to 2010. J Am Coll Cardiol. 2012;60(7):599–606.
171. Oliva RV, Bakris GL. Blood pressure effects of sodium–glucose co-transport 2 (SGLT2) inhibitors. J Am Soc Hypertens. 2014;8(5):330–9.
172. Ogden CL, Carroll MD, Kit BK, Flegal KM. Prevalence of childhood and adult obesity in the United States, 2011–2012. JAMA. 2014; 311(8):806.
173. Buse JB, Rosenstock J, Sesti G, Schmidt WE, Montanya E, Brett JH, et al. Liraglutide once a day versus exenatide twice a day for type 2 diabetes: a 26-week randomised, parallel-group, multinational, open-label trial (LEAD-6). Lancet. 2009;374(9683): 39–47.
174. Wang B, Zhong J, Lin H, Zhao Z, Yan Z, He H, et al. Blood pressure-lowering effects of GLP-1 receptor agonists exenatide and liraglutide: a meta-analysis of clinical trials. Diabetes Obes Metab. 2013;15(8): 737–49.
175. Ferdinand KC, Nasser SA. Racial/ethnic disparities in prevalence and care of patients with type 2 diabetes mellitus. Curr Med Res Opin. 2015;31(5): 913–23.
176. Xia Y, Kelton CML, Guo JJ, Bian B, Heaton PC. Treatment of obesity: pharmacotherapy trends in the United States from 1999 to 2010: pharmacotherapy treatment of obesity. Obesity. 2015;23(8): 1721–8.
177. Khan LK, Serdula MK, Bowman BA, Williamson DF. Use of prescription weight loss pills among US adults in 1996–1998. Ann Intern Med. 2001;134(4): 282–6.
178. Apovian CM, Aronne LJ, Bessesen DH, McDonnell ME, Murad MH, Pagotto U, et al. Pharmacological management of obesity: an endocrine society clinical practice guideline. J Clin Endocrinol Metab. 2015;100(2):342–62.
179. Zhuo X, Zhang P, Barker L, Albright A, Thompson TJ, Gregg E. The lifetime cost of diabetes and its implications for diabetes prevention. Diabetes Care. 2014;37(9):2557–64.
180. The Diabetes Prevention Program. Reduction in the incidence of type 2 diabetes with lifestyle intervention or metformin. N Engl J Med. 2002;346(6): 393–403.
181. Pan X-R, Li G, Hu Y-H, Wang J-X, Yang W-Y, An Z-X, et al. Effects of diet and exercise in preventing NIDDM in people with impaired glucose tolerance: the Da Qing IGT and Diabetes Study. Diabetes Care. 1997;20(4):537–44.
182. Delahanty LM, Pan Q, Jablonski KA, Aroda VR, Watson KE, Bray GA, et al. Effects of weight loss, weight cycling, and weight loss maintenance on diabetes incidence and change in cardiometabolic traits

in the diabetes prevention program. Diabetes Care. 2014;37(10):2738–45.
183. Diabetes Prevention Program Resea. 10-year follow-up of diabetes incidence and weight loss in the Diabetes Prevention Program Outcomes Study. Lancet. 2009;374(9702):1677–86.
184. Long-term effects of lifestyle intervention or metformin on diabetes development and microvascular complications over 15-year follow-up: the Diabetes Prevention Program Outcomes Study. Lancet Diabetes Endocrinol [Internet]. 2015 Sep [cited 2015 Oct 7]; Available from: http://linkinghub.elsevier.com/retrieve/pii/S2213858715002910
185. Ali MK, Echouffo-Tcheugui JB, Williamson DF. How effective were lifestyle interventions in real-world settings that were modeled on the diabetes prevention program? Health Aff (Millwood). 2012;31(1):67–75.
186. Kahn R, Davidson MB. The reality of type 2 diabetes prevention. Diabetes Care. 2014;37(4):943–9.
187. Samuel-Hodge CD, Johnson CM, Braxton DF, Lackey M. Effectiveness of diabetes prevention program translations among African Americans: African Americans and DPP translations. Obes Rev. 2014;15:107–24.
188. Ackermann RT, Liss DT, Finch EA, Schmidt KK, Hays LM, Marrero DG, et al. A randomized comparative effectiveness trial for preventing type 2 diabetes. Am J Public Health. 2015;105(11):2328–34.
189. Katula JA, Vitolins MZ, Morgan TM, Lawlor MS, Blackwell CS, Isom SP, et al. The healthy living partnerships to prevent diabetes study. Am J Prev Med. 2013;44(4):S324–32.
190. Faridi Z, Shuval K, Njike VY, Katz JA, Jennings G, Williams M, et al. Partners reducing effects of diabetes (PREDICT): a diabetes prevention physical activity and dietary intervention through African-American churches. Health Educ Res. 2010;25(2): 306–15.
191. Parikh P, Simon EP, Fei K, Looker H, Goytia C, Horowitz CR. Results of a pilot diabetes prevention intervention in East Harlem, New York City: project HEED. Am J Public Health. 2010;100 Suppl 1:S232–9.
192. Perez A, Alos VA, Scanlan A, Maia CM, Davey A, Whitaker RC, et al. The rationale, design, and baseline characteristics of PREVENT-DM: a community-based comparative effectiveness trial of lifestyle intervention and metformin among Latinas with prediabetes. Contemp Clin Trials. 2015;45:320–7.
193. Jiang L, Manson SM, Beals J, Henderson WG, Huang H, Acton KJ, et al. Translating the diabetes prevention program into American Indian and Alaska native communities: results from the special diabetes program for Indians diabetes prevention demonstration project. Diabetes Care. 2013;36(7): 2027–34.
194. Kaholokula JK, Wilson RE, Townsend CKM, Zhang GX, Chen J, Yoshimura SR, et al. Translating the diabetes prevention program in native Hawaiian and pacific islander communities: the PILI 'ohana project. Transl Behav Med. 2014;4(2):149–59.
195. Islam N, Zanowiak J, Wyatt L, Kavathe R, Singh H, Kwon S, et al. Diabetes prevention in the New York City Sikh Asian Indian community: a pilot study. Int J Environ Res Public Health. 2014;11(5):5462–86.
196. Leake AR, Bermudo VC, Jacob J, Jacob MR, Inouye J. Health is wealth: methods to improve attendance in a lifestyle intervention for a largely immigrant Filipino-American sample. J Immigr Minor Health. 2012;14(3):475–80.
197. Islam NS, Zanowiak JM, Wyatt LC, Chun K, Lee L, Kwon SC, et al. A randomized-controlled, pilot intervention on diabetes prevention and healthy lifestyles in the New York City Korean community. J Community Health. 2013;38(6):1030–41.
198. Dunkley AJ, Bodicoat DH, Greaves CJ, Russell C, Yates T, Davies MJ, et al. Diabetes prevention in the real world: effectiveness of pragmatic lifestyle interventions for the prevention of type 2 diabetes and of the impact of adherence to guideline recommendations: a systematic review and meta-analysis. Diabetes Care. 2014;37(4):922–33.
199. Chou C-H, Burnet D, Meltzer D, Huang E. The effectiveness of diabetes prevention programs in community settings [Internet]. 2015 [cited 15 Dec 2015]. Available from: http://198.246.124.29/diabetes/pdfs/data/2014-report-acknowledgments.pdf.
200. Knowler WC, Ackermann RT. Preventing diabetes in American Indian communities. Diabetes Care. 2013;36(7):1820–2.
201. Gaede P, Vedel P, Larsen N, Jensen GV, Parving H-H, Pedersen O. Multifactorial intervention and cardiovascular disease in patients with type 2 diabetes. N Engl J Med. 2003;348(5):383–93.
202. Moore SH, Martin DP, Richardson WC. Does the primary-care gatekeeper control the costs of health care? Lessons from the SAFECO experience. N Engl J Med. 1983;309(22):1400–4.
203. de Sonnaville JJ, Bouma M, Colly LP, Devillé W, Wijkel D, Heine RJ. Sustained good glycaemic control in NIDDM patients by implementation of structured care in general practice: 2-year follow-up study. Diabetologia. 1997;40(11):1334–40.
204. Hirsch IB, Goldberg HI, Ellsworth A, Evans TC, Herter CD, Ramsey SD, et al. A multifaceted intervention in support of diabetes treatment guidelines: a cont trial. Diabetes Res Clin Pract. 2002;58(1): 27–36.
205. Legorreta A, Peters A, Ossorio C, Lopez RJ, Jatulis D, Davidson MB. Effect of a comprehensive nurse-managed diabetes program: an HMO prospective study. Am J Manag Care. 1996;2:1024–30.
206. Sadur CN, Moline N, Costa M, Michalik D, Mendlowitz D, Roller S, et al. Diabetes management in a health maintenance organization. Efficacy of care management using cluster visits. Diabetes Care. 1999;22(12):2011–7.
207. Majumdar SR, Guirguis LM, Toth EL, Lewanczuk RZ, Lee TK, Johnson JA. Controlled trial of a

multifaceted intervention for improving quality of care for rural patients with type 2 diabetes. Diabetes Care. 2003;26(11):3061–6.
208. California Medi-Cal Type 2 Diabetes Study Group. Closing the gap: effect of diabetes case management on glycemic control among low-income ethnic minority populations: the California Medi-Cal type 2 diabetes study. Diabetes Care. 2004;27(1):95–103.
209. Polonsky WH, Earles J, Smith S, Pease DJ, Macmillan M, Christensen R, et al. Integrating medical management with diabetes self-management training: a randomized control trial of the Diabetes Outpatient Intensive Treatment program. Diabetes Care. 2003;26(11):3048–53.
210. Gaede P, Lund-Andersen H, Parving H-H, Pedersen O. Effect of a multifactorial intervention on mortality in type 2 diabetes. N Engl J Med. 2008;358(6):580–91.
211. Shea S, Weinstock RS, Starren J, Teresi J, Palmas W, Field L, et al. A randomized trial comparing telemedicine case management with usual care in older, ethnically diverse, medically underserved patients with diabetes mellitus. J Am Med Inform Assoc. 2006;13(1):40–51.
212. Ko S-H, Song K-H, Kim S-R, Lee J-M, Kim J-S, Shin J-H, et al. Long-term effects of a structured intensive diabetes education programme (SIDEP) in patients with Type 2 diabetes mellitus – a 4-year follow-up study. Diabet Med J Br Diabet Assoc. 2007;24(1):55–62.
213. Chin MH, Zhang JX, Merrell K. Specialty differences in the care of older patients with diabetes. Med Care. 2000;38(2):131–40.
214. Martin DP, Diehr P, Price KF, Richardson WC. Effect of a gatekeeper plan on health services use and charges: a randomized trial. Am J Public Health. 1989;79(12):1628–32.
215. Kivimäki M, Virtanen M, Kawachi I, Nyberg ST, Alfredsson L, Batty GD, et al. Long working hours, socioeconomic status, and the risk of incident type 2 diabetes: a meta-analysis of published and unpublished data from 222 120 individuals. Lancet Diabetes Endocrinol. 2015;3(1):27–34.
216. McKenzie B. Modes less traveled—bicycling and walking to work in the United States: 2008–2012. US Census Bur N Y [Internet]. 2014 [cited 15 Dec 2015]. Available from: https://www.census.gov/content/dam/Census/library/publications/2014/acs/acs-25.pdf.
217. Lachat C, Nago E, Verstraeten R, Roberfroid D, Van Camp J, Kolsteren P. Eating out of home and its association with dietary intake: a systematic review of the evidence: eating out and diet. Obes Rev. 2012;13(4):329–46.
218. Moore LV, Diez Roux AV, Nettleton JA, Jacobs DR, Franco M. Fast-food consumption, diet quality, and neighborhood exposure to fast food: the multi-ethnic study of atherosclerosis. Am J Epidemiol. 2009;170(1):29–36.
219. Roux AVD, Smith AE, Gore LD. Associations of fast food restaurant availability with dietary intake and weight among African Americans in the Jackson heart study, 2000–2004. Am J Public Health. 2011;101(S1):S301.
220. Block JP, Scribner RA, DeSalvo KB. Fast food, race/ethnicity, and income. Am J Prev Med. 2004;27(3):211–7.
221. Hicks RA, Lucero-Gorman K, Bautista J, HICKS GJ. Ethnicity, sleep duration, and sleep satisfaction. Percept Mot Skills. 1999;88(1):234–5.
222. Lauderdale DS. Objectively measured sleep characteristics among early-middle-aged adults: the CARDIA study. Am J Epidemiol. 2006;164(1):5–16.
223. Gangwisch JE, Heymsfield SB, Boden-Albala B, Buijs RM, Kreier F, Pickering TG, et al. Sleep duration as a risk factor for diabetes incidence in a large US sample. Sleep. 2007;30(12):1667.
224. Buxton OM, Pavlova M, Reid EW, Wang W, Simonson DC, Adler GK. Sleep restriction for 1 week reduces insulin sensitivity in healthy men. Diabetes. 2010;59(9):2126–33.
225. Broussard JL, Ehrmann DA, Van Cauter E, Tasali E, Brady MJ. Impaired insulin signaling in human adipocytes after experimental sleep restriction A randomized, crossover study. Ann Intern Med. 2012;157(8):549–57.
226. Cappuccio FP, D'Elia L, Strazzullo P, Miller MA. Quantity and quality of sleep and incidence of type 2 diabetes: a systematic review and meta-analysis. Diabetes Care. 2009;33(2):414–20.
227. Knutson KL, Ryden AM, Mander BA, Van Cauter E. Role of sleep duration and quality in the risk and severity of type 2 diabetes mellitus. Arch Intern Med. 2006;166(16):1768.
228. Beihl DA, Liese AD, Haffner SM. Sleep duration as a risk factor for incident type 2 diabetes in a multiethnic cohort. Ann Epidemiol. 2009;19(5):351–7.
229. Matthews CE, Chen KY, Freedson PS, Buchowski MS, Beech BM, Pate RR, et al. Amount of time spent in sedentary behaviors in the United States, 2003–2004. Am J Epidemiol. 2008;167(7):875–81.
230. Bodenheimer T, Wagner EH, Grumbach K. Improving primary care for patients with chronic illness. JAMA. 2002;288(14):1775–9.

Index

S. Dagogo-Jack (ed.), *Diabetes Mellitus in Developing Countries and Underserved Communities*,
DOI 10.1007/978-3-319-41559-8

D

MIX
Papier aus verantwortungsvollen Quellen
Paper from responsible sources
FSC® C105338

If you have any concerns about our products,
you can contact us on
ProductSafety@springernature.com

In case Publisher is established outside the EU,
the EU authorized representative is:
Springer Nature Customer Service Center GmbH
Europaplatz 3, 69115 Heidelberg, Germany

Printed by Libri Plureos GmbH
in Hamburg, Germany